MECHANISMS OF CARDIAC MORPHOGENESIS AND TERATOGENESIS

Perspectives in Cardiovascular Research
Volume 5

Perspectives in Cardiovascular Research

Series Editor:

Arnold M. Katz

Chief, Division of Cardiology
University of Connecticut School of Medicine
Farmington, Connecticut

Vol. 1: Developmental and Physiological Correlates of Cardiac Muscle, *edited by M. Lieberman and T. Sano.* 322 pp., 1975.

Vol. 2: Neural Mechanisms in Cardiac Arrhythmias, *edited by P. J. Schwartz, A. M. Brown, A. Malliani, and A. Zanchetti.* 460 pp., 1978.

Vol. 3: Ischemic Myocardium and Antianginal Drugs, *edited by M. M. Winbury and Y. Abiko.* 256 pp., 1979.

Vol. 4: Prophylactic Approach to Hypertensive Diseases, *edited by Y. Yamori, W. Lovenberg, and E. D. Freis.* 606 pp., 1979.

Vol. 5: Mechanisms of Cardiac Morphogenesis and Teratogenesis, *edited by Tomas Pexieder.* 526 pp., 1980.

Mechanisms of Cardiac Morphogenesis and Teratogenesis

Perspectives in Cardiovascular Research
Volume 5

Editor

Tomas Pexieder, M.D.
Associate Professor
Institute of Histology and Embryology
University of Lausanne
Lausanne, Switzerland

Raven Press ▪ New York

Raven Press, 1140 Avenue of the Americas, New York, New York 10036

Made in the United States of America

Library of Congress Cataloging in Publication Data

Main entry under title:

Mechanisms of cardiac morphogenesis and tera-
    togenesis.

    (Perspectives in cardiovascular research; v. 5)
    Includes bibliographical references and index.
    1.   Heart—Abnormalities. 2.   Heart—Anatomy.
3.   Morphogenesis. I.   Pexieder, Tomas, 1941–
[DNLM: 1.   Heart—Embryology—Congresses.
2.   Heart—Growth and development—Congresses.
3.   Heart defects, Congenital—Etiology—Congresses.
4.   Myocardium—Cytology—Congresses. W1 PE871AL
v. 5 /WG201 M486 1979]
RC687.M43   616.1′2043   79–65503
ISBN 0–89004–460–0

Preface

Although several centuries have passed since the first description of embryonic heart by Malpighi (1673) and von Haller (1758), only recently has research on cardiovascular embryology and teratology approached maturity.

In the last decade, research teams involved in systematic studies of heart morphogenesis and teratogenesis have developed throughout the world. The rising number of international meetings on heart morphogenesis and teratogenesis (Dayton, 1970; Tokyo, 1974; Leiden, 1977; Grand Canyon, 1977; Munich, 1978; Tokyo, 1978; Macclesfield, 1979) reflects the progress in this particular field of biology and medicine.

Present and future research efforts in the field of cardiovascular embryology can be characterized as follows:

1. Standardization of the nomenclature used to describe the morphogenesis of the heart and great vessels

2. Standardization and normalization of new techniques introduced in the investigation of cardiac development (e.g., scanning electron microscopy)

3. Initiation of research on early (embryonic) and late (fetal) morphogenesis of the *human* cardiovascular system

4. Search for the best animal model of normal human cardiovascular organogenesis with precise description of its limitations

5. Identification of new animal models of human congenital heart disease

6. Detailed step-wise organ-level studies on pathogenesis of congenital heart disease of genetic and epigenetic etiology

7. Analysis of cellular and subcellular mechanisms that realize and regulate morphogenesis and teratogenesis of the cardiovascular system.

Cardiac development is a very complex process. The normal development of the heart as an organ requires integration of many cellular and subcellular processes: Data on this topic are presented in this volume. Chapters are arranged in three main thematic blocks: organogenesis of the heart, cellular and subcellular mechanisms, and regulatory aspects.

The mechanisms of the normal and abnormal development of the heart are further elaborated in sections on cell proliferation, cell death, extracellular matrix, cell surface, and cell physiology and interactions. In addition to established subjects such as the extracellular matrix, there are newly arising topics such as cell surface or cell proliferation. The elementary mechanisms of development are active in all vertebrates and show very small, if, any interspecific differences at the cellular and subcellular level. The modulation of those elementary mechanisms is responsible for the differences observed in hearts of various species at the organ level.

The factors governing heart morphogenesis are analyzed in sections on genetic and epigenetic control. Each section is introduced by an expert in that particular field and also includes a discussion of the chapters to follow. Thus, a true multidisciplinary approach of the problem of normal and abnormal heart development is presented.

Recent clinical trials to apply embryological principles in classification of cardiovascular malformations and in studies of their pathogenesis emphasize the clinical relevance of the data reported in this volume. The presented, essentially basic research-produced knowledge is the indispensable prerequisite for any further development of new therapeutic, diagnostic, and especially preventive measures.

The analysis of cellular and subcellular mechanisms and their effect on the morphogenesis and the teratogenesis of the cardiovascular system was the topic of a workshop organized under the auspices of International Society of Developmental Biologists and the International Society and Federation of Cardiology in Lausanne, Switzerland. Because of the widespread coverage of the different aspects of the cardiovascular morphogenesis and teratogenesis, we decided to make the contributions and the discussions held at this workshop available to the international scientific community.

This volume will be of interest to cell biologists, developmental biologists, embryologists, teratologists, anatomists, cardiac pathologists, pediatric cardiologists, and cardiac surgeons.

T. Pexieder

Acknowledgments

We would like to acknowledge gratefully the generous financial help to the Workshop organization from the following institutions:

Swiss National Science Foundation
Union of Swiss Societies of Experimental Biology
Swiss Academy of Medical Sciences
Faculty of Medicine, The University of Lausanne

Interpharma, Basel
Institute of Histology and Embryology, Lausanne

Kontron, Zürich
Wild & Leitz, Zürich
Bobst, Lausanne
Contraves, Zürich

GAN Vie, Pully
Swissair, Zürich
Helvetia Vie, Genève
IBM Suisse, Zürich
Bâloise Assurances, Basel
Suisse Assurances, Lausanne

Crédit Foncier, Lausanne
Banque Aufina, Lausanne
Ch. Veillon, Lausanne
Kodak Suisse, Lausanne
Banque Vaudoise de Crédit, Lausanne
Caisse d'Epargne, Lausanne
Banque Lambert, Lausanne
Bender & Hobein, Zürich

Contents

ORGANOGENESIS OF THE HEART

3 The Importance of Cardiac Embryology for Cardiac Pathology
and Surgery
P. A. deVries

7 Synopsis of Normal Cardiac Development
P. Krediet and H. W. Klein

17 Morphogenesis of the Ventricular Flow Pathways in Man (Bulbus Cordis and Truncus Arteriosus)
F. Orts-Llorca, J. Puerta Fonollá, and J. Sobrado Pérez

31 Evolution of Precardiac and Splanchnic Mesoderm in Relationship
to the Infundibulum and Truncus
P. A. deVries

49 Quantitative Analysis of the Shape Development in the Chick Embryo Heart
T. Pexieder and Y. Christen

General Discussion

CELL PROLIFERATION

71 Introduction
D. A. Fischman

73 Patterns of Proliferation during the Organogenetic Phase of Heart
Development
N. Paschoud and T. Pexieder

89 DNA Synthesis and Polyploidization of Chicken Heart Muscle
Cells in Mass Culture
E. Bogenmann and H. M. Eppenberger

CELL DEATH

93 Introduction
T. Pexieder

101   Establishment of the Tubular Heart Role of Cell Death
      J. L. Ojeda and J. M. Hurle

115   Comparative and Morphometric Study on Genetically Pro-
      grammed Cell Death in Rat and Chick Embryonic Heart
      *Y. Satow, N. Okamoto, N. Akimoto, N. Hidaka, S. Miyabara and
      T. Pexieder*

127   Role of Cell Death in Conal Ridges of Developing Human Heart
      N. Okamoto, N. Akimoto, Y. Satow, N. Hidaka, and S. Miyabara

139   Formation of Foramina Secunda in the Chick
      D. E. Morse

151   Some Early Effects of Retinoic Acid on the Young Hamster Heart
      I. M. Taylor

EXTRACELLULAR MATRIX

165   Introduction
      F. J. Manasek

167   The Importance of Extracellular Matrix Components in Develop-
      ment of the Embryonic Chick Heart
      C. Argüello López and M. Servín Martínez

181   Synthesis and Distribution of Glycopeptides and Glycosaminogly-
      cans in Cultures of Embryonic Heart Cells
      F. J. Manasek, J. Lacktis, J. Aiton, and M. Lieberman

197   Localization of Fucose-Containing Substances in Developing
      Atrioventricular Cushion Tissue
      D. A. Hay and R. R. Markwald

213   Localization of Collagen Types in the Embryonic Heart and Aorta
      Using Immunohistochemistry
      M. J. C. Hendrix

227   Endocardial Shape Change in the Truncus During Cushion Tissue
      Formation
      T. P. Fitzharris

237   Structural Analyses of 6-Diazo-5-Oxo-L-Norleucine Effects Upon
      Early Cushion Tissue Morphogenesis
      R. R. Markwald and D. H. Bernanke

CELL SURFACE

255 Introduction
J. A. Los

267 Development and Fusion of Endocardial Structures in the Arterial
Pole of the Heart of Chick, Rat, and Human Embryos
H.-M. Laane and J. A. Roest-Wagenaar

CELL PHYSIOLOGY AND INTERACTIONS

283 Introduction
R. L. DeHaan

285 Assembly of Gap Junctions in Developing Mouse Cardiac Muscle
D. Gros, J. P. Mocquard, J. Schrével, and C. E. Challice

299 Intercellular Coupling of Embryonic Heart Cells
R. L. DeHaan, E. H. Williams, D. L. Ypey, and D. E. Clapham

317 Differentiation of Cellular Electrical Properties in the Developing
Embryonic Chick Heart
G. H. Le Douarin and D. Renaud

331 Role of Fibroblasts in Synchronizing the Beat Rhythm of Isolated
Heart Muscle Cells in Culture
W. O. Gross

337 Mechanisms of Pacemaker Activity in Embryonic Cardiac Muscle
*R. D. Nathan, P. C. Houck, S. J. Fung, D. M. Stocco, and
R. R. Markwald*

349 Coaggregation of Embryonic Chick Sympathetic Neurons with
Cardiac Myocytes: Evidence for Functional Synaptic Development
in Vitro
D. A. Fischman and N. G. Culver

367 Myofibrillogenesis in Vitro: Implications for Early Cardiac Morphogenesis
R. R. Kulikowski

GENETIC CONTROL

383 Genetic Aspects of Congenital Heart Disease
T. Pexieder

389 Congenital Heart Disease in Experimental (Fetal) Mouse Trisomies: Incidence
T. Pexieder, S. Miyabara, and A. Gropp

EPIGENETIC CONTROL OF CARDIAC MORPHOGENESIS

403 Introduction
Z. Rychter

407 Cardiac Function in the Embryonic Chick
R. R. Ruckman, R. J. Cassling, E. B. Clark, and G. C. Rosenquist

419 Spectrum of Pulmonary Venous Connections Following Lung Bud Inversion in the Chick Embryo
E. B. Clark, D. R. Martini, and G. C. Rosenquist

431 Angio- and Myoarchitecture of the Heart Wall Under Normal and Experimentally Changed Morphogenesis
Z. Rychter and V. Rychterová

453 Cono-Truncal Torsions and Transposition of the Great Vessels in the Chick Embryo
X. Dor and P. Corone

473 The Role of Catecholamines and Other Cardiac Stimulants in Cardiovascular Teratogenesis: Recent Observations and Proposed Mechanisms
E. F. Gilbert, H. J. Bruyere, Jr., S. Ishikawa, and M. O. Cheung

485 Teratogenic Considerations Regarding Aortic Arch Anomalies Associated with Cardiovascular Malformations
A. Oppenheimer-Dekker, R. J. Moene, A. J. Moulaert, and A. C. Gittenberger-De Groot

501 *Subject Index*

Contributors

J. Aiton. *Department of Physiology, Duke University Medical Center, Durham, North Carolina 27706*

N. Akimoto. *Department of Geneticopathology, Research Institute for Nuclear Biology and Medicine, Hiroshima University, Hiroshima, Japan*

Carlos Argüello-Lopéz. *Istituto Venezolano de Cardiologia, Caracas 104, Venezuela*

D. H. Bernanke. *Department of Anatomy, Texas Technical University School of Medicine, Lubbock, Texas 74909*

E. Bogenmann. *Institut für Zellbiologie, Eidgenössische Technische Hochschule, Hönggerberg, CH- 8049 Zürich, Switzerland*

H. J. Bruyere, Jr. *Department of Pathology, University of Wisconsin Clinical Science Center, Madison, Wisconsin 53792*

R. J. Cassling. *Department of Pediatrics and Cardiology, University of Nebraska Medical Center, Omaha, Nebraska 68105*

C. E. Challice. *Department of Physics, Faculty of Arts and Science, The University of Calgary, Calgary, Alberta, Canada T2N 1N4*

M. O. Cheung. *Department of Pathology, University of Wisconsin Clinical Science Center, Madison, Wisconsin 53792*

Y. Christen. *Institut d'Histologie et d'Embryologie, CH-1011 Lausanne-CHUV, Switzerland*

D. E. Clapham. *Department of Anatomy, Emory University, Atlanta, Georgia 30322*

E. B. Clark. *Department of Pediatrics and Cardiology, University of Nebraska Medical Center, Omaha, Nebraska 68105*

P. Corone. *Laboratoire d'Anatomie et d'Organogenèse, C.H.U. Pitié-Salpétrière, F-75013 Paris, France*

N. G. Culver. *Department of Medicine, University of Chicago Pritzker School of Medicine, Chicago, Illinois 60637*

R. L. DeHaan. *Department of Anatomy, Emory University, Atlanta, Georgia 30322*

P. A. DeVries. *Carnegie Laboratories of Embryology and Department of Surgery, University of California, Davis, California 95616*

X. Dor. *Laboratoire d'Anatomie et d'Organogenèse, C.H.U. Pitié-Salpétrière, F-75013 Paris, France*

H. M. Eppenberger. *Institut für Zellbiologie, Eidgenössische Technische Hochschule, Hönggerberg, CH - 8049 Zürich, Switzerland*

D. A. Fischman. *Department of Anatomy and Cell Biology, SUNY-Downstate Medical Center, Brooklyn, New York 11203*

T. P. Fitzharris. *Department of Anatomy, Medical University of South Carolina, Charleston, South Carolina 29403*

S. J. Fung. *Department of Physiology, Texas Technical University School of Medicine, Lubbock, Texas 79430*

Enid F. Gilbert. *Department of Pathology, University of Wisconsin Clinical Science Center, Madison, Wisconsin 53706*

A. C. Gittenberger-De Groot. *Institute of Embryology and Anatomy, State University Leiden, NL-2300 RC Leiden, The Netherlands*

A. Gropp. *Institut für Pathologie, Medizinische Hochschule Lübeck, D-24 Lübeck, FRG*

Daniel Gros. *Laboratoire de Zoologie et de Biologie Cellulaire, F-86002 Poitiers, France*

W. O. Gross. *Institut d'Histologie et d'Embryologie, CH-1011 Lausanne-CHUV, Switzerland*

D. A. Hay. *Department of Anatomy, University of New Mexico, Albuquerque, New Mexico 87131*

M. J. C. Hendrix. *Department of Anatomy, Harvard University, School of Medicine, Boston, Massachusetts 02115*

N. Hidaka. *Department of Geneticopathology, Research Institute for Nuclear Biology and Medicine, Hiroshima University, Hiroshima, Japan*

P. C. Houck. *Department of Physiology, Texas Technical University School of Medicine, Lubbock, Texas 79430*

J. M. Hurle. *Department of Anatomy, Faculty of Medicine, Santander, Spain*

S. Ishikawa. *Department of Pathology, University of Wisconsin Clinical Science Center, Madison, Wisconsin 53792*

H. W. Klein. *Afdeling Anatomie en Embryologie, Medische Fakulteit, Rotterdam, NL-Rotterdam 3002, The Netherlands*

P. Krediet. *Afdeling Anatomie en Embryologie, Medische Fakulteit Rotterdam, NL-Rotterdam 3002, The Netherlands*

Robert R. Kulikowski. *University of Chicago, Department of Anatomy, Chicago, Illinois 60637*

H. M. Laane. *Anatomisch Embryologisch Laboratorium, Universiteit van Amsterdam, NL-Amsterdam 020, The Netherlands*

J. Lacktis. *University of Chicago, Department of Anatomy, Chicago, Illinois 60637*

G. Le Douarin. *Laboratoire de Physiologie Animale et Cellulaire, Faculté dès Sciences, F-44037 Nantes, France*

M. Lieberman. *Department of Physiology, Duke University Medical Center, Durham, North Carolina 27706*

J. A. Los. *Anatomisch Embryologisch Laboratorium, Universiteit van Amsterdam, NL-Amsterdam 020, The Netherlands.*

F. J. Manasek. *University of Chicago, Department of Anatomy, Chicago, Illinois 60637*

R. R. Markwald. *Department of Anatomy, Texas Technical University School of Medicine, Lubbock, Texas 74909*

D. M. Martini. *Cardiopulmonary Embryology Laboratory, Department of Pediatrics, University of Nebraska Medical Center, Omaha, Nebraska 68105*

S. Miyabara. *Department of Geneticopathology, Research Institute for Nuclear Biology and Medicine, Hiroshima University, Hiroshima, Japan*

J. P. Mocquard. *Laboratoire de Physiologie et de Génétique des Crustacés. U.E.R. Sciences Fondamentales et Appliquées, F-86022 Poitiers, France*

R. J. Moene. *Department of Paediatric Cardiology, Free University Amsterdam, NL-1081 HV Amsterdam, The Netherlands*

D. E. Morse. *Department of Anatomy, Medical College of Ohio, Toledo, Ohio 43699*

A. J. Moulaert. *Wilhelmina Children's Hospital, State University Utrecht, NL-3512 LK Utrecht, The Netherlands*

R. D. Nathan. *Department of Physiology, Texas Technical University, School of Medicine, Lubbock, Texas 79409*

J. L. Ojeda. *Department of Anatomy, Faculty of Medicine, Santander, Spain*

N. Okamoto. *Department of Geneticopathology, Research Institute for Nuclear Biology and Medicine, Hiroshima University, Hiroshima, Japan*

A. Oppenheimer-Dekker. *Anatomisch Embryologisch Laboratorium der Rijksuniversiteit te Leiden, NL-Leiden, The Netherlands*

F. Orts-Llorca. *Faculdad de Medicina, Departamento anatomico, Ciudad Universitaria, Madrid, Espana*

N. Paschoud. *Hôpital St-Loup, Ch-1349 Pompaples, Switzerland*

T. Pexieder. *Institut d'Histologie et d'Embryologie, CH-1011 Lausanne-CHUV, Switzerland*

J. Puerta-Fonollá. *Faculdad de Medicina, Departamento Anatomico, Ciudad Universitaria, Madrid, Spain*

D. Renaud. *Laboratoire de Physiologie Animale et Cellulaire, Université de Nantes, Faculté des Sciences, F-44072 Nantes, France*

J. A. Roest-Wagenaar. *Anatomisch Embryologisch Laboratorium, Universiteit van Amsterdam, NL-Amsterdam 020. The Netherlands*

G. C. Rosenquist. *Department of Pediatrics, Cardiology, University of Nebraska Medical Center, Omaha, Nebraska 68105*

R. R. Ruckman. *Department of Pediatrics, Cardiology, University of Nebraska Medical Center, Omaha, Nebraska 68105*

Z. Rychter. *Department of Histology, Faculty of General Medicine, Charles University, Praha, Czechoslovakia*

V. Rychterová. *Department of Pathology, Faculty of Medical Hygiene, Charles University, Praha, Czechoslovakia*

Y. Satow. *Department of Geneticopathology, Research Institute for Nuclear Medicine and Biology, Hiroshima University, Hiroshima, Japan*

J. Schrevel. *Laboratoire de Zoologie et Biologie cellulaire, (L.A. CNRS 290), U.E.R. Sciences Fondamentales et Appliquées, F-86022 Poitiers, France*

Marta Servín-Martínez. *Instituto Venezolano de Cardiologia, Caracas 104, Venezuela*

J. Sobrado-Pérez. *Faculdad de Medicina, Departamento Anatomico, Ciudad Universitaria, Madrid, Spain*

D. M. Stocco. *Department of Biochemistry, Texas Technical University School of Medicine, Lubbock, Texas 79430*

I. Taylor. *Department of Anatomy, University of Toronto, Toronto, Ontario, Canada M53 1A8.*

E. H. Williams. *Department of Anatomy, Emory University, Atlanta, Georgia 30322*

D. L. Ypey. *Department of Anatomy, Emory University, Atlanta, Georgia 30322*

Organogenesis of the Heart

Perspectives in Cardiovascular Research, Vol. 5,
Mechanisms of Cardiac Morphogenesis and Teratogenesis,
edited by Tomas Pexieder. Raven Press, New York © 1981

The Importance of Cardiac Embryology for Cardiac Pathology and Surgery

P. A. de Vries

*Carnegie Laboratories of Embryology and Department of Surgery, University of California,
Davis, California 95616*

I feel most honored to be asked to provide an introduction regarding the interrelationship between cardiac embryology, pathology, and surgery. Over 200 years ago in Lausanne, Albertus von Haller made his epochal contributions to cardiac embryology in his descriptions of the formation of the heart of the chick (1). Von Haller's study of several hundred living chick embryos at various stages enabled him to describe accurately not only static form but the blood streaming through the living heart. Subsequently, von Baer (2) pointed out the significance of two apparent streams of blood coursing through the evolving heart and commented on their relationship to the aorta and pulmonary artery. Since that time, several theories and studies have attempted to define the relationship between the two apparent blood streams and to describe the development of septation in both normal and abnormal hearts (3–7).

Von Rokitansky's (8) 1875 publication of "Die Defecte der Scheidewände des Herzens" not only brought to cardiac pathology a comprehensive view of septal defects and the various forms of transposition but also discussed their pathogenesis. Unfortunately, in the 200 and 100 years, respectively, since the publication of these great works, problems associated with terminology have increased as both embryologists and pathologists have attempted to describe the development of the chambers, outflow tracts, and septa of the normal heart and to define these structures in the abnormal. The use of different names for supposed homologous parts from one class of animal to another has compounded the problem, and it is my hope that some of these difficulties will now be resolved.

Maude Abbott's "Atlas of Congenital Heart Disease," published in 1936 (9), renewed the interest of pathologists in this century. In 1938, success in the surgical management of congenital heart disease was heralded by Gross' closure of a patent ductus arteriosus (10). In the same year, Helen Taussig was unsuccessful in her attempts to interest Gross in the creation of an artificial ductus arteriosus as a palliative measure for infants and children with cyanotic heart disease (11). Within six years, however, her association with Alfred Blalock brought about the anastomotic shunt which improved the lives of so many afflicted

children (12). Operations rapidly followed for successful resection and reanasto-
mosis of coarctation of the aorta (13,14) and the "correction" of various types
of vascular rings. These and other procedures involving the great vessels, although associated with congenital heart disease, can more properly be viewed
as pericardiac surgery.

The advent of intracardiac surgery for congenital heart disease first came
about in 1948 (15) with Brock's successful "closed" operation for both pulmonary
valvular and infundibular stenosis. Now, for the first time, it was necessary
for the surgeon to have a greater understanding of the morbid anatomy of
the heart. My own first exposure to these problems occurred when, as a surgical
house officer, I participated in Gross' first attempt at closure of an atrial septal
defect by the ingenious insertion, through a well in the right atrium, of a prosthe-
sis which he affixed to either side of the atrial septum. Open operations on
the valves and atrial septum were shortly thereafter carried out under hypother-
mia and inflow occlusion.

The beginning of a whole new era, however, commenced in 1953 when Gibbon,
after years of pioneering laboratory work, successfully closed a large atrial septal
defect using a heart–lung machine which he and his wife had developed (16).
In surgical circles the rush was on. For the next several years the greatest
amount of energy was expended on development and improvement of pump
oxygenators and the establishment and control of operating teams. For the
surgeons during these early years of cardiac surgery, preoccupation with the
problems, both mechanical and physiological, associated with cardiorespiratory
bypass took preference over the obvious need for in-depth study of congenital
cardiac pathology. Perhaps many agreed with Park (11), who stated in 1947
that Dr. Taussig had "done for the clinician what Dr. Maude Abbott did for
the pathologist, namely, made the malformations of the heart understandable
and accessible." Nonetheless, the last 30 years have brought forth a vast literature
of interest to both the clinician and the pathologist dealing with congenital
heart disease. Yet only a few pathologists have developed any in-depth knowledge
of congenital hearts, among them Jessie Edwards and Maurice Lev. Some of
us have remained diverted from our initial interest in cardiac pathology and
teratology by the recognition of a need for further study and understanding
of normal development, so as to have a better basis for evaluating the variant
forms. I believe that it is all but impossible to understand pathologic hearts
without a knowledge of normal cardiogenesis.

In the last 25 years, many ingenious and successful operations have come
into common use for the "correction" of congenital cardiac defects. Still, even
recently, I have seen an expert cardiac surgeon inadvertently resect the ventricular conduction system as a result of failure to identify that portion of the trabecular muscle that constitutes the crest of the structure von Rokitansky termed
the "septum inferius" of the interventricular septum. As the more complex
congenital anomalies, particularly those involving the ventricles and outflow
tracts, come under more frequent surgical attack, success or failure will increas-

ingly depend on a knowledge of the pathologic variations. Further definition of these pathological entities remains the unfinished work of those engaged in the study of the mechanisms and structural changes of cardiac morphogenesis and teratology.

REFERENCES

1. von Haller, A. (1758): *"Sur la Formation du Coeur."* M. M. Bousquet, Lausanne.
2. von Baer, K. E. (1828): *Entwickelungsgeschichte der Thiere.* Vol. 1. Königsberg.
3. Spitzer, A. Uber die Ursachen und den Mechanismus der Zweiteilung des Wirbeltirherzens. *Arch Entwicklungsmech. Organismen,* 45:686.
4. Beneke, R. Uber Herzbildung und Herzmissbildung als Funktionen primarer Blutstromfor-mem. *Beitr. Pathol. Anat. Allg. Pathol.,* 67:1.
5. Bremer, J. L. The presence and influence of two spiral streams in the heart of the chick embryo. *Am. J. Anat.,* 49:408.
6. Goerttler, K. Hämodynamische Untersuchul über die Entstehung der Missbingdungen des arter-iellen Herzendes. *Virch. Arch.,* 328:391.
7. deVries, P. A., and Saunders, J. B. D. M. (1962): Development of the ventricle and spiral outflow tract in the human heart. A contribution to the development of the human heart from age group IX to age group XV. *Carnegie Inst. Wash. Publ. Contrib. Embryol.,* 37:89.
8. von Rokitansky, C. F. (1875): "Die Defecte der Scheidewände des Herzens" Braumüller, Vienna.
9. Abbott, Maude (1936): Atlas of Congenital Heart Disease. American Heart Association, New York.
10. Gross, R. E., and Hubbard, J. P. (1938): Surgical ligation of patent ductus arteriosus. *J.A.M.A.,* 112:729.
11. Taussig, H. B. (1947): Congenital malformations of the heart. The Commonwealth Fund, New York.
12. Blalock, A., and Taussig, H. (1945): Surgical treatment of malformations of the heart in which there is pulmonary stenosis or pulmonary atresia. *J.A.M.A.,* 129:189.
13. Crafoord, C., and Nylon, G. (1944): Congenital coarctation of the aorta and its surgical treat-ment. *J. Thoracic Surg.,* 14:347.
14. Gross, R. E., and Hufnagel, C. A. (1945): Coarctation of the aorta. *N. Engl. J. Med.,* 233:287.
15. Brock, R. C. (1948): Pulmonary valvulotomy for the relief of congenital pulmonary stenosis. *Br. Med. J.,* 1:1121.
16. Gibbon, J. H. (1954): Application of a mechanical heart and lung apparatus to cardiac surgery. *Minnesota Med.,* 37:171, 185.

Perspectives in Cardiovascular Research, Vol. 5,
Mechanisms of Cardiac Morphogenesis and Teratogenesis,
edited by Tomas Pexieder. Raven Press, New York © 1981

Synopsis of Normal Cardiac Development

P. Krediet and H. W. Klein

Department of Anatomy and Embryology, Erasmus University, Rotterdam, Netherlands

In our collection, consisting of 400 congenitally malformed and 100 normal hearts, we have measured the diameters of all ostia of the heart and the arterial stems at different sites (6,7,8). Since the capacity of blood vessels is directly related to their cross-sectional area, for which the formula reads πr^2, for purposes of comparison we can eliminate π and simply square the diameters. By doing this, it becomes clear that the sum of the squared diameters of the arterial branches is equal to the square of the diameter of the arterial stem itself. This holds true for the aorta ascendens, arcus aortae, and aorta descendens, for the pulmonary trunk with its branches, and for other large arteries.

It can be concluded from this observation that the cross-sectional area of an artery is proportional to the amount of blood passing. We can call this the flow-dependence rule. This rule holds true in the adult as well as in the newborn and the fetus, and even during the period of transformation of the aortic arch system (embryo length 7 to 17 mm) (3). The latter is demonstrated by the way the aortic arch system reacts to abnormal blood flow in malforming embryonic hearts (12 and unpublished data, 11,9), especially by persistence of parts that normally vanish. It is also clearly demonstrated after birth by the configuration of the derivatives of the aortic arch system in congenitally malformed hearts.

We strongly believe, therefore, that during septation processes the different parts of the heart and arterial trunks are strongly influenced by the way blood flow from the sinus venosus is divided at the atrial level and is pumped through the left and right heart, to be reunited in the descending aorta as the aortic and pulmonary arches join. For this reason, one can assume that during normal development a balance must be maintained between the amounts of blood pumped through the left and right heart. We must keep in mind, however, that neither the embryo nor the fetus gains any advantage or disadvantage from septation and division of the heart, whether these processes take place correctly or incorrectly. Circulation before birth will function as well with a simple single pump as with a more complex double pump. But function must take place without hindrance from the different structures under formation. The problem, therefore, is not primarily how malformations of the heart can develop, but rather how and why so often the balance between all processes involved is maintained, usually resulting in a "normal" heart, that is, a heart built up by structures within the normal range of individual variation. Deviation from normal development beyond a certain degree (the threshold between normal and abnormal is not yet known) will lead to alterations of blood flow through the dividing heart and consequently to adaptations which, in a cumulative way, may disturb septation and further outgrowth of the heart and arterial trunks (2,6). This leads to the conclusion that the heart develops according to two leading principles:

1. Formation of the tubular heart, its bending, and the onset of formation of septa, cushions, and ridges, are genetically determined.
2. Outgrowth of the different parts of the heart and the induced structures are both influenced by the moulding force of the bloodstream, and are thus the result of both genetic and epigenetic forces.

The consequence of the second principle is that normal development is also the result of reciprocal influences between structure and function. In other words, septa reach their destination only when the blood flow along them does not disturb their outgrowth beyond a certain, although unknown, point. Blood flow through both developing halves of the heart must maintain a kind of equilibrium, i.e., must be of more or less equal volume, to allow balanced further development, a condition without which creation of a normal heart is not possible.

All blood reaches the heart by way of the sinus venosus. During bending of the tubular heart and outgrowth of the atrium commune, this sinus is relocated to the right and dorsal side. The ostium atrioventriculare commune, at first situated on the left side, brings the blood into the ventricular loop. During atrial septation, the direction of flow undergoes great changes (9). The atrioventricular canal shifts toward a midposition and the atrium commune becomes divided into two parts by the atrial septum primum. This septum, in combination with the atrioventricular cushions and the infolding of the dorsal ventricular wall, will interfere primarily with blood flow via the foramen interatriale primum, directed to the left side of the atrioventricular canal. Formation of the foramen interatriale secundum (ovale) will restore the possibility of blood flow to the left side of the atrium and so to the left ventricle. It is of great importance that not only a flow to the left side is allowed, but blood flow to the left atrium and ventricle must be of approximately equal volume to that on the right side in order to create pairs of atria, ostia atrioventricularia, and ventricles that are of approximately equal size. This also depends on the direction of the bloodstream incoming from the sinus venosus. Later on, it is clear that the two laminar blood streams from the vena cava inferior, O_2-poor blood from the caudal part of the embryo and O_2-rich blood from the placenta, are predominantly directed towards the foramen ovale into the left atrium, while blood from the vena cava superior remains predominantly in the right atrium. This change in direction of the bloodstream, from foramen primum to foramen secundum (ovale) during formation of the atrial septum is a most important feature.

However, in reconstructions of embryonic hearts there is little substantially quantified information regarding this point (4).

Given a more or less equal division of the amount of blood between the atria, both atrioventricular canals transport about the same amounts of blood into the two outgrowing ventricles. In this balanced situation, both ventricles will become of similar size, with a septum interventriculare in the midposition. During outgrowth of the ventricular loop and the formation of left and right ventricles the truncus arteriosus becomes situated at the cranio-ventral side of the prospective right ventricle. The left ventricle also has an outflow tract through the foramen interventriculare into the truncus arteriosus. In the normal situation, the bloodstream from the right ventricle enters the cono-truncus along the right cranio-ventral side; the bloodstream from the left ventricle enters along the left caudo-dorsal side. Since the flow of both streams differs in direction, they will twist around each other in a clockwise manner in the cono-truncus and will thereby change their position on their way to the saccus aorticus (1,2). It is remarkable that in all mammals about which embryonic development is fairly well understood, these septation processes take place in embryos of about the same size, 7 to 17 mm CR length, although they may differ widely in conceptional age. This twisting enables the bloodstream from the right ventricle to reach the saccus aorticus in a left caudal position and the stream from the left ventricle in a right cranial position. In this way, blood from the vena cava inferior, passing the foramen ovale, reaches the saccus aorticus ventral to the fourth and third pair of aortic arches. It enters the saccus from the right side, passing the saccus towards the left fourth aortic arch, which will consequently become the aortic arch (in mammals, not in birds).

The only way the truncus arteriosus can be divided by a septum into two independent trunks is in between the two bloodstreams twisting around each other. Only in that position will the septum grow without struggle against the moulding force of the two bloodstreams. This is of crucial importance when the septum reaches the conus (or bulbus). The conus ridges will eventually elevate from the wall and finish septation with the aid of atrioventricular cushion tissue, separating definitively the right and the left ventricular bloodstreams. The pars membranacea septi will be formed. Serially reconstructed embryonic hearts in this phase of septation show in detail the sequence of events (5). However, they do not show the bloodstreams in the two arterial trunks. During normal development both bloodstreams and the septum under construction do not hinder each other. Expansion of the blood flow through one part of the heart—and consequent diminution of the flow through the other part—will direct a greater stream into one of the trunks, which will therefore enlarge. The lower edge of the septum under formation must, in order to stay in between the streams, give way to the enlarged stream and deviate from the midline position towards the lesser stream. In the conus region, this means that the ridges are under stress from the enlarged blood stream which will greatly hinder the endocardial cushion tissues in their task of closing the last opening (9).

There is a strong possibility, the more the imbalance increases, that closure of the foramen interventriculare secundum will be prevented. A VSD, a "foramen interventriculare persistens," is born. This would imply that persistence of the foramen interventriculare might be caused by any irregularity disturbing the balance between the two bloodstreams in the heart. This could be malposition of the sinus venosus, delayed formation or incorrect position of the foramen ovale, unequal division of the atrioventricular canal as well as unequal ventricular outgrowth, malposition of the conus in relation to the ventricular septum, or incorrect twisting of left and right ventricular outflow streams in the cono-truncus region. These deviations from normal development will influence one another. Even in detailed reconstructions of malformed embryonic hearts, it will be impossible to tell what initiated the imbalance.

SYNOPTIC DIAGRAM (FIG. 1)

In order to illustrate in a practical and visual way our concept of the processes involved in normal cardiovascular development as well as those of maldevelopments and their interrelations, we have drawn a synoptic diagram. The diagram is subdivided into zones which, from left to right, represent developmental periods. In each zone, those primordia and developmental processes are indicated which are considered to play essential roles in the sequence of events leading to a normal or to an abnormal heart. On the left side, we have put in the first column the cardiac tube with primitive sinus venosus and truncus arteriosus. In the second and third columns the cardiac tube has looped.

To read the diagram, one must simply follow the lines connecting the different items, thus tracing the development of "adult" structures from the primordia. Each step will influence the next and other subsequent steps. These influences are indicated by interconnecting lines in a horizontal, vertical, and/or oblique direction. Where septation results in two parallel parts involved in left–right balance, a vertical rectangle, divided by a diagonal line into two triangles, appears to the left of the item. The triangle with base upward indicates a part belonging to the left heart and the one with base downward a part belonging to the right heart. All processes with a balance sign may become unbalanced. This will influence most of the other processes with a balance sign in one way or another.

During the septation processes, or even earlier, there are critical zones and critical times at which equal distribution of blood between both parts of the heart may become impaired. These critical points include:

1. Looping of the cardiac tube
2. Repositioning of the sinus venosus (L/R)

———————————————————————▶

FIG. 1. *Synoptic diagram of cardiovascular development.* The most important relationships between essential structures and/or processes are symbolized by interconnecting lines. Structures strongly depending on left-right balance are marked by the sign L/R (see also pps. 10 and 14).

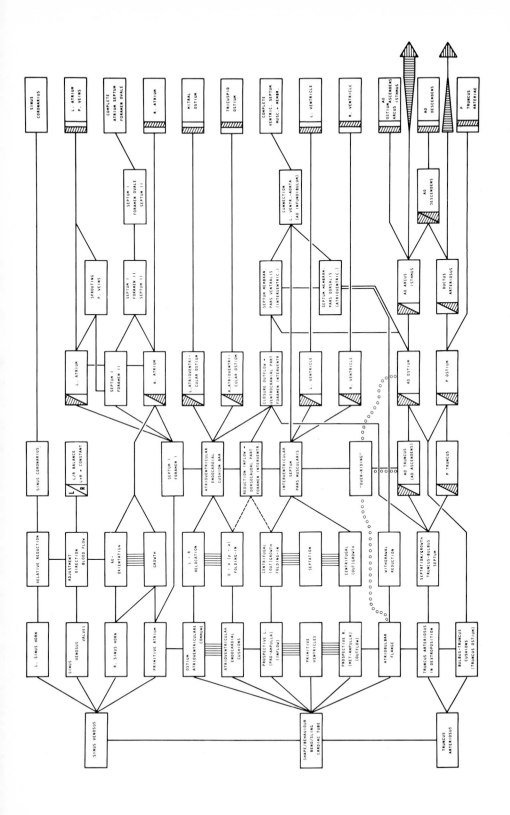

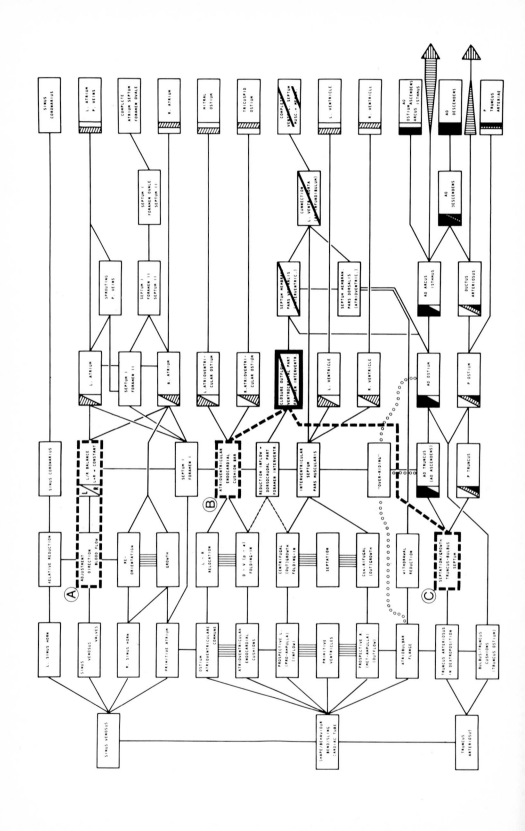

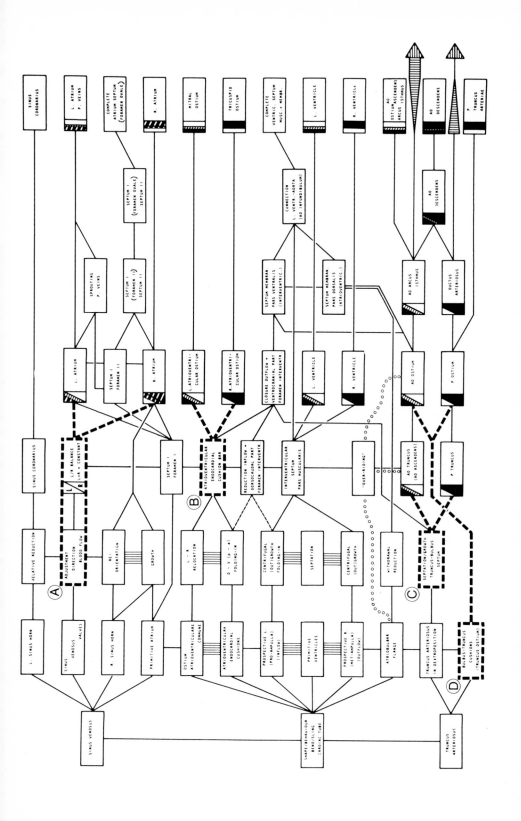

FIG. 2. (p. 12) Example in which a disturbance starting at three different points (A,B,C) in each case may lead to failure of formation of the pars ventralis septi membranacei (foramen interventriculare persistens)—maintenance of overriding of aorta = favored position—aortopulmonary unbalance in disfavour of pulmonary trunk L/R—*Fallot's tetralogy* (see also pps. 9, 10, and 14).

FIG. 3. (p. 13) Starting at four different points (A,B,C,D), unbalance in favour of the right heart L/R may lead to a hypoplastic left heart syndrome; unbalance in favour of the left heart L/R would result in a *hypoplastic right heart syndrome* (see also pps. 10 and 14).

3. Relocation of the ostium atrioventriculare commune
4. Formation of the septum atriorum primum, including formation and location of the foramen secundum (ovale) (L/R)
5. Formation and location of the atrioventricular endocardial cushion bar (L/R)
6. Outgrowth of both ventricles, including formation of the septum interventriculare (L/R)
7. Partition of the truncus and bulbus arteriosus (L/R)
8. Positioning of the bulbus ridges connecting the inferior margin of the truncus septum and the superior margin of the septum interventriculare (L/R)
9. Allotment of the bulbus (truncus) cushions to valvulae semi-lunares (L/R)

We feel it necessary to state that each small deviation from normal blood flow at one level of the heart will immediately have adaptational consequences at the same and other levels upstream and downstream. Deviations at any point of the path from sinus venosus to descending aorta may influence the features of the total path in the left as well as in the right heart. Disturbance of balance between left and right heart is the first consequence which, in its turn, causes deviations in the further progress of septation and growth. Nevertheless, if septation is achieved, a predilectional way of flow may result, with one half of the heart acting more and more as the main pump while the other half acts as an accessory pump only. Extreme examples of such an unbalanced condition are the hypoplastic left and right heart syndromes.

Many conditions of unbalance have obvious consequences for the great arterial stems. To illustrate, we offer two examples, leading to the tetralogy of Fallot and to a hypoplastic heart syndrome. In Fig. 2 three starting points are indicated, leading to failure of formation of the pars membranacea septi interventricularis; the aorta will remain in an overriding position. In Fig. 3 four means of starting imbalance are given, in the extreme of which the heart will become hypoplastic. The figure indicates formation of the hypoplastic left heart syndrome; reversal of imbalance will result in a hypoplastic right heart syndrome.

REFERENCES

1. Bremer, J. L. (1932): The presence and influence of two spiral streams in the heart of the chick embryo. *Am. J. Anat.*, 49:409-440.

2. Jaffee, O. C. (1978): Hemodynamics and cardiogenesis: The effect of physiologic factors on cardiac development. *Birth Defects: Original Article Series XIV,* 7:393-404.
3. Krediet, P. (1962): Anomalies of the arterial trunks in the thorax and their relation to normal development. *Thesis.* Pressa Trajectina, Utrecht.
4. Los, J. A. (1972): The heart of the 5-day chick embryo during dilatation and contraction. A functional hypothesis based on morphological observations. *Acta Morphol. Neerl. Scand.,* 9:309-335.
5. Los, J. A. (1978): Cardiac septation and development of the aorta, pulmonary trunk and pulmonary veins: Previous work in the light of recent observations. *Birth Defects: Original Article Series XIV,* 7:109-138.
6. Meurs-van Woezik, H. van, and Klein, H. W. (1974): Calibres of aorta and pulmonary artery in hypoplastic left and right heart syndromes: Effect of abnormal blood flow? *Virchows Arch. A. Pathol. Anat.,* 364:357-364.
7. Meurs-van Woezik, H. van, Klein, H. W., and Krediet, P. (1977): Normal internal calibres of ostia of great arteries and of aortic isthmus in infants and children. *Br. Heart J. (Lond.),* 8:860-865.
8. Meurs-van Woezik, H. van, Klein, H. W., and Krediet, P. (1979): Tunica media of aorta and pulmonary trunk in relation to internal calibres in transposition of great arteries, in hypoplastic and in normal hearts. *Virchows Arch. A. Pathol. Anat. (submitted for publication).*
9. Pexieder, T. (1975): Cell death in the morphogenesis and teratogenesis of the heart. *Adv. Anat. Embryol. Cell Biol.,* 51(3):1-100.
10. Pexieder, T. (1978): Cellular changes accompanying the pathogenesis of experimental hemodynamically induced ventricular septal defects in the chick embryo. *Birth Defects: Original Article Series XIV,* 7:452-455.
11. Rychter, Z. (1962): Experimental morphology of the aortic arches and the heart loop in chick embryo. *Adv. Morphogen.,* 2:333-371.
12. Schenk, V. W. D., Geene, M. J., Klein, H. W., Krediet, P., and Stefanko, S. (1976): A human embryo of 28 mm crown-rump length with cerebral, esophagotracheal, and cardiovascular malformations. *Anat. Embryol.,* 150:53-62.

DISCUSSION

De Haan: Would the heart not adapt to the increased resistance to flow by pumping larger amounts of blood?

Krediet: We believe that if one half of the heart is not used, it is missing its stimulation and will become hypoplastic. Because of the communication between ventricles and eventually the outflow tracts, the developing embryo has normally no reason to make one of the ventricles pump harder.

De Vries: As blood pressure seems to have something more to do with morphogenesis, have you looked at the relationships between the cross-section of the vessel, blood flow, and blood pressure?

Krediet: We think that in embryonic and fetal hearts the interconnection of systemic and pulmonary circulation by the way of the ductus arteriosus equalizes the pressures in both halves of the heart.

Oppenheimer-Dekker: You said that if there is some imbalance in the heart during morphogenesis, the interventricular septum will not complete. How can you then explain the intact interventricular septum in the left heart hypoplasy?

Krediet: This is a question of timing of the imbalance relative to the timing of the closure of the foramen interventriculare. Many of the underdeveloped hearts have finished septation before an imbalance started.

Challice: Are you suggesting that a primary deviation can cause or accentuate a secondary deviation, or are you suggesting that a genetic error produces a geometric disorder and that these two, combined, make the anomaly progressively worse?

Klein: I think that there is a competition between developing structures and the heart function. The result of this interplay will decide if a deviation will be enforced or overcome.

Krediet: I would like to stress that the imbalance may start anywhere, at the arterial as well as at the venous side of the heart.

Clark: In the mammalian fetus, there is good evidence that the right and left heart flows are not equal. There is, rather, a right heart predominance. The fact that the incidence of left-sided defects is more frequent would support your hypothesis.

Krediet: I compared the development of pig and cow hearts. The right heart predominance in the cow is accompanied by a very strong isthmus, whereas the left heart predominance in the pig coincides with the absence of isthmic interruption of the aortic arch.

Dor: I would like to bring to your attention that Dr. Rychter was able to get similar kinds of malformations by clipping off the atria.

Krediet: Yes, because as deduced from our observations, even a temporary narrowing of the AV canal will produce a malformed heart.

Dor: This is to stress that not every cause is genetic.

Pexieder: There are some links we have to mention. First: the primary aberrations of the heart development are followed by functional adaptation producing other structural anomalies. The message we try to pass to pathologists, especially, is that they never can say from the malformed heart what happened 8 months ago. Second: an interference at the proximal (venous) or distal (arterial) part of the developing heart may alter its development. Third: I would like to recall our previous work on the blood pressure changes in relationship to the disappearance or persistence of an aortic arch [Pexieder, T. (1969): *Folia Morphologica (Prague)*, 17:273-290].

De Vries: You will see variations in cardiac structure because even in homozygous twins there will be some variations in cardiac function. Often twins homogenous for certain genetic defects have dissimilar cardiac defects.

Challice: My understanding of your response is that we have both a genetic and a mechanical effect here. Under some circumstances, a genetic effect that is not corrected by the feedback mechanism can be made worse by the mechanical effect which is thus introduced.

De Haan: Is it true that if the vectorial flow decreases, the vessel diminishes in size?

De Vries: This is true and has even been analogized to the angle of ductus arteriosus and isthmus in relationship to its function.

Perspectives in Cardiovascular Research, Vol. 5,
Mechanisms of Cardiac Morphogenesis and Teratogenesis,
edited by Tomas Pexieder. Raven Press, New York © 1981

Morphogenesis of the Ventricular Flow Pathways in Man (Bulbus Cordis and Truncus Arteriosus)

F. Orts Llorca, J. Puerta Fonollá, and J. Sobrado Pérez

Faculdad de Medicina, Ciudad Universitaria, Madrid, Spain

On the basis of our observations and of the work of other investigators, we believe that there are several fundamental points that cause confusion when we attempt to elucidate the mechanisms by which septation of the bulbus cordis (conus), of the truncus, and of the ventricles is accomplished. Among these are the following:

1. Rotation of the cardiac loop
2. Formation of the interventricular septum and displacement of the atrioventricular foramen toward the right
3. Absorption of the conus
4. Fusion of the atrioventricular cushions
5. Independence of the bulbus cordis and truncus arteriosus
6. The bulbar ridges and closure of the interventricular communication.

The first two sections will be the subject of another publication.

This work has been carried out by studying embryos from the Orts Llorca Collection of Madrid, and from the Chair of Anatomy of Cádiz (Professor López Rodriguez). The specimens were drawn from stages 12 to 19 (22 to 39 ± 2 days; 4.5 to 21 mm). They were fixed in 10% neutral formol and embedded in paraffin. Serial sections were made on different planes, and were stained with hematoxyline, azan, Bielschowsky "in toto," and V.O.F.

Total or partial reconstructions of the external morphology, as well as of the cardiac cavities and the lumen of the truncus arteriosus of some specimens, were made by the three-dimensional method of Born (Table 1).

FUSION OF THE ATRIOVENTRICULAR CUSHIONS

The descriptions given in the majority of embryology books regarding the fusion of the middle part of the superior and inferior atrioventricular cushions to form the septum intermedium, which will separate the right (tricuspid) and left (mitral) atrioventricular orifices, do not correspond to reality. Such books state that in very early stages (13, 5 mm to 17, 11 mm) the superior and inferior cushions have fused, forming the so-called "septum intermedium" which will

TABLE 1. *Material used in this study*

Embryo	Length	Reconstruction	Collection
GV-5	4.5 mm	× 123 (total)	Madrid
Oy-4	6.0 mm	× 100 (")	Madrid
F-8	6.7 mm		Cádiz
Mta	10.5 mm	× 100 (")	Madrid
Cn-4	11.5 mm	× 100 (")	Madrid
Mar-4	12.0 mm		Madrid
Mte	13.0 mm	× 111 (")	Madrid
Faus	13.6 mm	Lumen × 50	Madrid
		Total × 50	
		Partial × 100	
HF	14 mm		Cádiz
No-15	15 mm	Partial × 100	Madrid
F-5	16 mm	Lumen × 100	Cádiz
Civ	16 mm		Madrid
Mar-2	18 mm		Madrid
Civ-2	18 mm		Madrid
Bot	21 mm		Madrid

separate the tricuspid orifice from the mitral orifice. In both the chick embryo and the human embryo, however, we have observed fusion of the atrioventricular cushions in the majority of embryos up to much later stages.

In human embryos of 11 to 14 mm, it can be observed that in most cases the superior and inferior cushions are still independent, a space or fissure existing between them (Fig. 1A). This is also observable in many embryos of 14 to 16 mm (Fig. 1B), and even in older embryos (21 mm and more) the line of fusion between the two can still be seen. This space will form a canal connecting the atrium dextrum with the aortic infundibulum, "canalis infundibulo–atrialis." As we shall see later, this will form the third root of the aortic infundibulum in the stages that precede complete closure of the interventricular communication.

Frazer (2) and Odgers (11) speak of the "bulbo-auricular canal." Odgers has noted it in a human embryo of 12.5 mm and has also observed it, as we have done, in one embryo of 14.5 mm and in another of 16 mm. He states that it will close because of the approximation and fusion of the right bulbar ridge with the right wall (tubercle) of the atrioventricular cushions, but he does not discuss its true significance.

Independence of the Bulbus and the Truncus with Respect to Each Other

The classic treatises on embryology describe the septation of the truncus and conus (bulbus) as a unitary process that commences cranially between the fourth and sixth arterial arches and advances in a caudal direction. However, Kramer (7) has already demonstrated that there is no continuity between the truncal and bulbar ridges, but that the interruption between the two is found immediately caudal to the region in which the sigmoid valves are formed.

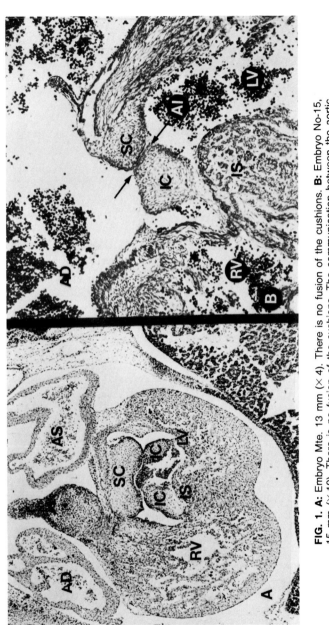

FIG. 1. A: Embryo Mte. 13 mm (× 4). There is no fusion of the cushions. **B:** Embryo No-15, 15 mm (× 10). There is no fusion of the cushions. The communication between the aortic infundibulum and the atrium dextrum is shown *(arrows)*. AD, atrium dextrum; AS, atrium sinistrum; IC, inferior cushion; SC, superior cushion; AI, aortic infundibulum; LR, left or septal ridge; IS, interventricular septum (pars muscularis); RV, right ventricle; LV, left ventricle.

Grant (6) has stated that septation of the truncus is an independent process from that of the bulbus, since the truncal ridges never fuse with the bulbar ridges. We agree with this viewpoint. In fact, if we study human embryos of 9 to 12 mm it is easy to confirm that septation between aorta and pulmonary artery is complete (Fig. 2A) at the level of the truncus while this septation does not yet exist in the bulbus, and the coni or infundibula of the aorta and of the pulmonary artery communicate with each other (Fig. 2B).

Today we know, especially as the result of experimental work with marking in the chick embryo carried out by V. de la Cruz et al. (1), that the truncus and the conus are two different embryological entities. This is important because the truncus, which lengthens considerably, continues with the right and left arterial arches (principally the third, fourth, and sixth) which "anchor" it to the ventral face of the pharynx. It therefore cannot undergo rotation.

When we consider the foregoing points, it seems remarkable that this distinction is not made in the excellent works of Los (9,10) on the chick. He speaks of truncal ridges when it can clearly be seen in his figures that it is the bulbus that is concerned. We consider that this distinction is of great importance for understanding cardiac septation, since the truncus does not properly belong to the heart but to the arterial system. It is derived from the lengthening, and from the visible dilation in somitic embryos, of the so-called "saccus aorticus" from which the arterial arches emerge. This is also an important consideration in seeking an explanation for the different varieties of truncus arteriosus persistens.

The Bulbar Ridges. Isolation of the Infundibulum of the Aorta from the Pulmonary Artery. Closure of the Interventricular Communication

Very early, while the processes described above are occurring, projections develop toward the lumen of the bulbus cordis, the so-called bulbar ridges. Because of their situation they are dorso-lateral (right for Grant; parietal for Los) and ventro-medial (left for Grant; septal for Los). They begin to form at the junction of the truncus and the bulbus where the rudiments of the sigmoid valves appear. From this point they advance in a proximal direction toward the trabeculated portion of the right ventricle. Their appearance in embryos of 10 to 11 mm is shown in Fig. 2B. They form an incomplete separation between a dorso-medial portion and a ventro-lateral portion. The former is the future aortic conus (infundibulum) and the latter the pulmonary infundibulum. Even in younger embryos of 6 to 7 mm (Horizon XIV, 28 days), before projections are formed in the lumen, the accumulation of cardiac jelly at this level can be seen on the dorso-lateral and medio-ventral faces of the bulbus.

If the bulbar ridges are followed carefully in a proximal direction in this and in successive stages, sections of embryos and reconstructions show that the right ridge continues and amalgamates with the right lateral part of the atrioventricular cushions (Fig. 3A and B). The left ridge arrives at the right

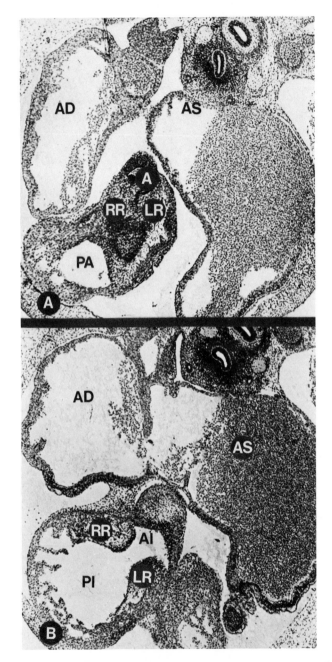

FIG. 2. A: Embryo Cn-4. 11 mm (× 4). The truncus arteriosus is septated. There is separation between the aorta and the pulmonary artery. **B:** Embryo Cn-4. 11 mm (× 4). The bulbus cordis is not septated. The aortic and pulmonary infundibula communicate amply. There are manifest bulbar ridges. A, aorta; AD, atrium dextrum; AS, atrium sinistrum; PA, pulmonary artery; AI, aortic infundibulum; PI, pulmonary infundibulum; RR, right ridge; LR, left ridge.

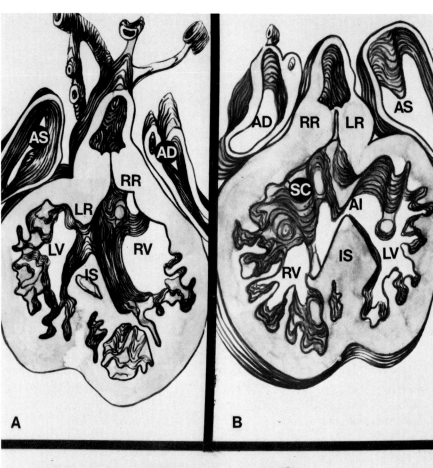

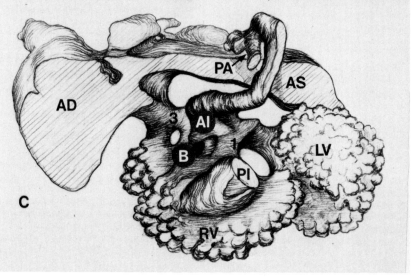

apical portion of the interventricular septum in a manner similar to that described some time ago by Odgers (11).

In the early stages (12 and 13, ± 5 mm) in which the atrioventricular foramen has not yet moved towards the right, there is an orifice, ample in relation to the size of the heart (1 mm maximum dimension), limited ventrally by the free edge of the rudimentary interventricular septum and dorsally by the bulbo-ventricular spur. The primitive ventricle (future left ventricle) makes contact with the bulbus, whose caudal portion, when it grows, will form the trabeculated portion of the right ventricle. This orifice is the bulboventricular foramen or interventricular foramen I as described by Goor et al. (3–5). It is obvious that this orifice cannot close. Instead, it will structure itself, as we shall see later, to form the outflow conus from the left ventricle, or aortic infundibulum.

When displacement of the atrioventricular foramen towards the right and disappearance of the bulboventricular spur take place, during stages 14 to 16 (29 to 33 days), the future right atrioventricular orifice (tricuspid) opens into the right ventricle.

The fundamental processes that lead to definitive septation of the aortic and pulmonary coni or infundibula and to separation of the two ventricles take place in human embryos of 13 to 18 to 20 mm (stages 17 to 19; 37 to 42 days). For this reason, we have made several reconstructions in these stages. In embryos of 13 to 14 mm, as a result of the disappearance of the bulboventricular spur and of the so-called absorption of the bulbus by the right ventricle, the bulbus forms the smooth nontrabeculated part of the ventricle. The portion of the bulbus from which the aortic conus will form overrides the interventricular septum (Fig. 3A and B).

In sections, and more clearly in solid reconstructions of the endocardiac lumen in embryos at these stages, we can see that the aortic infundibulum has three sources of origin (Fig. 3C). The first of these is an origin or root that proceeds from the left ventricle, which will be the aortic infundibulum and which is a restructured bulboventricular foramen (interventricular I), so that this orifice never closes, as noted by Odgers (11) and Orts Llorca et al. (13). This orifice therefore does not decrease in size during these stages; its diameter will later expand to form the aortic infundibulum (Fig. 3C).

The second root (Figs. 3A and B) proceeds from the right ventricle. This is

---

FIG. 3. A–B: Drawing of reconstruction in plastic by the method of Born of the heart of embryo Mte, 13 mm (× 111). A. Cranial–ventral segment of the reconstruction. The left ridge contacts the superior portion of the interventricular septum. B. Inferior dorsal–caudal portion of the reconstruction. The right ridge contacts the superior cushion. **C:** Diagram of the reconstruction of the lumen of the heart and great vessels of embryo F-5, 16 mm (× 100). The truncus pulmonalis has been sectioned in order to observe the aortic infundibulum with its three roots: (1) left ventricular root; (2) right ventricular root; (3) atrial infundibular root. AD, atrium dextrum; AS, atrium sinistrum; PA, pulmonary artery; SC, superior cushion; AI, aortic infundibulum; PI, pulmonary infundibulum; RR, right ridge; LR, left ridge; IS, interventricular septum (pars muscularis); RV, right ventricle; LV, left ventricle.

the interventricular foramen II, which has not yet "closed." This root progressively decreases in size in successive stages. Grant (6) believes that this foramen has a constant dimension of 0.5 mm, and that it will continue thus during the fetal period.

What are the limits of this orifice? The limits are formed to a great extent by the dorso-lateral and ventro-medial bulbar ridges, which descend from the vicinity of the aortic valves where they form an inferiorly concave arch that will be the future crista supraventricularis. In the reconstruction and in the sections it can be seen how the medial ridge moves downward and forward to situate itself on the right part of the free edge of the interventricular septum on its anterior part. This is the septal ridge of Los (8) (Fig. 3A and B).

The lateral ridge continues with the right lateral part of the atrioventricular cushions, limiting the tricuspid foramen laterally (Fig. 3A and B). At this level, the posterior part of the interventricular septum is the very large inferior cushion which limits the orifice. The lateral bulbar ridge becomes lost in the muscular wall of the right ventricle, hence the name "parietal" that Los gave it (Fig. 4).

The third root of the aortic infundibulum is very small in these stages, but is always present in embryos of up to 15 to 16 mm; the remains of it are visible in some specimens of 21 mm. In the solid reconstruction of the endocardial lumen of embryo F-5, a long but fine communication is observed between the aortic infundibulum and the atrium dextrum in the vicinity of the tricuspid orifice. This is the foramen infundibulo-atrialis (Figs. 1B, 3C, and 4A). Odgers (11) observed that it was still present in embryos of 14.5 to 16 mm, but he does not discuss its true significance. Los (8) demonstrated it in an embryo of 7.6 mm and the remnants of its fusion in one embryo of 19.8 mm and in another of 21 mm.

If the sections that pass through this region in embryos of 12 to 15 mm are carefully studied, several interesting facts are observed. In an embryo of 12 mm the right ridge occupies the concavity formed between the superior and inferior atrioventricular cushions, not yet fused to each other (Fig. 4A). In an embryo of 14 mm (Fig. 4B) the arrangement is very similar, although the superior and inferior cushions are in contact with each other. In an embryo of 15 mm the space described earlier (Fig. 1B) exists between the two; in another embryo of 16 mm it is readily apparent, and in the reconstruction it is clearly seen (Fig. 3C). This is what we have called the "third root of the aortic infundibu-

---

FIG. 4. A: Embryo Mar-4, 12 mm (× 10). The third root of the aortic infundibulum is seen between the two cushions *(arrow).* **B:** Embryo HF, 14 mm (×4). Disposition of the endocardial cushions and the right bulbar ridge. **C:** Diagram of the aortic infundibulum, based on reconstructions of embryos Mte, Mar-4, HF, No-15, and F-5 (16 mm): (1) atrial infundibular root; (2) interventricular foramen II; (3) foramen atrioventriculare dextrum. AD, atrium dextrum; AS, atrium sinistrum; IC, inferior cushion; SC, superior cushion; AI, aortic infundibulum; RR, right ridge; LR, left ridge; IS, interventricular septum (pars muscularis); RV, right ventricle; LV, left ventricle.

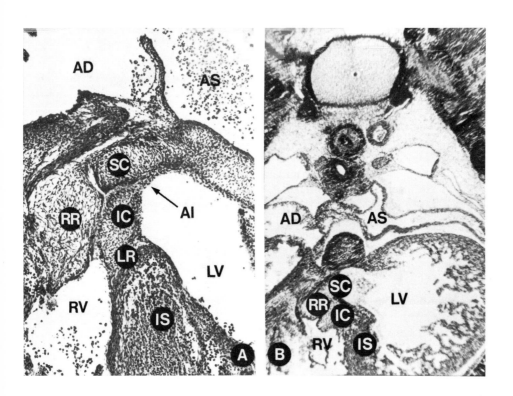

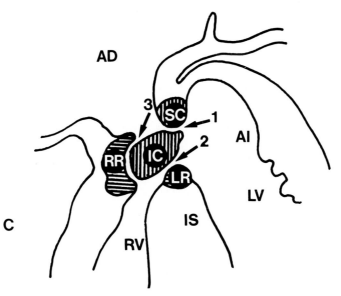

lum" and the communication with the right ventricle between the bulbar ridges. These structures limit the aortic infundibulum on the right.

If we attempt to schematize what we have just described (Fig. 4C), we see that the above-mentioned structures limit the aortic infundibulum on the right. Two communications start from it in these stages. One connects the aortic infundibulum with the right ventricle, limited at this level between the left bulbar ridge and the inferior cushion, and more posteriorly between the inferior cushion and the interventricular septum. This is the interventricular foramen II, on the point of disappearing. The other, the atrial infundibulum, results from the non-fusion of the superior and inferior cushions that terminate in the right atrium on the aspect that leads to the tricuspid foramen.

Los (8) described two human embryos, one of 19.8 mm and the other of 27 mm, with a defect in the interventricular septum. It is evident that in other cases the infundibulo–atrial communication may be preserved (1 of Fig. 4C) together with the interventricular communication. The persistence of a right atrium–left ventricle communication has been observed in 1% of cardiac malformations and, curiously, more frequently in the female sex. Several of these cases were published by Perloff (14), and the first case was described by Thurnham (15) in 1838. This communication is caused by posterior enlargement of what we have described as the "third root" of the aortic infundibulum, as a consequence of the non-fusion of the right part of the atrioventricular cushions (Fig. 4C).

It is very interesting to recall that during these stages (embryos of 11 to 16 mm) the inferior cushion undergoes considerable growth and is inclined in such a way that it adheres to the right aspect of the interventricular septum, forming an angle that is almost a right angle with the superior cushion. The importance of a hypoplasia at this level can easily be deduced.

Closure of the Interventricular Communication. "Pars Membranacea" of the Interventricular Septum

What structures contribute to the closure of the interventricular communication, which of them form the "pars membranacea," and what is their evolution? These problems have interested many investigators. In our work of 1970 (12) we reviewed the literature up to that time.

It is clear that the primary interventricular or bulboventricular communication cannot close as Frazer (2) suggested. Absorption or inhibition of growth of the posterior part of the conus places it in contact with the mitral foramen. Muscle fibers do not develop at this level, a fibrous continuity being established between the aorta and the foramen mitrale. Goor (4) observed the continuity of the two valves, aortic and mitral, in human embryos of stage 22.

With regard to the closure of the interventricular communication, therefore, the interventricular foramen II is referred to. The original idea that the septum bulbi, formed by the fusion of the two ridges (lateral and medial) would fuse with the free edge of the interventricular septum when it descends, thus closing the interventricular communication, cannot be accepted. On the contrary, the atrioventricular cushions, which undergo considerable development, will make an important contribution to septation.

The opinions of different investigators vary with regard to the proportion and importance of the materials (right and left ridges) of the bulbus cordis, superior and inferior atrioventricular cushions, that take part in definitive closure of the interventricular communication and in the formation of the "pars membranacea." Our observations allow us to describe the processes that lead to the closure of the interventricular communication.

Both in reconstructions and in sections of embryos of these stages, it is possible to follow the course of the bulbar ridges with precision. The medial ventral ridge (left or septal) descends through the anterior and medial part of the bulbus to reach the free edge of the interventricular septum on its anterior part (Fig. 3A and B). The lateral dorsal ridge (right or parietal) reaches the right part of the atrioventricular cushions, occupying the concavity that they form (Figs. 4A and B). The tricuspid foramen is thus limited laterally, and becomes lost in the muscle wall of the right ventricle. Both ridges proceed from the concave inferior edge of the septum bulbi, from which the crista supraventricularis will be formed. The atrioventricular cushions grow considerably toward the endocardial lumen and will contribute to formation of a large part of the pars membranacea (Fig. 1B, 4A and B, and 5A).

The inferior cushion reaches the posterior part of the free edge of the interventricular septum, the extension of the left ridge (Figs. 4A and C) being placed between the two. In some specimens a communication at this level can still be observed. In almost all the embryos studied at these stages, no fusion of the superior and inferior cushions still exists. However, the so-called atrial infundibular duct (Fig. 4C) does exist. With this diagram it is easy to understand how, when the above-mentioned orifices close, the closures will originate principally with the material of both cushions (Fig. 4C). When this occurs, two portions may be distinguished in the future pars membranacea, one being the right superior atrial infundibular portion and the other the inferior interventricular portion. This portion joins the aortic infundibulum to the right ventricle when the inferior cushion develops in the manner shown in Fig. 4C. Later, when the septal valve of the tricuspid is formed by delamination, the insertion of this valve in the pars membranacea will separate the atrial infundibular portion from the bulboventricular portion (Fig. 5A).

The only point in doubt is the possible contribution of the bulbar ridges in the inferior portion of the pars membranacea. In this respect, we feel that it is important to analyze the works of Wenink (16,17) and of Los (8) and to compare them with our results. Wenink believes that all of the membranaceous portion situated below the insertion of the septal valve of the tricuspid derives from the left ridge which, growing in the form of a hook in a backward and downward direction along the length of the free edge of the interventricular

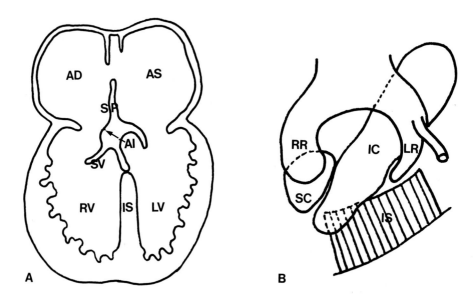

FIG. 5. A: Definitive constitution of the aortic infundibulum. The *arrow* separates the atrial infundibular portion from the bulboventricular portion of the pars membranacea of the interventricular septum. **B:** Diagram based on our observations. The left or septal bulbar ridge occupies only the superior and anterior part of the muscular septum. AD, atrium dextrum; AS, atrium sinistrum; IC, inferior cushion; SC, superior cushion; AI, aortic infundibulum; RR, right ridge; LR, left ridge; IS, interventricular septum; SP, septum primum; RV, right ventricle; LV, left ventricle; SV, septal valve of the tricuspid.

septum, separates it from the atrioventricular cushions. However, we observed that we could follow this ridge on the free edge of the interventricular septum only for a short course, limited to its anterior and superior part (Figs. 4A and 5B).

Los, who, like Wenink, has studied embryos belonging to the University of Leiden, reaches the conclusion that the "final closure of the interventricular communication is due to the fact that the right superior extremity of the inferior cushion is situated in such a way as to fuse with the concave edge of the right (parietal) ridge of the conus (bulbus); with the left (septal) ridge, and the neighbouring part of the interventricular portion of the pars membranacea. The right extremity of the superior cushion forms the portion that separates the right atrium from the pars membranacea of the aortic infundibulum, sending an extension in the form of a tongue up to the level of the aortic sigmoids."

We agree with Los that it is evident that all the posterior part of the interventricular septum comes into contact with and fuses with the inferior cushions. However, we agree with Wenink that the left (septal) ridge makes contact with the anterior part of the interventricular septum and forms a small wedge between it and the inferior cushion (Fig. 4A and 5B), and that it must therefore contribute to formation of a small part of the pars membranacea (interventricular portion). The septal valve of the tricuspid undoubtedly derives from the inferior cushion and not from the left bulbar ridge as Wenink believes.

REFERENCES

1. de la Cruz, M. V., Sanchez Gomez, C, Arteaga, M., and Arguello, C. (1977): Experimental study of the development of the truncus and the conus in the chick embryo. *J. Anat.,* 123:661-666.
2. Frazer, J. E. (1932): Development of the heart and vessels of the anterior part of the embryo. In: *Manual of Embryology,* p. 306. William Wood and Company, New York.
3. Goor, D., Edwards, J. W., and Lillehei, C. W. (1970): The development of the interventricular septum of the human heart; correlative morphogenetic study. *Chest,* 58:453-459.
4. Goor, D. A., Dische, R., and Lillehei, C. W. (1972): The cono-truncus. I. Its normal inversion and conus absorption. *Circulation,* 46:375-382.
5. Goor, D., and Edwards, J. E. (1973): The spectrum of transposition of the great arteries; with specific reference to developmental anatomy of the conus. *Circulation,* 48:406-410.
6. Grant, R. P. (1962): The morphogenesis of transposition of the great arteries. *Circulation,* 26:819.
7. Kramer, T. C. (1942): The partitioning of the truncus and conus and the formation of the membranous portion of the interventricular septum in the human heart. *Am. J. Anat.,* 71:3431-3471.
8. Los, J. A. (1970/1971): A case of heart septum defect in a human embryo of 27 mm R.R. length, as a helpful record in studying the components participating in the heart septation. *Acta Morphol. Neerl. Scand.,* 8:161-181.
9. Los, J. A., and Van Eijndthoven, R. (1972): Electronmicroscopical study of the fusion of the atrioventricular endocardial cushion in the embryonic chick heart. *Acta Morphol. Neerl. Scand.,* 10:391-392.
10. Los, J. A. (1971/1972): The heart of 5 days chick embryo during dilation and contraction. A functional hypothesis based on morphological observation. *Acta Morphol. Neerl. Scand.,* 9:309-315.
11. Odgers, P. N. B. (1938): The development of the pars membranacea septi in the human heart. *J. Anat.,* 72:247-279.
12. Orts Llorca, F., Lopez Rodriguez, A, and Garcia Garcia, J.: Morfogenesis del tabique interventricular. Paper given at the VII *Congress of the Spanish Anatomical Society.* Cádiz, 1970.
13. Orts Llorca, F., and Puerta Fonolla, J. (1979): Rotation of the cardiac loop and formation of the interventricular septum. (Unpublished work.)
14. Perloff, J. K. (1971): Therapeutics of nature. The invisible sutures of "spontaneous closure." *Am. Heart J.,* 82:581-586.
15. Thurnam, J. (1838): Aneurysms of the heart. *Med. Chir. Trans. Roy. Med. Chir. Soc.,* 21:187-215.
16. Wenink, A. C. G. (1971): Some details on the final stages of the heart septation in the human embryo. *(Thesis.)* Leyden.
17. Wenink, A. C. G. (1974): La formation du septum membranaceum dans le coeur humain. *Bull. Assoc. Anat. (Nancy),* 58:1127-1129.

DISCUSSION

Klein: As far as the third root of aortic infundibulum is concerned, do you not believe that this cleft will close every time blood is ejected into the aortic ostium?

Orts Llorca: I agree with you. Both the communication between the aortic vestibulum and the right atrium and that between the aortic vestibulum and the right ventricle do not function. However, they may be of importance under abnormal hemodynamic conditions. Also, in the truncus arteriosus of normal 6 to 8.5 mm human embryos there is always a communication between the aorta and the pulmonary artery. This may be important for the pathogenesis of the aorticopulmonary window.

Los: In my opinion, the left septal truncus ridge does not reach as far as you have described. I also do not agree with you that the fusion of all cushions takes place at the 17 mm stage.

Perspectives in Cardiovascular Research, Vol. 5,
Mechanisms of Cardiac Morphogenesis and Teratogenesis,
edited by Tomas Pexieder. Raven Press, New York © 1981

Evolution of Precardiac and Splanchnic Mesoderm in Relationship to the Infundibulum and Truncus

Pieter A. deVries

*Department of Surgery, University of California, Davis Medical Center,
Sacramento, California 95817*

The origins of the right ventricle, interventricular septum, infundibulum (conus, bulbus), and arterial trunks have remained controversial both ontogenetically and phylogenetically. If we are to understand abnormal morphogenesis, we must first have a clearer understanding of the normal.

In our earlier description of the development of the ventricles and outflow tract of the human heart (7), we were unable in early cardiogenesis to histologically distinguish myocardial primordia from nonmyogenic prepharyngeal tissues. This limitation resulted in our rather ambiguous use of the term "truncus arteriosus." Between 4 somites, stage 10, and 30 somites, the end of stage 12, we viewed it as morphologically synonymous with Davis' aortic bulb (4), a part of the epimyocardial mantle which admittedly became undefinable during stages 13 and 14, whereas in stage 15 we identified the presumed same segment derived from "epimyocardial mantle" as an apparently nonmyocardial portion of the outflow tract beyond the tricuspid valve primordia and between the myocardial infundibulum and the extracardiac prepharyngeal spur of tissue dividing the confluences of the fourth and sixth arterial arches. This obvious ambiguity appeared resolvable only by employing histologic techniques which would both define the endomyocardial layer and differentiate, throughout cardiogenesis, myocardial from nonmyocardial tissue. I will use the term "truncus arteriosus" for that segment of the outflow tract beyond the heart seen in mammalia from stage 13 to 17, which is similar to that designated by Greil (8) as truncus arteriosus in the developing reptile heart.

METHODS AND MATERIALS

Observations of human embryos were made largely from serially sectioned specimens in the Carnegie Collection, many of which are listed in *Developmental Horizons in Human Embryos* (10,19,20,21) and *Developmental Stages in Human Embryos* (18), together with plaster reconstructions in the collection or plastic sheet and glass plate reconstructions made by this author from enlarged photomicrographs of sections. Stages 8 and 9 are defined by O'Rahilly and are not synonymous with *Horizons* (18).

Primate serially sectioned embryos are from either the Carnegie Collection or Dr. Hendrickx's collection; the latter are listed by age and stage in *Embryology of the Baboon* (9).

Reptile embryos are *Xantusia vigilis,* a viviparous lizard provided by Dr. Malcomb Miller. The stage of development has been compared with Lacerta as described by Greil (8).

Serially sectioned Long-Evans strain rat embryos are from the author's collection; most were stained with alcian blue and P.A.S. (3; F.J.A. McManus, personal communication).

EMBRYOLOGIC OBSERVATION

Stage 8, Human

Presomite embryos, 0.5 to 2 mm, 17 to 19 days estimated age, are characterized by the evolution of the primitive pit, notochordal canal, and the neurenteric canal (18). The primitive node, notochordal process (head process), and prechordal plate (endoderm thickening) are present at the beginning of this stage. Bartelmez (1) pointed out in older embryos that those with the same number of somites may have varying degrees of development in different systems. Therefore, although I could find no clearly recognizable pericardial coelom in 5960, with the most advanced neural development, all embryos in stage 8 were examined. In 5960, as in other stage 8 embryos, the anterior and lateral intraembryonic mesoblast has vesicular areas which can be confused with coelmic primordia (Fig. 1A). No precardiac splanchnic cells could be identified in relation to such cysts which were lined with a squamous epithelium. Beneath the embryonic disc anterior to the prechordal plate, there is a crescent of mesoblast containing cuboidal, presumptive cardiogenic cells. They extend anteriomedially across the midline. More laterally, they are aggregated in clumps, as described by De Haan in the chick (5). Near the posterior lateral tip of the crescent at the level of the prechordal plate, there are areas in which ventral cuboidal cells are laminated to dorsal squamous cells without intervening space. These areas appear to be the sites of beginning differentiation into splanchnic and somatic mesoderm, and are the regions in which the beginning of the pericardial coelom is seen in more advanced rat and human embryos.

FIG. 1. (A) Cross-section of human embryo 5960, × 150, pre-somite, stage 8, at the level of the prechordal plate (EPP); cysts are in extra-embryonic mesoderm **(C)**. **(B)–(D)** Rat embryo E 4-6, stage 9, 9.5 days, × 240. **(B)** Cross-section at anterior end of pericardial cavity (PCC); ventrally splanchnic mesoderm (Spl) is stained with P.A.S.; the pericardium (P.C.) is dorsal. **(C)** Section halfway between sections B and D with pericardium (SOMPC) above pericardial cavity (PCC) and ventricular myocardium (Spl) below. **(D)** Cross-section at level of prechordal plates showing infundibular myocardium (Inf) and extra-embryonic cysts (C).

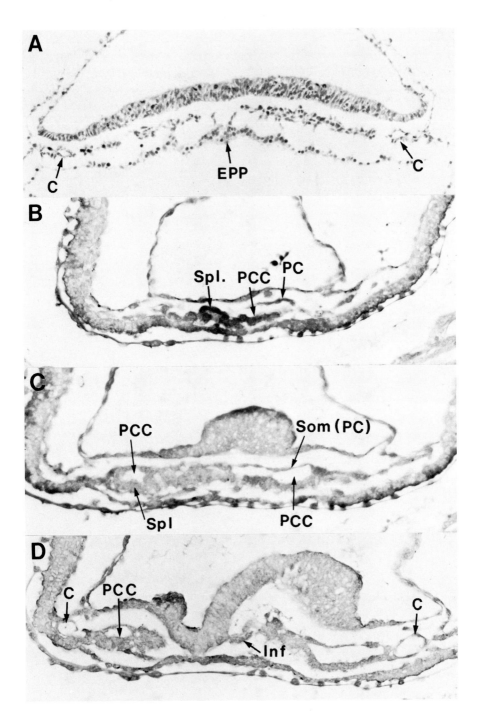

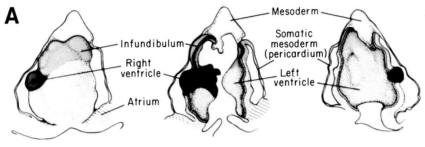

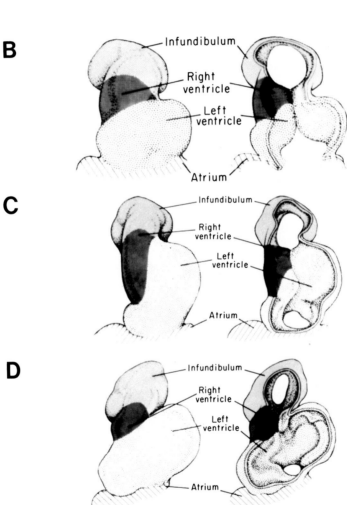

Surprisingly, in none of the stage 8 embryos could I identify with certainty any pericardial coelom. The McIntyre embryo (16) is said to have a pericardial coelom.

Rhesus embryo C473 is very similar in precardiac development to human embryo 5960, and lacks a pericardial coelom.

Stage 8, Rat

Nine-day rat embryos are developmentally similar to primates in stage 8. By 9.5 days, before formation of the first somite, however, the pericardial coelom is well formed laterally. Although there is some bridging (intimate contact) between splanchnic and somatic mesoderm, delamination has taken place across the anterior midline, beneath the embryonic disk in front of the evolving head fold (Fig. 1B). Burlingame and Long (2) stated that the "right and left mesodermal plates" were still separate at 9.25 days, and illustrated the point with a dorsal photograph in which lines were drawn in to show the coelomic spaces. No section in the midsagittal plane or cross-sectional plane documented their finding. Our embryos E4, 5 through E4, 14, either presomite or first somite forming, have continuity of splanchnic, precardiac mesoderm across the midline (Fig. 3B). Embryo E4, 6 lacks a foregut diverticulum and the short prechordal plate barely makes contact with the ectoderm at the anterior tip of the neural groove posterior to the precardiac splanchnic mesoderm (Fig. 1D).

Embryo E4, 5 first somite forming, 9.5 days is more advanced and has a significant foregut diverticulum. The ventral part of the cardiogenic plate is seen on parasagittal section (Fig. 3A). Beneath the myocardium, stained with P.A.S., the endothelium and myoendocardial glycosaminglycan (G.A.G.) of the endocardium is demonstrable. Medially, the presumed preinfundibular portion of the cardiogenic mantle has ascended dorsally with the foregut diverticulum and joins in an obtuse angle with presumed ventricular myocardium, still further anteriorly (Fig. 3B).

Cardiac development appears to be more precocious in the rat than in primates, relative to somite development.

Stage 9, Human

There are only ten stage 9 embryos, 1 to 3 somites, 1.5 to 3 mm, estimated age 19 to 21 days, reported in the literature, three of which are in the Carnegie

FIG. 2. Illustrated reconstructions of evolving myocardial tubes in human embryos, stages 9 and 10. **(A)** Stage 9 embryo 7650, 2-3 somites. Left figure: frontal view. Center figure: frontal view of inner surface after removal of ventral third of reconstruction. Right figure: inner surface view of ventral third. **(B)** Right frontal interior and exterior views of embryo 4216, 7-somite. **(C)** and **(D)** Similar views of embryos 4439, 9 somites and 3707, 12 somites. Note progressive dorsal fusion of fold, both anteriorly and posteriorly. There is segmental asymmetry in each of the four primordial hearts. Beginning "loop" formation seen in these hearts is not observable in straight frontal views of the same or similar embryos illustrated by Davis.

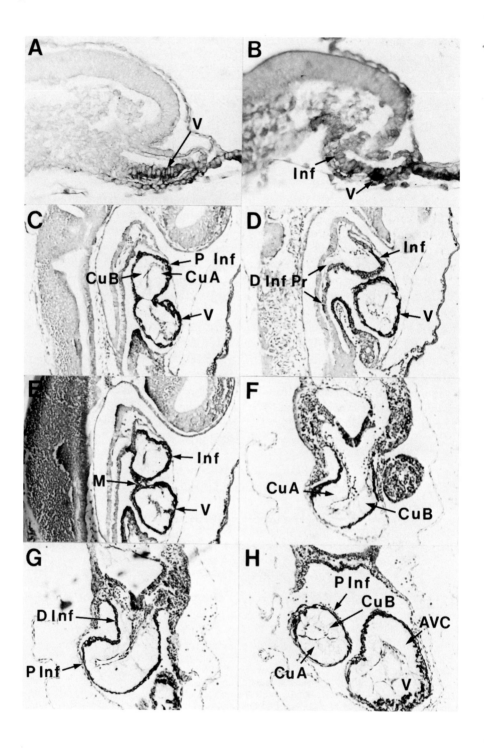

Collection (5080, 1878, and 7650). Only 5080, with one somite, has had the cardiac region described in detail; unfortunately, its poor histologic quality precludes further description than given by Davis for this earliest embryo of the stage. There is only a suggestion of some segmentation.

Da 1, Carnegie 5982. Examination of the photographs of cross-sections in the Carnegie Collection shows the pericardial coelom above the head fold, anterioventral to the foregut diverticulum and also in front of the head fold between the ectoderm and endoderm. Coalescing cystic areas show clearly the evolving pericardial coelom where the splanchnic and somatic mesoderm are well defined. The coelomic cavity extends posteriorly on either side to the level of the first somite formation.

The precardiac splanchnic mesoderm is bent around the head fold, accentuating a ventral infolding at the ventriculo-infundibular junction. The ectal grooves and bulges denoting these two primordial segments are clearly observable in each fold, whereas the ventricular primordia of each fold shade into their respective atrial primordia. Dorsal to the ventricle and the pericardial coelom, the lateral mesoderm is delaminating, and the medial portion appears to represent the future retrocardiac prepharyngeal wall. Right ventricular primordia could not be identified; however, one can see segments which we now view as proximal and distal infundibulum, respectively.

Embryo 1878, 2 somites, first described by Ingalls (11), was viewed by Davis (4) as more advanced than the 4-somite, stage 10 embryo 3709. The right lateral and left oblique illustrations in Ingalls' work appear to represent the configuration of the heart as seen in the sections better than Davis'. Neither shows clearly the dorsal and ventral contours as seen in the reconstructions and sections; however, I cannot dismiss Ingalls' suggestion that the specimen could represent ventricular situs inversus.

Number 7650 is a 2- to 3-somite embryo whose cardiac primordium has not previously been described. Illustrations were made from the reconstructions (Fig. 2A).

The splanchnic folds of the myocardial mantle are united ventrally without trace of fusion in the ventricular and proximal infundibular regions. There is ventrally a deepening sulcus between the folds of the distal infundibulum as

---

FIG. 3. (A) and **(B)** Sagittal sections, $\times$ 250, of rat embryo, E4,5, 9.5 days, stage 9, 96 μm apart. **(B)** Medial section shows infundibular (Inf) and ventricular (V) myocardium stained with P.A.S. **(A)** Lateral section showing only ventricular myocardium. **(C)–(E)** Rat embryo E3-5, 10.5 days, stage 11, sagittal sections, $\times$ 88. **(C)** Left border of junction between ventricle (V) and proximal infundibulum (P Inf). Cushions A and B (Cu A) and (Cu B) are seen in the proximal infundibulum, above ventricle (V). **(D)** Midsagittal section showing posterior prolongation of the distal infundibular wall (D Inf Pr) and G.A.G. **(E)** Section between **(C)** and **(D)** which shows bilaminar mesentery (M) lying in frontal plane between infundibulum and ventricle. **(F)–(H)** Transverse sections, $\times$ 88, anterior to posterior, of rat embryo EA-8, 11 days, stage 12. **(F)** Shows anterolateral walls of distal infundibulum extending to junction with transverse limb of proximal infundibulum. **(G)** Transverse limb of proximal infundibulum. **(H)** Shows distal infundibulum prolongation dorsally and ventricle (V) at atrioventricular canal (AVC).

they extend dorsally to fuse laterally with the pericardium and medially with the unsplit mesoderm. The folds are not approximated dorsally, but are closest at the interventricular region, and are segmentally asymmetrical. The infundibular region lacks a dorsal wall. Most noteworthy is a structural bulging between what I interpret to be the left ventricular primordium and the proximal infundibulum of the right fold. There is no similar structure in the left fold. After a restudy of all stage 10 to 14 embryos, I concluded that in all likelihood it was the right ventricular primordium. This is a departure from our previous view that the right ventricle was predominantly derived from the right fold, with the left major sulcus, the interventricular sulcus. The right trabeculated ventricle in both crocodilia and mammalia appears to have evolved from a part of a single ventricle rather than from a "bulbus cordis." In neither my study of *Xantusia vigilis* nor a review of Greil's descriptions of Lacerta can I find support for the idea of either "absorption" of the bulbus cordis into the right ventricle or "undermining" of the right infundibulum by trabeculae to effect its inclusion within the right ventricle. From the beginning the infundibulum is, on its greater curvature, continuous with the ventricle.

The horizontal septum of the lizard does indeed represent the left bulboventricular ridge corresponding to the left bulboventricular sulcus, and marks the anteroventral junction of the right ventricle and infundibulum in mammals.

Stage 10, Human

There is considerable variation in embryos, 4 to 12 somites, 2 to 3 mm in length, estimated age 22 to 23 days; in general. The asymmetry first seen in some specimens of stage 9 (Fig. 2A) progresses so that by the end of this stage the atrioventricular canal is toward the left border of the atrium, and the sulcus in the left fold between the infundibulum and ventricle has markedly deepened (Fig. 1D). Dorsal fusion of the folds first takes place at the junction of the infundibulum and ventricular segments (Fig. 1B), progressing both anteriorly and posteriorly (Fig. 1B-D). Segmental growth of the dorsally fusing folds is predominantly ventral, so that a lesser curvature is established along the line of fusion.

The cardiac mesentery is derived from the splanchnic mesoderm of the cardiac mantle dorsal to the line of myogenic fusion and extends, in embryos of 8 to 10 somites, from the more tubular proximal infundibulum to the atrium. It is bilaminar, one layer contributed by each of the folds. By 10 somites, the mesentery has broken down at the interventricular–infundibular junction, the apex of a ventral curve resulting from linear growth of the partially tubular heart. Thereafter, above and below this apex, cystic remnants of the mesentery appear as further interruption of its continuity occurs. The lateral bulbus folds of the distal infundibulum are unfused at the beginning of this stage, and become progressively narrowed by fusion. In embryos of 8 to 12 somites, the most anterior portions of the saccular infundibulum, above and partially ventral to the diverging first arterial arches, fuse and develop a bilaminar mesentery, while dorsally progressive fusion adds to the proximal tubular portion by incorporating the large unfused lateral saccular portions. The infundibular primordium does not terminate at the level of the first arterial arches, but extends progressively caudally in subsequent stages in front of the first three arterial arches having both a myogenic wall and underlying cardiac jelly or G.A.G. in the myoendocardial space. Reexamination of embryo 3709, a 4-somite human embryo previously described by Davis (4) shows it to be the youngest of this stage. It is not symmetrical, and one can see in the sections, reconstructions, and in Davis' Fig. 12, Plate 1, a segment of the right fold dorsally between infundibular and left ventricular primordia similar to that seen in the stage 9 embryo 5650, which I interpreted as the right ventricular primordium. Davis described a pair of sulci in the left fold, but I am able to identify only one deep sulcus, at the junction of the infundibular and ventricular primordia. The folds are of equal length and the asymmetry is with regard to the differences in length of the segments.

The asymmetric segmental growth and overall doubling of the cardiac length in embryos between 7 somites, stage 10, and 16 somites, stage 11, represents the period of "loop" formation. We have illustrated reconstructions of the myocardium and coelom of three stage 10 embryos, right frontal views (Fig. 2A-D).

Other Primate Embryos

In baboon embryo A65-142, 5 somites, there is a deep infundibular ventricular sulcus in the left fold and a definite segment of the right fold, identical to that which, in the human, I interpreted to be the right ventricular primordium. The heart has already started an S-shaped looping as a result of increased overall length and asymmetrical segmental growth of the folds.

The dorsal folds of the proximal infundibulum are closely approximated with a short mesentery forming, which extends largely from the right fold. The distal infundibulum has two bulbar lateral components, one from each of the ventrally fused folds. They are similar in appearance to late stage 9 and stage 10 human embryos.

Cardiac development in rhesus embryos is similar to that seen in human embryos having two to three fewer somites.

Stage 10, Rat

In the 10-day, 5-, 6-, and 7-somite rat embryo, the cardiac primordium, though segmentally asymmetric, is vertical without ventral or lateral bending. The proximal infundibulum narrows posteriorly where it joins the ventricle in the 5-somite embryo. Anteriorly, it is a clefted midline segment, which extends dorsally into a right-sided saccular distal infundibulum. The left distal infundibulum has virtually disappeared. There is an outpouching of the dorsal lateral wall of the right fold above the atrioventricular junction and below the infundibulum, which is similar to that seen in the human and baboon and is, therefore, interpreted as the right ventricular primordium. No truncus arteriosus is present as we have defined it. The segmental asymmetry described in this embryo progresses during stage 10. Loop formation commences before 9 somites, and the beginnings of the second arterial arches are observable. Cardiac development in the rat during the remainder of this stage resembles that of the primates, although somewhat more precocious relative to somite development.

It is not within the scope of this chapter to present in detail sequential changes and measurements in subsequent stages. However, comparison of the human embryo with the more appropriately stained rat embryos has provided some new insights which need description.

Stage 11, Human

The hearts of human embryos, 13 to 20 somites, about 23 to 26 days (12) correspond to those of rat embryos 10.5 days. During this stage, the cardiac length doubles and the axis between the lesser and greater curvature of the proximal infundibulum and ventricular segments shifts, as denoted by the remnants of the dorsal mesentery. In the human 20-somite embryo, this axis in the ventricular region has come to lie largely in a transverse plane, with the A.V. canal on the left and the right ventricular primordium on the right—a rotation of 90 degrees. The mesentery of the lesser curve of the elongated tubular proximal infundibulum extends dorsally to the left, having rotated 90 degrees. The short, now tubular, distal infundibulum still projects ventrally in front of the first and evolving second arterial arches, and its myocardium still extends laterally and caudally over the medial confluence of these lateral arches (Fig. 3C-E). The distribution of the myoendocardial G.A.G. is asymmetric, and in

---

Figure 4. Sections stained with P.A.S.–alcian blue to show myocardium and G.A.G. of myoendocardial space. **(A)** and **(B)** Sagittal sections, × 88, of rat embryo EP-9, 11 days, early stage 12. **(A)** Shows distal infundibular prolongation (D Inf Pr) above atrium (At) and distal infundibulum (Inf) above ventricle (V), just to right of atrioventricular canal. **(B)** Section to right of (A) showing interrupted mesentery (M), and mesenteric cyst at lesser curvatures of infundibulum (Inf) and ventricle (V). **(C)–(E)** Sagittal sections, × 88, of rat embryo EB-7, 11.5 days, late stage 12. **(C)** Left side of distal infundibulum above atrioventrioventricular canal (AVC). **(D)** Right side of distal infundibulum with proximal transverse infundibulum (P Inf) and its prominent cushion A (Cu A) above ventricle (V). **(E)** Central section through distal infundibulum and junction of distal and proximal segments ventrally. Evolving truncus arteriosus (TA) seen best anteriorly. **(F)** Sagittal section, × 88, of rat embryo EB-1, 12 days, stage 13, with increased length of truncus arteriosus (TA) anteriorly above and posteriorly below central confluence of arterial arches. **(G)** and **(H)** transverse sections, × 88, through mid and posterior portions of distal infundibulum in rat embryo at same stage as **(F)**; distal infundibular truncal junction is marked with arrows; the segments have started counterclockwise rotations as noted by the location of dorsal fusion cyst of the distal infundibulum above atrioventricular canal (AVC) and between atria (RA and LA). Note absence of cells in cushion G.A.G. in early stage 12 and increasing proximal cellular population in myoendocardial space in stage 13.

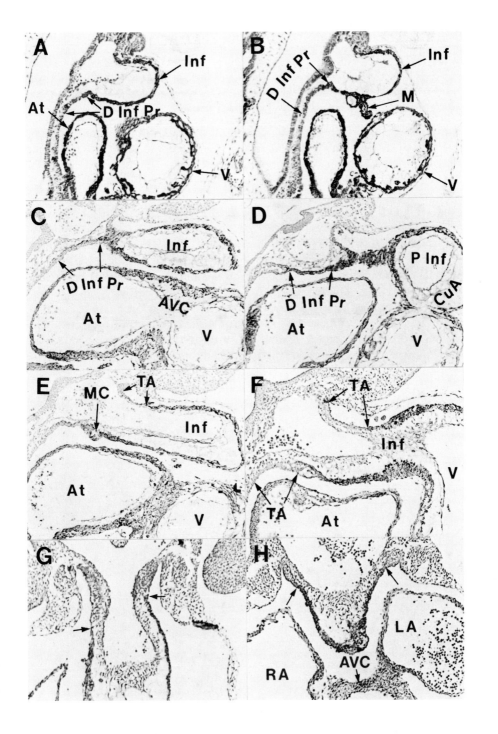

the proximal infundibulum the primordia of the spiral cushions A and B are clearly identifiable.

Stage 12, Human, 21 to 29 Somites, About 26 to 30 Days. Rats: 11 to 11.5 Days

A trabecular layer grows into the G.A.G. of the myoendocardial space in the ventricular regions, while the tubular length of the distal infundibulum increases with further incorporation of the lateral and posterior extensions of the infundibular primordium seen in the previous stages (Fig. 3F-H). There is concomitant growth, by cellular proliferation, of the prepharyngeal mesoderm where it joins the infundibulum, so that as the third arterial arches evolve one can now identify the beginning of the truncus arteriosus, particularly anteriorly (Fig. 4A-B). By the end of this stage, the third arches have so enlarged that the flow of blood is directly into these dominant vessels. The second arches are now anterior, while the development of the fourth arches is just beginning. In prior stages, the infundibular primordium of the myocardial mantle constituted the ventral wall of the aortic sac. Now anterior and ventral to the second arch, prepharyngeal truncus arteriosus primordium lies within the pericardial coelom and progressively becomes a part of the outflow tract. Posteriorly, just above the level of the primordial fourth arches, the myocardium of the infundibular primordium is split into two layers marking the distal termination of the infundibulum and the beginning of the truncus arteriosus. The infundibulum's linear growth, most marked in the previous stage, is now accompanied by increasing circumferential growth and some reduction of the acute angle between its proximal and distal portions.

Figure 5. A–D frontal sections, × 88, of rat embryo EA-6, 13 days, stage 15, from ventral to dorsal. **(A)** Shows infundibulum at level of semilunar valve formation. Aortic (Ao) and pulmonary (P) channels on either side of approximating infundibular cushions A and B; primordia of the six leaflets are distinguishable when compared with **(E)**, late stage 16. **(B)** is distal to **(A)** at infundibular–truncal junction. The lateral flanges of infundibular myocardium extend distally; protruding truncus arteriosus (TA) extends ventrally farther anteriorly than posteriorly. Note split in myocardial wall of distal infundibulum seen in earlier stages and the clockwise rotation of infundibular cushions relative to counterclockwise rotation of infundibular (Inf) and truncal (TA) walls. **(C)** is further distal with intrapericardial (TA) leading into arterial arches 2–6. **(D)** is just distal and posterior to **(C)** showing within the truncus arteriosus (TA) extracardiac connective tissue between confluence of fourth and sixth arches, the aortic pulmonary system (A–PS) in a transverse plane; the dividing connective tissue between right and left sixth arches is in a sagittal plane. **(E)** and **(F)** are frontal sections, × 88, of rat embryo EC-3, 14 days, late stage 16. The infundibular cushions A and B have fused; pulmonary and aortic semilunar valves (PSLVs) and (AoSLVs) are surrounded by distal infundibulum in **(E)**. In more distal section **(F)** the asymmetric elongation of infundibulum (P Inf) can be seen on the left surrounding a portion of the pulmonary semilunar valves (PSLVs), whereas to the right and anterior the separated aortic trunk is seen. In the 13.5 day rat embryo at the time of cushion fusion, cushions A and B terminate anteriorly posteriorly at the proximal extension of the aortic pulmonary septum, whereas earlier they terminated on the right and left walls.

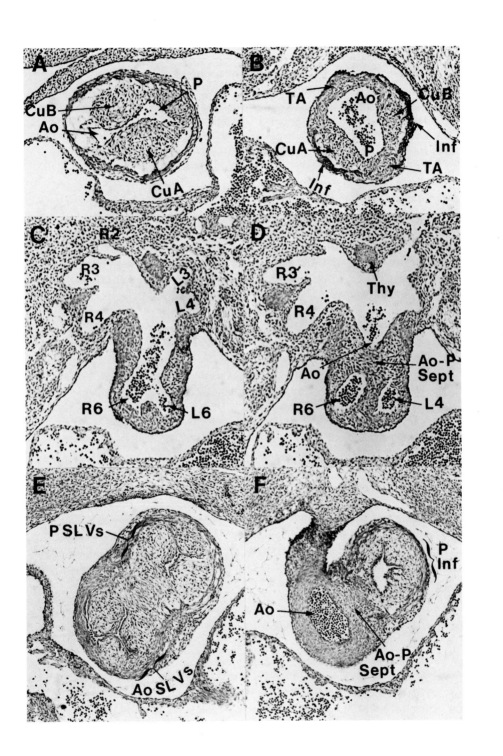

Stage 13, Human Embryos, 4 to 6 mm with Four Limb Buds, Lens Disc, and Otic Vesicle: Estimated Age 28 to 32 Days. Rats: 12 Days

At the beginning of this stage mesenchymal cells from the prepharyngeal mesoderm, between the endothelium and the evolving truncus wall, invade the G.A.G. of the infundibular myoendocardial space (Fig. 4F-H). This was described and illustrated by Greil 75 years ago in the 1.5 mm Lacerta embryo (8), and recently in the chick by Thompson and Fitzharris (22). This proximal migration and proliferation from cells beyond the heart tube is followed shortly thereafter by that from the endothelium within the heart tube as we showed previously in man (7) and as was shown by Markwald et al. in chick and rats (14, 15). With the cellular invasion, the cardiac jelly of previous stages is converted to cardiac mesenchyme in this and subsequent stages. The expansive growth of myocardium results in a shifting of the A.V. canal to the right, particularly of the left atrium. With increasing circumferential growth of the infundibulum there is further straightening of the angle between the segments, which now come to lie in an interatrial groove. These changes are significant, because rats treated with the teratogen trypan blue on day 9, who developed transposition, atrial localization to one side, tricuspid atresia, and a sinuous infundibulum and truncus, apparently do not manifest normal growth in this stage. Monie (17) was unable to observe abnormalities prior to e.d. 13; however, I believe further studies of trypan blue-treated embryos prepared in the manner of our normal specimens will permit earlier detection of abnormal changes and greater insight concerning both the time and targets of the teratogen.

Stage 14, Human, Estimated Age 31 to 35 Days. Rat: 12.5 Days

Continued ventricular growth, especially of the trabecular layers seen in stage 13, results in a clearly definable trabecular component of the interventricular septal primordium extending from the right wall of the atrioventricular canal to the infundibular ventricular crest. The establishment of the sixth arterial arches is accompanied by the further linear growth of the truncus arteriosus, now shaped rather like a truncated cylinder with its greatest length anterior. Cushions A and B spiral through 180 degrees in the infundibulum from the trabeculated right ventricle to the truncal infundibular junction.

Stage 15, Human, Estimated Age 35 to 38 Days. Rat: 13 Days

The expansive growth of the infundibulum and mesenchymal spiral cushions of stage 14 continues in stage 15. At the beginning of the stage, cushion A terminates on the right wall of the distal infundibulum, and cushion B terminates on the left wall (Fig. 5B). The common trunk, truncus arteriosus, between the terminal infundibulum and the transverse spur of connective tissue dividing the origins of the fourth and fifth arches, is now intrapericardial (Fig. 5C).

Its walls share in a counterclockwise torsion of the infundibular wall which, during this stage, results in a rotation of 45 degrees at their junction. The mesenchymal primordia of the semilunar pulmonary and aortic valves is identifiable within the infundibulum's myocardial wall (Fig. 5A).

Stage 16, Human, Estimated Age 37 to 42 Days. Rat: 13.5 to 14 Days

During this stage, fusion of the infundibular cushions occurs distally. In the 13.5-day rat, rotation of the distal infundibular and truncal walls has undergone further torsion. Now the formerly long anterior truncal wall has rotated 90 degrees and is situated on the right side, and the former short posterior wall is on the left; the longer distal infundibular myocardial wall is now on the left side and the short wall on the right; the extracardiac mesenchymal spur, between the fourth and sixth arches, the aortic pulmonary septum, lies in a sagittal plane, having rotated 90 degrees. The fusion of the two infundibular cushions has occurred and is at the site of the forming valve leaflets.

In rat embryos of 14 days, late stage 16, there is no longer a truncus arteriosus. Proliferative growth of the fused infundibular cushions resulted in their fusion with the aorticopulmonary septum of the truncus, and thereafter, separate arterial trunks.

SUMMARY AND CONCLUSIONS

It was found that the infundibular (bulbus, conus), ventricular, and atrial portions of the lateral cardiogenic folds derived from splanchnic mesoderm are distinguishable and partially fused anteriorly in stage 9 (0 to 3 somites), as the pericardial coelom forms. The distal infundibulum (Davis' aortic bulb) is a part of the heart; its primordium is definable anteriorly in stages 9 to 10, and continues to differentiate distally through stage 13. Cardiac asymmetry develops in stage 10 (4 to 12 somites) by asymmetric segmental growth, as the right proximal infundibular segment (Davis' bulbus cordis) and the ventricular segments become tubular by dorsal fusion, while the left distal infundibular segment disappears. From stage 11 (13 to 22 somites), as additional arterial arches evolve, the "aortic sac" develops. Its ventral wall is the primordium of the distal infundibulum until the truncus arteriosus evolves. The distribution of "cardiac jelly", the configuration of the endomyocardial G.A.G., is established in stage 11. The "truncus" evolves from extracardiac, prepharyngeal mesoderm beginning in stage 12, about 25 somites, peripheral to the distal infundibular primordium. Division of the outflow tract starts in the heart by fusion of the infundibular cushions distally at the site of the semilunar valves in stage 16, following torsion of the "truncus" and distal infundibular walls through 90 degrees.

The view of de la Cruz et al. (6) that the conus (infundibulum) and truncus are not present at the start of (dorsal) fusion of the myocardial folds is correct as regards the truncus, but is acceptable only in a limited sense with regard to the infundibulum, at least in mammals. She has apparently overlooked the anterolateral placement of the infundibular primordia. Her view of the site of semilunar valve formation suggests a definition of the truncus more akin to that of Laane (13).

ACKNOWLEDGMENT

Original illustrations by Kathryn P. Marr.

REFERENCES

1. Bartelmez, G. W., and Evans, H. M. (1926): Development of the human embryo during the period of somite foundation including embryos with two to sixteen pairs of somites. *Carnegie Inst. Wash. Publ.* 362, *Contrib. Embryol.*, 17:1-69.
2. Burlingame, P. I., and Long, J. A. (1939): The development of the heart in the rat. *Univ. of California Publ. in Zool.*, 43:249-320.
3. Chiquoine, A. D. (1957): The distribution of polysaccharides during gastrulation and embryogenesis in the mouse embryo. *Anat. Rec.*, 129:495-510.
4. Davis, C. L. (1927): Development of the human heart from its first appearance to the stage found in embryos of 20 paired somites. *Carnegie Inst. Wash. Publ.* 380, *Contrib. Embryol.*, 19:245-284.
5. De Haan, R. L. (1963): Migration patterns of the precardiac mesoderm in the early chick embryo. *Exp. Cell. Res.*, 29:544.
6. de la Cruz, M., Gomez, C. S., Arteaga, M. M., and Arguello, C. (1977): Experimental study of the development of the truncus and conus in the chick embryo. *J. Anat.*, 123:661-686.
7. de Vries, P. A., and Saunders, J. B. de C. M. (1962): Development of the ventricles and spiral outflow tract in the human heart. *Carnegie Inst. Wash. Publ.* 621, *Contrib. Embryol.*, 37:87-114.
8. Greil, A. (1903): Beiträge zur vergleichenden Anatomie und Entwicklungsgeschichte des Herzens und des Truncus Arteriosus der Wirbelthiere. *Morph. Jahrb.*, 31:123-310.
9. Hendrickx, A. G. (1971): *Embryology of the baboon.* University of Chicago Press, Chicago.
10. Hensen, C. H., and Corner, G. W. (1957): Developmental horizons in human embryos. Description of age group X, 4 to 20 somites. *Carnegie Inst. Wash. Publ.*, 611, *Contrib. Embryol.*, 36:29-39.
11. Ingalls, N. W. (1920): A human embryo at the beginning of segmentation with special reference to the vascular system. *Carnegie Inst. Wash. Publ.*, 274, *Contrib. Embryol.*, 11:61-90.
12. Jirasek, J. E. (1971): *Development of the genital system and male pseudohermaphroditism.* Johns Hopkins Press, Baltimore.
13. Laane, H. M. (1974): The nomenclature of the arterial pole of the embryonic heart I-IV. *Acta Morphol. Neerl. Scand.*, 12:167-210.
14. Markwald, R. R., Fitzharris, T. P., and Manasek, F. (1977): Structural analysis of cardiac mesenchyme (cushion tissue) development. *Am. J. Anat.*, 148:85-120.
15. Markwald, R. R., Fitzharris, T. P., and Adams Smith, W. N. (1975): Endocardial cytodifferentiation: Structural analysis correlated with sulfated mucopolysaccharide synthesis. *Dev. Bio.*, 42:160-180.
16. McIntyre, D. (1926): The development of the vascular system in the human embryo prior to the establishment of the heart. *Trans. R. Soc. Edinburgh,* 55:77-113.
17. Monie, I. W., Takacs, E., and Warkany, J. (1966): Transposition of the great vessels and other cardiovascular abnormalities in rat fetuses induced by trypan blue. *Anat. Rec.*, 156:175-190.
18. O'Rahilly, R. (1973): Developmental stages in human embryos. Part A: Embryos of the first three weeks (stages 1-9). *Carnegie Inst. of Wash. Publ.*, 631.
19. Streeter, G. L. (1948): Developmental horizons in human embryos. Description of age groups XV, XVI, XVII, and XVIII, being the third issue of a survey of the Carnegie Collection. *Carnegie Inst. Wash. Publ.*, 575, *Contrib. Embryol.*, 32:133–203.

20. Streeter, G. L. (1945): Developmental horizons in human embryos. Description of age group XIII, embryos about 4 to 5 millimeters long, and age group XIV, period of indentation of the lens vesicle. *Carnegie Inst. Wash. Publ.*, 557, *Contrib. Embryol.*, 31:27-63.
21. Streeter, G. L. (1942): Developmental horizons in human embryos. Description of age group XI, 13 to 20 somites and age group XIII, 21-29 somites. *Carnegie Inst. Wash. Publ.*, 541, *Contrib. Embryol.*, 30:211-245.
22. Thompson, R. P., and Fitzharris, T. P. (1979): Morphogenesis of the truncus arteriosus of the chick heart: The formation and migration of mesenchyme tissue. *Am. Jour. Anat.*, 154:545-556.

DISCUSSION

De Haan: Is it true that there is no contribution from the left side?

De Vries: I am unable to find one.

De Haan: If you remember our studies on cardia bifida in chick embryos, we have also seen much a larger contribution to the left ventricle on the right side. However, there is clearly some contribution to the right ventricle on the right side. I do not know if it is a species difference or a result of a more sensitive method in asking the question.

De Vries: How do you know that this is a right ventricular primordium? How far have you followed this?

De Haan: You are right. I do not absolutely know.

De Vries: I did not see it in many more embryos. I do not see any reason why there needs to be a contribution from the left side, other than the fact that you and others have interpreted it in the bifid heart as a right ventricular component.

Los: In the absence of a congress on the nomenclature of the developing heart, I would like to suggest changing of the term "aortic sac" to "aortic sinus" (analogous to venous sinus). I consider the outgrowth of pulmonary veins as analogous to the outgrowth of branchial arteries. As far as the persistence of ventral mesocardium is concerned, it has been illustrated by Dankmeijer, Oppenheimer-Dekker and Snellen in some abnormal human hearts. You can also see one in my poster.

De Vries: In abnormal hearts I have seen more of the mesocardial structures as the infundibulum has not progressed in them.

Rychter: Did you study the number and distribution of mitoses in relation to the sudden increase in the length of the heart tube between stages 11 and 13? Is it reasonable to speak about the cushions of the infundibulum before the immigration of mesenchyme? Or is it better to say that this is the region where, in later stages, the bulbar cushions will develop or not? The immigration of mesenchyme may be the causative factor explaining the different fate of cardiac jelly in bulbar and ventricular positions on the heart tube.

De Vries: Unhappily, I do not agree with your thesis, on the whole. I try hard to avoid any teleology. When I wrote my '61 paper I wished to confirm the spiral streams causing outflow tract spiralling. Therefore, I was not willing to see in stage 11 embryos the primordia of the cushions. Even if it is more difficult to see them in the transverse portion of the infundibulum in human than in rat and chick embryonic hearts, the primordia are there. The asymmetric distribution of the primordia is genetically there before the streams appear, and even before cellular proliferation.

De Haan: The whole-mount staining of the chick embryo will suggest that P.A.S. stains both glycogen and surface glycosaminoglycans.

De Vries: Are you concerned that we may be showing something other than the epimyocardium mantle with the glycogen?

Bogenmann: I am more concerned with the issue of whether the glycogen content is a true measure of what you are calling myocytes.

Fitzharris: If you look at P.A.S. positive areas, identified by light microscopy, with the electron microscope you will find cells with basal lamina, heavy glycosaminoglycan and glycoprotein aggregates, and circular to this myofibrils and glycogen, etc., which look to be by definition genuine myocytes.

Challice: We have done alternate sections, one for electron microscopy, the next one using P.A.S. reaction.

Perspectives in Cardiovascular Research, Vol. 5,
Mechanisms of Cardiac Morphogenesis and Teratogenesis,
edited by Tomas Pexieder. Raven Press, New York © 1981

Quantitative Analysis of Shape Development in the Chick Embryo Heart

Tomas Pexieder and Yves Christen

Institut d'Histologie et d'Embryologie, Université de Lausanne, Lausanne, Suisse

In prenatal cardiac ontogenesis, after looping of the heart tube, four fundamental events modify the external appearance of the embryonic heart. These events are:

1. Medial shift of the atrioventricular canal to the right
2. Medial shift of the conotruncus to the left
3. Effacement of the conoventricular fold
4. Absorption of the conus.

They have been observed and described under various names and in different fashions in almost every authoritative study on cardiac embryology and/or teratology (1–11,15–18,21–34,36,41,43,44,46,47,50–54).

Particular attention has been paid to the medial shift of the conotruncus, which is considered by some as one of the key steps in the so called "transfer of the aortic component of the distal bulbus to the left ventricle" (1). The following interpretations of the causes and mechanisms of this shift have been formulated:

a. displacement of the atria (17,46)
b. AV canal migration and expansion (3,27,33,50)
c. expansion of the right ventricle (17)
d. rotation of the right ventricle (11,17,32)
e. growth of the conus (6,7,29,41,47)
f. shift of the bulbus (2,5,17,26,28,30,36,44,50,51)
g. vectorial bulbus rotation (9,10,15,18,22,24,25)
h. resorption of the conoventricular flange (44,47,51).

Among these various interpretations the vectorial bulbus rotation (18) occupies a special place. Widely known and accepted within the German literature, this ·concept was recently claimed (15) to share many common points with the ideas developed in the 1970s by Goor et al. (27) and even more recently by Anderson et al. (3) concerning the morphogenesis of transposition of great vessels. In its original form (18), the theory of vectorial bulbus rotation states that the medial shift of the bulbus (conotruncus) is a complex process composed of:

a. displacement (Wanderung) of the conotruncus (bulbus) from a right to a ventral position
b. torsion (Drehung) of the arterial end of the heart around its longitudinal axis
c. angular shortening of the bulbus from right and ventral to left and dorsal.

Later, Bersch (10) and Chuaqui (15) presented a slightly modified version of this theory (Fig. 1):

a. leftward shift of the bulbus together with bulbar shrinkage and a displacement of the truncus
b. 45-degree clockwise bulbar torsion of the ostium bulbometampullare (cono-ventricular)
c. 150-degree counterclockwise torsion of the truncus at the bulbotruncal (cono-truncal) orifice.

On the assumption of the existence of this vectorial bulbus rotation, Doerr (18) and his pupils (10,15,24,25) have built up an important pathogenetic and classification concept. According to this concept, the varying extent of arrest of the rotation (torsion) will result in heterotropies of the great vessels, the individual forms of which constitute a "teratological series" including Eisenmenger's complex, Fallot's tetralogy, Taussig–Bing anomaly, and complete transposition (Fig. 1).

As experimental work did not confirm the existence of any torsion or rotation of the conotruncus other than that imposed on the heart tube during its looping (38), we decided to determine whether the leftward shift of the bulbus does really exist or whether it is only an optical illusion.

MATERIALS AND METHODS

White Leghorn fertilized eggs from the Institute's flock were incubated at 37.5°C and 60% relative humidity in a forced-draft incubator. The embryos were sampled between 2nd e.d. and 7th e.d. at intervals of 8 h. After perforation of the shell overlying the air chamber, the eggshell was opened by the windowing technique. The shell membrane was removed. After opening of the vitelline and embryonic membranes, the beating hearts were perfused *in situ* using beveled micropipets with the tip diameter in the range of 60 to 120 μm. The perfusion fluid was a fixation mixture containing 2% glutaraldehyde and 1% formaldehyde in 0.1 M cacodylate buffer. The buffer osmolarity was adjusted by NaCl to stage-dependent value (13,37,42), e.g., 280 mOsm on the 4th e.d. The initial perfusion was followed by the removal of the whole embryo from the egg. Fixation was continued by 1½ h immersion in the same fixative mixture. 0.1 M cacodylate buffer with osmotic pressure adjusted by NaCl to stage-related isotonicity was used for a 60-minute rinse. This was followed by 1 h postfixation in 1% osmium tetroxide in 0.1 M isotonic cacodylate buffer. Thereafter the embryos were stored in isotonic 0.1 M cacodylate buffer.

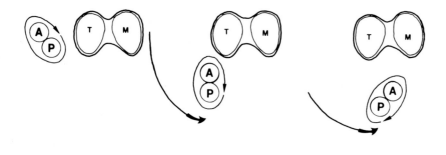

a

Initial situation

Normal heart

Aortic ventricle

Arrest

b

Corrected transposition   Transposition

FIG. 1. Conception of the vectorial bulbar torsion (twist) and its pathogenetic significance. **a:** Torsion and angular displacement of the conotruncus during normal development. **b:** Teratological series produced by alterations of the vectorial bulbar torsion. A = aorta; P = pulmonary artery. (Based on Doerr, 1955, 1978).

Preparation for scanning electron microscopy (SEM) began with microdissection of the heart. The pericardial cavity was opened and the heart exposed for three principal views: frontal, right lateral, and left lateral. For the right and left lateral views the atria were removed if they masked the outflow tract and/or great vessels. The remaining cephalic and abdominal portions of the embryo were then removed, leaving a thoracic block. The separating cuts were placed at the level of entrance of the truncus arteriosus into the branchial arches and beneath the septum transversum, perpendicularly to the neural tube.

The microdissected thoracic blocks were dehydrated by increasing concentrations of ethanol and transferred through series of ethanol–Freon 113 mixtures into 100% Freon 113. The latter was used as an intermediate fluid for critical point drying from Freon 13 using Bomar SPC 900/EX CPD apparatus. Dried specimens were attached to SEM subs using colloidal silver in three essential orientations: en face, right profile, and left profile. They were sputter coated with 300 nm gold in an Edwards S150 sputter coater. Subsequently, they were observed in JSM-35 SEM at 25 kV. At each stage, there were at least five hearts for each of the three principal orientations investigated. When taking the SEM micrographs, care was taken to use constant magnification (x 12) and maintain identical orientation of embryonic torsa, the guiding line being the axis of the neural tube.

Standard magnification prints (x 2.8) were overlayed by transparent paper on which the axis of the neural tube, as reference system, and the contours of the heart were copied. The overlays were used to draw the distances to be measured (Fig. 2 and 3). The overlays were then placed on a HP 9864A digitizer for measurement. In the frontal view we have quantified (Fig. 2) the distance of the right and left bulbar borders from the axis of the body, the distance of the bulbar midpoint from the axis of the body, and the distance of the left ventricular border from this axis. In the right profile (Fig. 3) the following parameters were measured: distance of the anterior and posterior bulbar borders from a line interpolating the neural tube, distances of the bulbar midpoint, anterior and posterior borders of the right ventricle and of the midpoint of the right ventricle from the same reference line.

The values obtained were entered into the HP 9845S desktop computer. Using this computer, secondary variables were calculated. For the en face views: bulbar width, ventricular width, and the ventriculo-bulbar index. In the series of right profile views, secondary variables computed were: bulbar width, right ventricular width, the ratio of right ventricular width/bulbar width, right bulboventricular index, and bulbar and right ventricular growth. The mathematical definitions of all these variables can be found in Appendix I.

The developmental changes of all parameters measured and computed were characterized by third degree polynomial regression against the developmental age computed by HP 9845S. Regression curves were plotted by the HP 9872A plotter.

RESULTS

I. En face views

A. Position changes of the right side of the bulbus and of the right ventricle
   (Fig. 4A)

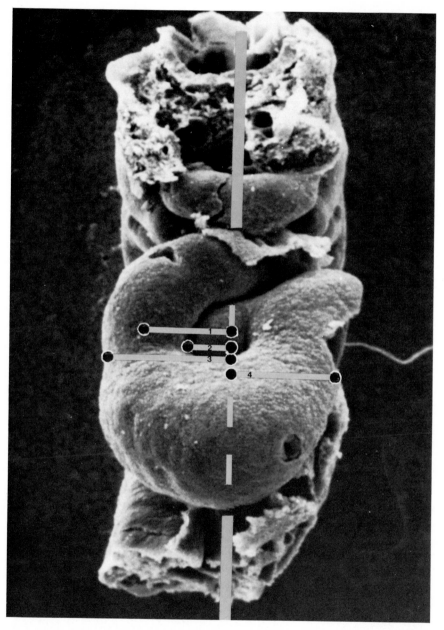

FIG. 2. SEM micrograph of a chick embryo heart in frontal orientation with superimposed sites of measurements. 2 e.d. 16 h, × 95. 1: Bulbar midpoint. 2: Left bulbar border. 3: Right bulbar border. 4: Left ventricular border.

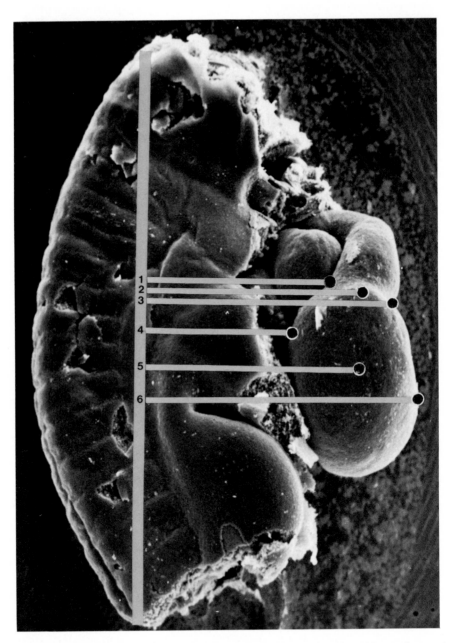

FIG. 3. SEM micrograph of a chick embryo heart in right profile orientation with superimposed sites of measurement. 3 e.d. 8 h, × 55. 1: Posterior border of the bulbus. 2: Bulbar midpoint. 3: Anterior border of the bulbus. 4: Posterior border of the right ventricle. 5: Ventricular midpoint. 6: Anterior border of the right ventricle.

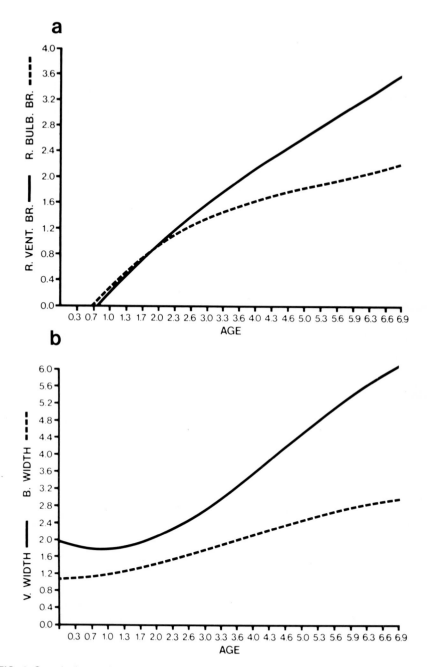

FIG. 4. Quantitative evaluation of the positional changes of the bulbus and the right ventricle in the frontal plane. **a:** Comparison of the right ventricular and right bulbar border positions. **b:** Comparison of the bulbar and ventricular width. Age in embryonic days.

The development of the embryo is accompanied by an increase in the distance separating the right borders of both bulbus and right ventricle from the axis of the body. This increase has the same pace in the bulbus and the ventricle until the 2 e.d. 8 h. Starting from this point, the displacement is much more pronounced in the ventricle than in the bulbus.

B. Position changes of the left side of the bulbus and of the right ventricle (Fig. 5A)

Between the 2nd e.d. and the 2nd e.d. 16 h the left border of the bulbus displaces first to the right. Thereafter, it regains the central position at 4 e.d. 16 h and crosses the axis of the body to the left. These positional changes are displayed in parallel also by the left border of the left ventricle which, however, never crosses the axis of the body to the right.

C. Development of bulbar and ventricular width (Fig. 4B)

There is a steady increase in both bulbar and ventricular width. However, the slope of the ventricular width growth curve is much steeper than that of the bulbar width.

D. Ventriculo-bulbar index (Fig. 5B)

Whereas on the 2nd e.d. bulbus width represents approximately 70% of ventricular width, its relative importance in the whole of the embryonic heart decreases steadily to 55%.

E. Position changes of the center of the bulbus

The center of the bulbus increases its distance from the reference line until the 3 e.d. 8 h. Thereafter, this distance continuously diminishes.

II. Right profile view

It is interesting that the six primary parameters display the same developmental trends (Fig. 6 and 7). They increase from the 2nd e.d. to 5 e.d. 16 h and thereafter they level off.

A. Position changes of the anterior border of the bulbus and the right ventricle (Fig. 6A)

Through all of the stages investigated, the anterior border of the right ventricle was situated more ventrally than the anterior bulbar border.

B. Position changes of the posterior border of the bulbus and the right ventricle (Fig. 7B)

Generally speaking, the difference between the antero-posterior distance of the bulbus and the right ventricle was smaller than that concerning their anterior borders. Until the 2 e.d. 16 h the posterior border of the right ventricle is more distant from the reference line than the posterior bulbar border. Starting with 3 e.d., it is the posterior bulbar border that is situated more anteriorly with respect to the reference line.

C. Position changes of the center of the bulbus and the right ventricle (Fig. 6B)

Through all of the stages studied, the center of the right ventricle was situated more anteriorly than the center of the bulbus in relationship to the reference line.

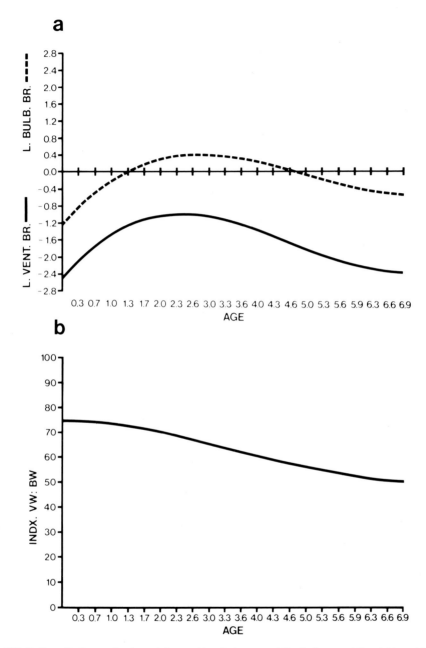

FIG. 5. Quantitative evaluation of the positional changes of the bulbus and the right ventricle in the frontal plane. **a:** Comparison of the left ventricular and left bulbar border positions. **b:** Bulbus width as percentage of the ventricular width. Age in embryonic days.

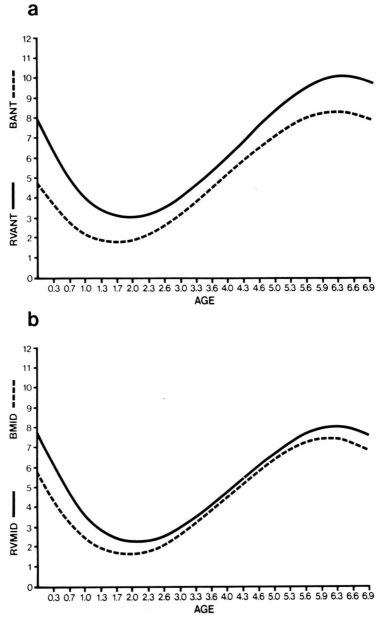

FIG. 6. Quantitative evaluation of the positional changes of the bulbus and the right ventricle in the right parasagittal plane. **a:** Comparison of positions of the anterior bulbar and ventricular border. **b:** Comparison of positions of the ventricular and bulbar midpoint. Age in embryonic days.

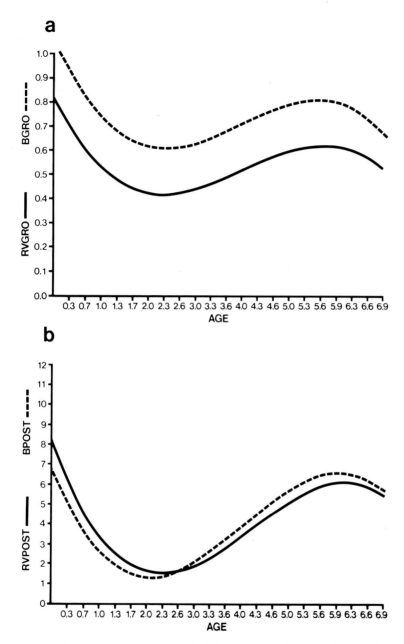

FIG. 7. Quantitative evaluation of the positional changes of the bulbus and the right ventricle in the right parasagittal plane. **a:** Comparison of the right ventricular and bulbar growth. **b:** Comparison of position of the posterior bulbar and ventricular border. Age in embryonic days.

D. Developmental changes in bulbar and ventricular growth (Fig. 7A)

Both the bulbus and the right ventricle showed a very similar rate and trend of growth in their size in this projection.

E. Development of bulbar and ventricular width

The antero-posterior width of the right ventricle increases almost linearly. The antero-posterior width of the bulbus was smaller than that of the right ventricle. It increases between the 2nd and 3rd e.d. This increase is followed by a slowing-down period until 5 e.d. 8 h. Thereafter, this parameter resumes its growth.

F. Ventriculo-bulbar index

This ratio decreases from 2.4 on 2nd e.d. to 2 on 3rd e.d. Subsequently, it increments its value to 2.3 at 6 e.d.

G. Right bulboventricular index

The relation of the bulbar and ventricular midpoints as described by this index increased from 0.7 on the 2nd e.d. to 0.93 at 4 e.d. 16 h and then continuously decreased to 0.85 on 7 e.d.

DISCUSSION

Studies of the conotruncus (bulbus) shift are obviously related to descriptions of the positional changes of the neighboring structures in the developing heart. The heart as a whole (39,45) and many of its parts permanently and more or less independently change their positions in space, so that we are faced with the problem of finding natural landmarks or providing artifical ones (12) and a coordinate system for objective evaluation of their positional changes. The vast majority of studies listed in the Introduction can be criticized for their lack of a reference frame independent of heart development. Moreover, the widely used serial sections and reconstructions of the embryonic heart are frequently unsuitable for a true three-dimensional assessment of these positional changes.

Our approach takes advantage of the technological progress brought about by scanning electron microscopy with its focus depth, and uses a reference structure independent of heart morphogenesis. Recently another arbitrary reference system was devised by Thompson and Fitzharris (48,49) with the aim of studying septation of the outflow tract and the accompanying tissue reorganization. We believe that, as far as the conotruncus (bulbus) positional changes are concerned, our method is superior, since it accounts for and reproduces the real development of the heart and its individual parts, whereas in the graphs of Thompson and Fitzharris' contributions (48,49), the "stations" are presented as equidistant throughout the heart morphogenesis studied.

Our investigations show that an objective, quantitative study of the development of heart shape is feasible. Because of the reported species differences in organogenesis of the heart (38), it will be extremely interesting and useful to apply our method to mouse, dog, and human embryonic hearts actually studied in our laboratory. Recent advances in macrophotography allow application of this nondestructive approach to rare specimens (e.g., human embryonic and fetal hearts, hearts of Keeshond dog embryos), which can subsequently be microdissected and study continued using SEM.

We interpret the measurements obtained as follows: as seen from the front of the embryo, the right ventricle expands to the right much more rapidly than the proximal bulbus (conus) (Fig. 4A), whose widening to the left parallels the development of the left ventricle (Fig. 5A). As a consequence of the concomitant growth of the left ventricle (Fig. 4B), the relative importance of the proximal bulbus (conus) decreases (Fig. 5B). Viewed from the right profile, the positional changes of both right ventricle and proximal bulbus (conus) show the same trend and pace (Fig. 6A, B, 7A). At no stage does the center of the proximal bulbus (conus) lie anteriorly to the center of the right ventricle (Fig. 6B). Greater posterior growth of the right ventricle and straightening of the angle at which the proximal bulbus (conus) leaves the right ventricle explain the crossing over of the two regression lines at 2 e.d. 16 h in Fig. 7B. This straightening was confirmed by measurements of angles (14) between the longitudinal axis of the right ventricle and the craniocaudal body axis on the one side and between the longitudinal axis of the proximal bulbus (conus) and the craniocaudal body axis on the other side. The angle of the right ventricular longitudinal axis decreases from 70 to 0 degrees, whereas the angle of the bulbar longitudinal axis increases from 0 to 60 degrees. At the same time, the angle between the longitudinal axis of the proximal bulbus (conus) and that of the right ventricle drops from 60 to 10 degrees.

As suggested by Christen (14), the existence of linear measurements in two perpendicular planes (frontal and parasagittal) allows us to consider the developmental changes of the proximal bulbus (conus) and the right ventricle in the transverse plane of the bulboventricular (conoventricular) orifice ("Ventilebene" of Doerr, 18). Again, there is no trace of vectorial bulbar rotation. The bulboventricular (conoventricular) orifice maintains its relative position with respect to the ventricular contours and the neural tube. The vectorial bulbus rotation is an optical illusion caused by an important expansive growth of the right ventricle to the right of the body axis, with the proximal bulbus (conus) maintaining at the same time its paracentral position. Of the different hypotheses suggested in Fig. 8 (differential growth of the right ventricle, bulbar (conal) shift, or their combination), it is the growth of the right ventricle that seems to hold true.

The probability that expansive growth of the right ventricle is responsible for the "medial shift" of the conotruncus is supported also by evidence from underlying cellular mechanisms. Our studies of the patterns of proliferation and DNA synthesis in the outflow tract (35,38) show that the proliferation center of the right ventricle is localized in the neighborhood of the right bulboventricular boundary. A further supporting element is the recent observation (40) that the initial event in pathogenesis of aortic dextroposition in the conoventricu-

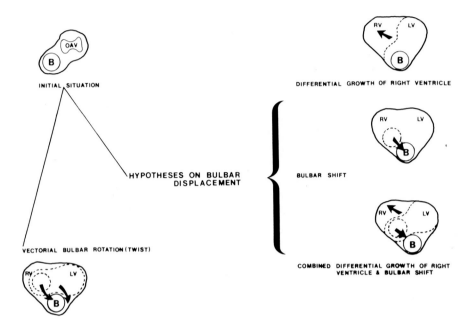

FIG. 8. Proposed hypotheses on the "median conotruncus (bulbus) shift."

lar malformation complex of Keeshond dogs is hypoplasia of the right ventricle.

Bankl (6,7,8), one of the traditional opponents in German literature of the vectorial bulbus rotation, recalls that in 1950 Doerr himself pointed out that he was uncertain as to whether or not the suggested bulbotruncal torsions really existed. Doerr and his pupils argued that they were developing purely formal and therefore absolute concepts. This approach singularly resembles the recent statement of Anderson (1): ". . . embryology can be applied . . . as platform for understanding both normal and abnormal morphology, but in all instances taking care to ensure that embryology plays a subordinate role." Even if we recognize the temporal practical relevance and sometimes stimulating influence of such a pragmatic approach, we are convinced that it is not eternally defensible.

We have also reported (38) that absorption of the conus, another fundamental morphogenetic event of prospective pathogenetic importance, seems to be an optical and interpretative illusion rather than a reality. It will therefore be more than desirable to subject the absorption of the conus, the effacement of the conoventricular fold, and the medial shift of the atrioventricular canal to a similar objective and exacting analysis.

ACKNOWLEDGMENT

This research was supported by Grant No. 3.162.0.77 from the Swiss National Science Foundation.

REFERENCES

1. Anderson, R. H. (1978): Another look at cardiac embryology. In: *Progress in Cardiology, Vol. 7*, edited by P. N. Yu and I. F. Goodwin, pp. 1-13. Lea & Febiger, Philadelphia.
2. Anderson, R. H., and Ashley, G. T. (1974): Anatomic development of the cardiovascular system. In: *Scientific Foundations of Pediatrics*, edited by J. Davies and J. Dobbing, pp. 165-198. Heinemann, London.
3. Anderson, R. H., Wilkinson, J. L., Arnold, R., and Lubkiewicz, K. (1974): Morphogenesis of bulboventricular malformations. I. Considerations of embryogenesis in the normal heart. *Br. Heart J.*, 36:242-255.
4. Anderson, R. H., Wilkinson, J. L., and Becker, A. E. (1978): The bulbus cordis—a misunderstood region of the developing human heart: Its significance to the classification of congenital cardiac malformations. In: *Morphogenesis and malformation of the cardiovascular system*, edited by G. C. Rosenquist and D. Bergsma, pp. 1-28. *Birth Defects:* Orig. Art. Ser., Vol. XIV, No. 7. Alan R. Liss, New York.
5. Asami, I. (1969): Beitrag zur Entwicklung des Kammerseptums im menschlichen Herzen mit besonderer Berücksichtigung der sogenannten Bulbusdrehung. *Z. Anat. Entwickl.-Gesch.*, 128:1-17.
6. Bankl, H. (1971): *Missbildungen des arteriellen Herzendes*. Urban & Schwarzenberg, Wien.
7. Bankl, H. (1977): *Congenital malformations of the heart and great vessels. Synopsis of pathology, embryology and natural history*. Urban & Schwarzenberg, Wien.
8. Bankl, H. (1979): Progress in the interpretation of pathogenesis of congenital cardiac malformations. *Wien. Klin. Wochenschr.*, 91:475-481.
9. Becker, A. E., and Anderson, R. H. (1978): Fallot's tetralogy—developmental aspects, anatomy and conducting tissues. In: *Paediatric Cardiology 1977*, edited by R. H. Anderson and E. A. Shinebourne, pp. 245-257. Churchill Livingstone, Edinburgh–London–New York.
10. Bersch, W. (1978): The formal morphogenesis of arterial transposition with special regard to the concept of homology and series formation. In: *Embryology and Teratology of the Heart and the Great Arteries*, edited by L. H. S. Van Mierop, A. Oppenheimer-Dekker, and C. L. D. C. Bruins, pp. 112-122. Leiden Univ. Press, The Hague.
11. Born, G. (1889): Beiträge zur Entwicklungsgeschichte des Säugetierherzens. *Arch. Mikr. Anat.*, 33:284-377.
12. Butler, J. K. (1952): *An experimental analysis of cardiac loop formation in the chick*. The Gen. Libraries, The Univ. of Texas at Austin, Austin.
13. Chavaz, P., and Pexieder, T. (1976): Quelle osmolarité choisir pour la fixation en microscopie électronique? *Acta Anat. (Basel)*, 95:142-143.
14. Christen, Y. (1980): *Analyse quantitative du développement de la forme du coeur embryonnaire*. Thèse, Université de Lausanne.
15. Chuaqui, B. (1979): Doerr's theory of morphogenesis of arterial transposition in light of recent research. *Br. Heart J.*, 41:481-485.
16. Corone, P. (1972): *Cardiopathies congénitales*. Maloine SA, Paris.
17. De Vries, P. A., and Saunders, C. M. (1962): Development of the ventricles and spiral outflow tract in the human heart. *Contrib. Embryol.*, 37:87-114.
18. Doerr, W. (1952): Ueber ein Prinzip der Koppelung von Entwicklungsstörungen der venösen und arteriellen Kammerostien. *Z. Kreisl.-Forsch.*, 41:269-284.
19. Doerr, W. (1955): Die formale Entstehung der wichtigsten Missbildungen des arteriellen Herzendes. *Beitr. Path. Anat.*, 115:1-32.
20. Doerr, W. (1977): Pathogenesis of cardiac infarction—few comments on some unanswered questions. *Virchows Arch.*, 373:177-191.
21. Dor, X. (1976): *Etude des torsions distales de l'ébauche cardiaque: Développement normal et malformations expérimentales réalisées chez l'embryon de poulet*. Thèse, Nantes.
22. Dor, X., and Corone, P. (1973): Le rôle du conus dans la morphogenèse cardiaque—Essai d'étude sur l'embryon de poulet. *Coeur*, 4:207-307.
23. Dor, X., Corone, P., and Cabrol, C. (1978): Création expérimentale de ventricules uniques chez l'embryon de poulet. Etude au microscope électronique à balayage. *Coeur*, 9:1131-1156.
24. Goerttler, K. (1958): Normale und pathologische Entwicklung des menschlichen Herzens. *Zwangl. Abhandl. Norm. Path. Anat.*, 5:1-123.

25. Goerttler, K. (1963): Entwicklungsgeschichte des Herzens. In: *Das Herz des Menschen,* edited by W. Bargmann and W. Doerr, pp. 21-87. G. Thieme, Stuttgart.

26. Goor, D. A., Dische, R., and Lillehei, C. W. (1972): The conotruncus. I. Its normal inversion and conus absorption. *Circulation,* 46:375-384.

27. Goor, D. A., Edwards, J. E., and Lillehei, C. W. (1970): The development of the interventricular septum of the human heart—correlative morphogenetic study. *Chest,* 58:453-467.

28. Goor, D. A., and Lillehei, C. W. (1976): *Congenital Malformations of the Heart—Embryology, Anatomy, and Operative Considerations.* Grune & Stratton, New York–San Francisco–London.

29. Keith, A. (1924): Schorstein lecture on the fate of the bulbus cordis in the human heart. *Lancet,* 2:1267-1273.

30. Kramer, T. C. (1942): The partitioning of the truncus and conus and the formation of the membranous portion of the interventricular septum in the human heart. *Am. J. Anat.,* 71:343-370.

31. Laane, H.-M. (1978): *The arterial pole of the embryonic heart.* Swets & Zeitlinger B. V., Amsterdam & Lisse.

32. Langer, A. (1895): Zur Entwicklungsgeschichte des Bulbus cordis bei Vögeln und Säugetieren. *Morph. Jb.,* 22:99-112.

33. Langman, J., and Van Mierop, L. H. S. (1968): Development of the cardiovascular system. In: *Heart Disease in Infants, Children and Adolescents,* edited by A. J. Moss and F. H. Adams, pp. 3-25. Williams & Wilkins, Baltimore.

34. Murray, H. A. Jr. (1919): The development of the cardiac loop in the rabbit, with special reference to the bulboventricular groove and origin of the interventricular septum. *Am. J. Anat.,* 26:29-39.

35. Paschoud, N., and Pexieder, T. (1980): Patterns of proliferation during the organogenetic phase of heart development. In: *Mechanisms of Cardiac Morphogenesis and Teratogenesis,* edited by T. Pexieder, pp. 73-88. Raven Press, New York.

36. Pernkopf, E., and Wirtinger, W. (1933): Die Transposition der Herzostien—ein Versuch der Erklärung dieser Erscheinung. Die Phoromonie der Herzentwicklung als morphogenetische Grundlage der Erklärung. I. Teil. Die Phoromonie der Herzentwicklung. *Z. Anat. Entwickl.-Gesch.,* 100:563-711.

37. Pexieder, T. (1976): The role of buffer osmolarity in fixation for SEM and TEM. *Experientia,* 32:806-807.

38. Pexieder, T. (1978): Development of the outflow tract of the embryonic heart. In: *Morphogenesis and Malformation of the Cardiovascular System,* edited by G. C. Rosenquist and D. Bergsma, pp. 29-68. *Birth Defects:* Orig. Art. Ser., Vol. XIV, No. 7. Alan R. Liss, New York.

39. Pexieder, T. (1979): Changing scene in cardiac embryology. *Herz,* 4:73-77.

40. Pexieder, T., Patterson, D. F., and Van Mierop, L. H. S. (1980): Pathogenesis of the hereditary cono-truncal defects in the Keeshond dog—an organ level study. *World Congr. Paed. Cardiol.,* London.

41. Robertson, J. (1913): The comparative anatomy of the bulbus cordis with special reference to abnormal positions of the great vessels in the human heart. *J. Pathol. Bact.,* 18:191-210.

42. Romanoff, A. L. (1967): *Biochemistry of the avian embryo.* J. Wiley & Sons, New York.

43. Rychter, Z. (1959): Vascular system of the chick embryo. II. To the problem of heart bulb and trunk septation by the chick embryo. *Čs. Morfol.,* 8:1-20.

44. Shaher, R. M. (1973): *Complete Transposition of the Great Arteries.* Academic Press, Inc., New York.

45. Sissman, N. J. (1970): On embryologic terminology and the truncus arteriosus. In: *Cardiac Development with Special Reference to Congenital Heart Disease,* edited by O. P. Jaffee, pp. 11-27. University of Dayton Press, Dayton.

46. Spitzer, A. (1923): Ueber den Bauplan des normaen und missbildeten Herzens (Versuch einer phylogenetischer Theorie). *Virchows. Arch.,* 243:81-272.

47. Tandler, J. (1911): Die Entwicklungsgeschichte des Herzens. In: *Handbuch der Entwicklungsgeschichte des Menschen,* edited by F. Keibel and F. P. Mall, pp. 517-551. Hirzel, Leipzig.

48. Thompson, R. P., and Fitzharris, T. P. (1979a): Morphogenesis of the truncus arteriosus of the chick embryo heart: Tissue reorganization during septation. *Am. J. Anat.,* 156:251-264.

49. Thompson, R. P., and Fitzharris, T. P. (1979b): Morphogenesis of the truncus arteriosus of the chick embryo heart: The formation and migration of mesenchymal tissue. *Am. J. Anat.,* 154:545-556.

50. Van Mierop, L. H. S. (1974): Anatomy and embryology of the right ventricle. In: *The Heart*, edited by J. E. Edwards, M. Lev, and M. R. Abell, pp. 1-16. The Williams & Wilkins Company, Baltimore.
51. Van Mierop, L. H. S. (1976): Embryology of the atrioventricular canal region and pathogenesis of endocardial cushion defects. In: *Atrioventricular Canal Defects*, edited by R. H. Feldt, pp. 1-12. W. B. Saunders Co., Philadelphia.
52. Van Mierop, L. H. S. (1979): Morphological development of the heart. In: *Handbook of Physiology, Section 2: The Cardiovascular System, Vol. 1: The Heart*, edited by R. M. Berne, pp. 1-28. Amer. Physiol. Soc., Bethesda.
53. Van Mierop, L. H. S., and Patterson, D. F. (1978): The pathogenesis of spontaneously occurring anomalies of the ventricular outflow tract in Keeshond dogs: embryologic studies. In: *Morphogenesis and Malformation of the Cardiovascular System*, edited by G. C. Rosenquist and D. Bergsma, pp. 361-375. *Birth Defects:* Orig. Art. Ser., Vol. XIV, No. 7. Alan R. Liss, New York.
54. Waterston, D. (1917): The development of the heart in man. *Trans. Roy. Soc. Edinburgh*, 52:257-302.

APPENDIX I

Definitions of Secondary (Computed) Variables

En face view:

Bulbar width = position of the right bulbar border + position of the left bulbar border

Ventricular width = position of the right ventricular border + position of the left ventricular border

$$\text{Ventriculo-bulbar index} = \frac{\text{ventricular width}}{\text{bulbar width}}$$

Right profile view:

Bulbar width = position of the anterior bulbar border + position of the posterior bulbar border

Right ventricular width = position of the anterior right ventricular border + position of the posterior right ventricular border

$$\text{Bulbar growth} = \frac{\text{Position of the anterior bulbar border}}{\text{Position of the posterior bulbar border}}$$

$$\text{Right ventricular growth} = \frac{\text{Position of the anterior right ventricular border}}{\text{Position of the posterior right ventricular border}}$$

$$\text{Right bulboventricular index} = \frac{\text{Position of the bulbar midpoint}}{\text{Position of the right ventricular midpoint}}$$

$$\text{Right ventriculo-bulbar index} = \frac{\text{Right ventricular width}}{\text{Bulbar width}}$$

DISCUSSION

Rychter: I would like to emphasize that this was the first time that this differential growth was quantitated. The heart-independent reference system is very important, as natural landmarks can be misleading. This consideration was also the reason for our choice of Seichert's labeling technique.

Pexieder: I have seen, in contact with clinicians, that the concept of vectorial bulbus rotation was very important, especially for classifying heart malformations. If I show that this idea is not correct, the clinician would have to change his classification, or else not argue with certain embryological terms in making his classification. We know something about the mechanism of differential growth of the right ventricle. As you will see in our paper with Dr. Paschoud, there is a distinct proliferation center at the right bulboventricular border on 3rd e.d. There is no similar proliferation in the bulbus at that time.

Fitzharris: We can see only relative shifts between different tissues, because even the different reference frames themselves can move. For the actual model of septation you must look inside the truncus. You will then see perhaps no rotation but certainly a downward movement of the myocardium along the length of the truncus in association with septation. This is the cause of septation, not the shifting of the right ventricle or a differential growth.

De Vries: I think both points are true. There is evidence on sections which are closely graded that there is a rotation. Furthermore, at the stages you are studying most of the rotations have already gone, except dorsally in regard to the infundibulum.

Pexieder: I would like to make precise two points. First: The presence or absence of torsions and rotations studied never represented a tentative of a unique explanation of heart septation. The positional relationships of the bulbus, right ventricle and atrioventricular canal are just single but equally important aspects of heart morphogenesis, which is a complex event. Second: The analysis of heart development should be approached on defined levels. I have shown here the organ level approach. On the basis of these quantitative observations, you can formulate hypotheses and analyze them at the cellular and even subcellular level. But the levels of analysis should not be mixed.

De Vries: I would like to stress the need for relating the stages of development of the different species we are working on.

Pexieder: It has been done by Sissman (1970). *Am. J. Cardiol.* 25:141-148.

Dor: I would like to present two arguments in favor of the existence of conal torsions. The first is the changing position of anlagen of the aortico-pulmonary septum, as seen on serial sections. The second is the possibility that the cushions rotate independently from the epimyocardial mantle (for details, see the contribution by Dor, *this volume*).

Hurle: Did you compare the growth of the AV canal with the growth of the bulbar region?

Pexieder: Not yet; these measurements require another kind of microdissection.

De Vries: I have measured some human and rat embryos, the transverse diameter of the AV canal and cross-section diameter as well as the length of the infundibulum and truncus arteriosus. The truncus arteriosus does not increase or decrease in length from stage 7 to stage 16.

GENERAL DISCUSSION

De Haan: We have all been talking about things like growth and movement. I would like to make a plea for an attempt to be more accurate in the terms we use. Cells can divide, move, adhere or de-adhere, pump fluids, change shape, die, etc. All these represent the repertoire of capabilities of individual cells directed at least at some level by the genetic mechanisms. So growth may be due to proliferation *in situ* or to immigration from outside. There is a second, external force—the hydrodynamic activity of the system. For us, as embryologists, it is important to begin to think about what repertoire of cell behavior is going into any particular change in the structure of the heart at any given stage.

Fitzharris: In looking at a static scanning electron microscopic picture, be it most beautiful, it is very difficult to derive a mechanism from that kind of observation.

Pexieder: The presence of an organogenesis section in the workshop on mechanisms is based on my personal experience. Until the Grand Canyon meeting in 1978, all of my interest was oriented toward the problems of cellular mechanisms of cardiac morpho-genesis and teratogenesis. I could obtain many precise quantitative data, especially where cell proliferation and cell death were concerned. I was profoundly disappointed when I tried to relate these data to the development of the heart as an organ. You cannot simply compare a quantitative description of cellular mechanisms with a qualitative description of heart organogenesis. The piece of evidence that is missing is the quantitative description of the development of the heart at the organ level, and this is what our work was aimed at. As far as the use of SEM is concerned, I am convinced that there are some features that you cannot read out from serial sections and their reconstructions. You need to see what a structure and its topography look like in actual three-dimensional views. It would lead to misunderstandings to try to explain heart morphogenesis or terato-genesis simply on the basis of our observations at the organ level. On the basis of those observations, we can make certain statements regarding the shape change. Then we can look to see what mechanism underlies this change. Is it a proliferation, an increase in the synthesis of the intercellular substance, or a decreased degeneration? The danger is either in confounding the different levels of analysis (organ, tissue, cellular, subcellular) or in overemphasizing an isolated factor.

Cell Proliferation

Perspectives in Cardiovascular Research, Vol. 5,
Mechanisms of Cardiac Morphogenesis and Teratogenesis,
edited by Tomas Pexieder. Raven Press, New York © 1981

Introduction

Donald A. Fischman

Downstate Medical Center
State University of New York
Brooklyn, New York 11203

Regulation of heart cell proliferation during embryogenesis, postnatal growth, cardiac injury, and hypertrophy must be acknowledged as a poorly understood field of experimental cardiology. In contrast to skeletal muscle, in which replicative DNA synthesis is limited to the undifferentiated, non-contractile myoblast population (2,7,8), proliferation within the heart, during most of embryonic life, occurs within myofibril-containing myocytes, which exhibit obvious contractile activity (10,15,19). Thus, skeletal muscle development is characterized by maintenance of a dividing pool of myogenic precursor cells, some of which remain in muscle tissue of adult vertebrates as "satellite cells" (12,13), capable of myogenesis during the regenerative response after muscle injury (1,9).

In the chick embryo, a functional heart can be observed after 48 hours of incubation. All of the myocardial cells contain myofibrils, and no satisfactory evidence has been presented for a population of myogenic precursor cells in the heart once its chambered, contractile structure has formed (11). Yet the number of heart cells (5) and the total DNA content (6) continue to increase throughout chick embryogenesis. In fact, significant cell replication of differentiated cardiac myocytes occurs after hatching in birds and is even more prominent in mammals after birth (17).

Myocyte cell division ceases before adolescence in birds and mammals, and no significant myocardial regeneration is evident after injury (15). A contrasting situation is evident in amphibians, in which significant cardiac regeneration has been conclusively demonstrated (14,16). The picture that is beginning to emerge suggests that cardiac myocytes are a determined cell population within the precardiac mesoderm even before the tubular heart is formed (3). Differentiation of this population becomes evident once the tubular heart begins to loop (18). The absolute number of cardiac myocytes increases by a defined number of cell divisions (still to be established) of this early myocyte population (4). The proliferative potential of these cells apparently decreases with progressive embryonic and postnatal development. We know very little about extrinsic factors which might regulate the mitotic program of the myocytes. But, for whatever solace it may provide, the same state of affairs is true of other cell types, most notably the neurons of the central nervous system.

Although cell and organ cultures have been used for many years to examine selected aspects of cardiac cytodifferentiation, there is still very little information regarding a number of questions. For example, what role does the extracellular matrix play in regulating cell division? Is intercellular contact important in this phenomenon? Is it significant that nerves enter the heart at a period when cardiac cell division decreases significantly (ca. stage 26 in the chick embryo). Does the workload of the embryonic heart stimulate or repress mitotic activity in the myocytes? What is the functional interaction between muscle and nonmuscle cell populations? It is not difficult to pose endless questions about this subject, but perhaps those I have mentioned will serve to focus attention for the papers to follow.

REFERENCES

1. Bischoff, R. (1975): Regeneration of single skeletal muscle fibers in vitro. *Anat. Rec.,* 182:215-236.
2. Buckley, P. A., and Konigsberg, I. R. (1977): The role of environment in the control of myogenesis in vitro. In: *Pathogenesis of Human Muscular Dystrophies,* edited by L. P. Rowland, pp. 779-798. Excerpta Medica, Amsterdam.
3. Chacko, S., and Joseph, X. (1974): The effect of 5-bromodeoxyuridine (BrdU) on cardiac muscle differentiation. *Dev. Biol.,* 40:340-354.
4. Clark, W. A., and Fischman, D. A. (1978): Cardiac growth: A comparison of cell proliferation in vivo and in vitro. In: *Proc. 3rd US–USSR Joint Symposium on Myocardial Metabolism,* edited by H. E. Morgan, pp. 211-226. DHEW (NIH) Publ. # 78-1457.
5. De Haan, R. L. (1971): Cardiac development. In: *Carnegie Inst. Washington Yearb.,* 70:72-76.
6. Doyle, C. M., Zak, R., and Fischman, D. A. (1974): The correlation of DNA synthesis and DNA polymerase activity in the developing chick heart. *Dev. Biol.,* 37:133-145.
7. Fischman, D. A. (1972): The development of striated muscle. In: *The Structure and Function of Muscle,* Vol. 1, 2nd ed, edited by G. Bourne, pp. 75-148. Academic Press, New York.
8. Holtzer, H. (1972): The cell cycle, cell lineage, and cell differentiation. In: *Current Topics in Developmental Biology,* Vol. 6, edited by A. A. Moscona and A. Monroy, pp. 229-256. Academic Press, New York.
9. Konigsberg, V. R., Lipton, B. H., and Konigsberg, I. R. (1975): The regenerative response of single mature muscle fibers isolated in vitro. *Dev. Biol.,* 45:260-275.
10. Manasek, F. J. (1968): Mitosis in developing cardiac muscle. *J. Cell Biol.,* 37:191-196.
11. Manasek, F. J. (1968): Embryonic development of the heart. I. A light and electron microscopic study of myocardial development in the early chick embryo. *J. Morph.,* 125:329-365.
12. Mauro, A. (1961): Satellite cells of skeletal muscle fibers. *J. Biophys. Biochem. Cytol.,* 9:493-495.
13. Mauro, A. (1979): *Muscle Regeneration.* Raven Press, New York.
14. Oberpriller, J. O., Bader, D. M., and Oberpriller, J. C. (1979): The regenerative potential of cardiac muscle in the newt, Notophthalmus viridesceus. In: *Muscle Regeneration,* edited by A. Mauro, pp. 323-333. Raven Press, New York.
15. Rumyantsev, P. P. (1975): Electron microscopic study of the myofibril partial disintegration and recovery in mitotically dividing cardiac muscle cell. *Z. Zellforsch.,* 129:471-499.
16. Rumyantsev, P. P. (1977): Interrelationships of the proliferation and differentiation processes during cardiac myogenesis and regeneration. In: *Int. Rev. Cytol.,* Vol. 51, edited by G. Bourne and J. F. Danielli, pp. 187-273. Academic Press, New York.
17. Sasaki, R., Watanabe, Y., Morishita, T., and Yamagato, S. (1968): Estimation of the cell number of heart muscles in normal rats. *Tohoku J. Exp. Med.,* 95:177-184.
18. Van Mierop, L. H. S. (1967): Location of pacemaker in chick embryo heart at the time of initiation of heartbeat. *Am. J. Physiol.,* 212:407-415.
19. Weinstein, R. B., and Hay, E. D. (1970): Deoxyribonucleic acid synthesis and mitosis in early chick embryogenesis. *J. Cell Biol.,* 47:310-316.

Perspectives in Cardiovascular Research, Vol. 5,
Mechanisms of Cardiac Morphogenesis and Teratogenesis,
edited by Tomas Pexieder. Raven Press, New York © 1981

Patterns of Proliferation During the Organogenetic Phase of Heart Development

Nicolas Paschoud and Tomas Pexieder

Institut d'Histologie et d'Embryologie, Université de Lausanne, Lausanne, Suisse

The advancement of our knowledge of cardiac embryology requires a comprehensive description of the morphogenesis of the heart. Its analysis may be approached at different levels: organ, tissue, and cell. As far as the cellular level of heart morphogenesis is concerned, one of the fundamental questions is: would the embryonic heart be better described as an assembly of individual cardiac cells, or does the concept of the presence of one or more cell populations hold true?

If we accept the concept of embryonic heart as an assembly of cell populations, this enables us to consider the hypothesis of mosaicism of the mechanisms of cardiac morphogenesis. This hypothesis expects the cells to behave in different ways during the organogenetic phase of the heart development. As a result of integration of individual cellular behaviors (9,10,11,12,13), changes do occur in the gross appearance of the developing heart. Most cells have the capacity to divide, to increase their size, to move, to metabolize, to secrete, and to die (1). From this spectrum of cellular activities, cell death (11), intercellular substance (4), and cell proliferation (8,12) began to be seriously studied in their relationship to development of the heart. As we actually know much more about the role of the first two aspects of cell physiology, we decided to investigate the contribution of DNA synthesis and mitosis to organogenesis of the heart.

To date, five major papers have dealt specifically with cell proliferation in the developing heart of the chick embryo. Goerttler (2) described variations of the mitotic index in the heart at different developmental stages. Units of analysis in his contribution were endocardium and mesenchyme, myocardium and epicardium, studied in the bulbus cordis, the ventricles, and the atria. The least amount of proliferation has been observed in the bulbus. At 5 e.d. the mitotic activity attained its maximum. Goerttler's pupil Grohman (3) broadened the initial study by Goerttler (2) and, in particular, confirmed the period from 36 hours of incubation to the 4th e.d. as the principal growth phase of the heart in the chick embryo (from the standpoint of cell division). Sissmann (15) was the first to use ³H-thymidine autoradiography in the study of embryonic hearts. His studies were limited to the earlier (35 hr to 3 e.d.) phases of heart organogenesis in the chick. Endocardium and myocardium were the only layers studied at bulbar, ventricular and atrial localizations. Sissmann has described interesting variations of the labeling index: an increase in the myocardium and a decrease in the endocardium. In spite of this, the endocardium was much more heavily labeled than he had expected. He speculated that this high labeling of endocardial cells is the basis of their role in "seeding" of the cardiac jelly. Stalsberg (16) studied the stathmokinetic index using colcemid in early chick embryo. Although he did not succeed in discovering any left–right asymmetry of the numbers of arrested mitoses, which might contribute to the explanation of cardiac looping, he was able to identify successive waves of mitoses descending the heart tube from its distal to proximal end. Recently, Thompson and Fitzharris (17) studied the mitotic index in the outflow portion of the heart, with the aim of describing tissue reorganizations accompanying separation of the aorta and the pulmonary artery. These authors analyzed the mitotic index in three different compartments (endocardium, mesenchyme, and myocardium) at five arbitrarily selected "stations."

MATERIALS AND METHODS

We used White Leghorn chick embryos incubated for 3, 4, 5, 6 and 7 days. At each day of incubation, 3 embryos were labeled with tritiated thymidine (specific activity 100 μc/ml). After windowing of the shell, 2, 5, 10, 14 or 50 μl of the isotope were injected by micropipets in the most accessible vitelline vein. The volume of the isotope injected was calculated so as to maintain the same concentration of tritiated thymidine per unit volume of the circulating blood. The eggs were closed and reincubated at 37.5°C for 30 minutes in the presence of injected and circulating isotope. Thereafter they were Bouin fixed, paraplast embedded and serially sectioned at 5 μm. The sections were dipped in Kodak NTB2 emulsion, exposed for 35 days, and developed in Kodak D-19 developer. After fixation, the sections were counterstained with Meyer's hematoxylin.

To avoid the problem of double counting of the same cell, each 4th section was considered. The cells were counted in categories of labeled and unlabeled interphase, mitotic, and dying cells, against the background. These counts were performed for the endocardium, the mesenchyme, and the myocardium separately in each of the 28 different localizations (Table 1) which we were able to identify on serial sections of the embryonic heart. Using a card punch connected to CCM-641 Fistronic-Weibel, the counts were done and directly transferred to punched cards. These were used as support media for entry to the Control Data Cyber 7326 computer at the Computing Center of the Federal Polytechnic School at Lausanne. Our data were analyzed using the analysis of variance, the nonparametric Man-Whitney test (6), and the cluster analysis (18). All significance thresholds were set at $\alpha \leq 0.05$. The results reported in the next section are based on counts of 670,224 cells realized on 2,725 serial sections.

TABLE 1. *Localizations identified in the out-flow tract*

Posterior	aorticopulmonary septum
Anterior	aorticopulmonary septum
Global	aorticopulmonary septum (APS)
Truncus mesenchyme (TME)	
Distal ventral	bulbar cushion (DVBC)
Distal dorsal	bulbar cushion (DDBC)
Pulmonary	valves (PV)
Aortic	valves (AV)
Left	intercushion zone
Right	intercushion zone
Left	proximal cushion (PLBC)
Right	proximal cushion (PRBC)
Ventral	intercushion zone
Dorsal	intercushion zone
Left	bulbus half
Right	bulbus half
Accessory anterior cushion	
Truncal myocardium (TMU)	
Distal ventral	myocardium (DVM)
Distal dorsal	myocardium (DDM)
Left	intercushion myocardium (LICM)
Right	intercushion myocardium (RICM)
Left	proximal myocardium (LPM)
Right	proximal myocardium (RPM)
Ventral	intercushion myocardium (IVM)
Dorsal	intercushion myocardium (IDM)
Accessory	anterior myocardium
Accessory	ventral myocardium

RESULTS

Rough results of our study represent thousands of computer printouts which cannot be presented in detail here and which will be the subject of a doctoral thesis (7). We would like to present here just a few selected examples showing the possibilities of different analytical approaches. Four kinds of evaluation will be shown:

I. Global outflow tract proliferation pattern
II. Comparison of proliferation patterns in selected localizations
III. Two-dimensional graphic reconstruction of proliferative activity
IV. Search for proliferation foci along the outflow tract.

I. Global outflow tract proliferation pattern (Fig. 1)

The percentage of labeled mitoses decreases significantly from 3 to 4 e.d. This drop is followed by a continuing significant increase until the 7th e.d. The

OUTFLOW TRACT GLOBAL LABELING INDEX

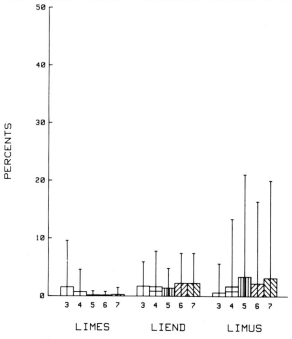

OUTFLOW TRACT GLOBAL LABELING INDEX

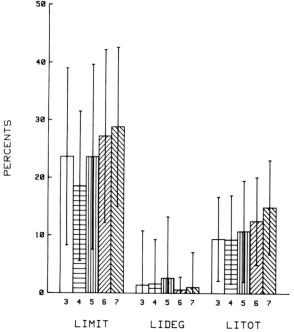

total labeling index increases steadily and significantly from the 4th to the 7th e.d. In the three principal compartments studied, thymidine incorporation into mesenchymal cells decreases significantly between the 4th and 5th e.d. Labeling of the endocardium increases significantly only at the end of the period investigated, whereas in the myocardium only the increase between the 4th and the 5th e.d. is significant.

II. Comparison of proliferation patterns in selected localizations (Figs. 2 and 3)

The design of this experiment allowed us to compare chosen localizations from the standpoint of their proliferative activity at different developmental stages. As an example, we present the distal ventral bulbar (dextrosuperior truncus) cushion and the proximal left (sinistroventral conus) cushion. Of the several variables displayed, only the presence of label in mitotic cells changes significantly. It decreases from 3rd e.d. to 4th e.d. in the distal ventral bulbar (dextrosuperior truncus) cushion. Similar statistically significant change is seen in the proximal left bulbus (sinistroventral conus) cushion, followed in this particular localization by significant increase from the 4th e.d. to the 5th e.d.

III. Two-dimensional graphic reconstruction (Fig. 4, 5 and 6)

In this approach, individual values were plotted in a scattergram against the sequence of serial sections from which they were read. The presented lines are third degree polynomial regression curves computed from the scattergram data.

A. Global labeling index (Fig. 4A)

On the 3rd e.d. there are two peaks. These peaks disappear on the 4th e.d. On the 5th e.d. there is a general increase in total labeling and two more maxima appear. On the 6th e.d. the heart increases in length, and the distal proliferative focus changes its localization. On the 7th e.d. a third (medial) proliferation peak appears.

B. Index of labeled mitoses (Fig. 6B)

There are similar patterns, with a more important decrease in the proximal portion of the outflow tract on the 4th e.d.

C. Index of labeled dying and dead cells (Fig. 6A)

On the 3rd e.d. there are no labeled dying cells. On the 4th e.d. they appear only in the distal part of the outflow tract. On the 5th e.d. maximum labeling is situated between the proximal bulbar (conus) and distal bulbar (truncus) cushions. The 6th e.d. is characterized by moderate labeling of dying and dead cells. During the 7th e.d. a proximal focus of labeled cell death appears.

D. Labeling index of endocardium (Fig. 4B)

There is a high level of thymidine incorporation in the distal part of the

---

FIG. 1. Developmental changes in ^{3}H-thymidine incorporation. 3, 4, 5, 6, 7 = embryonic days. LIMES = labeling index of mesenchyme; LIEND = labeling index of endocardium; LIMUS = labeling index of myocardium; LIMIT = labeling index of mitosis; LIDEG = labeling index of dying and dead cells; LITOT = total labeling index (m ± s).

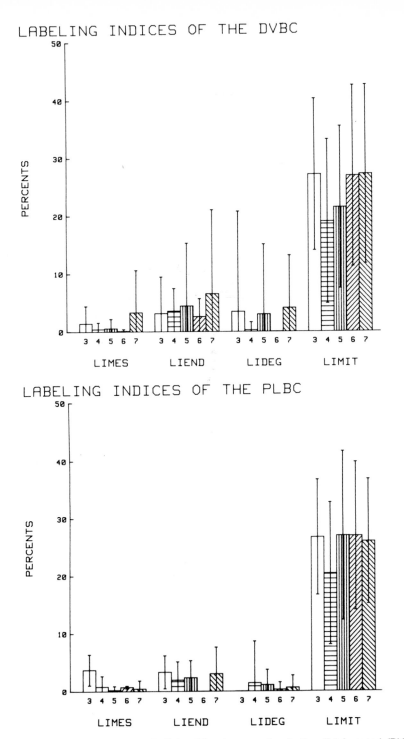

FIG. 2. Comparison of evolution of ³H-thymidine incorporation in the distal ventral (DVBC) and proximal left (PLBC) bulbar cushions. For abbreviations, see text to Fig. 1 (m ± s).

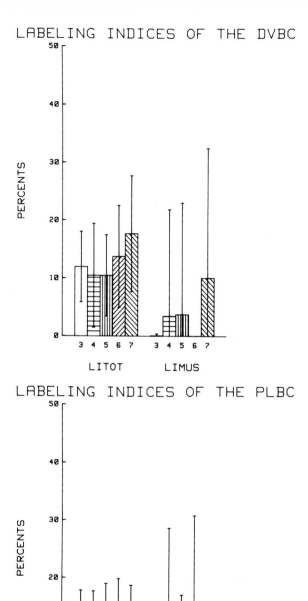

FIG. 3. Comparison of evolution of ³H-thymidine incorporation in the distal ventral (DVBC) and proximal left (PLBC) bulbar cushions. For abbreviations, see text to Fig. 1 (m ± s).

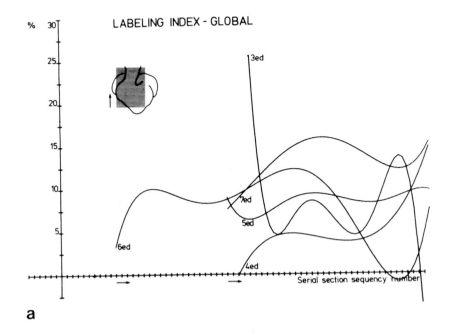

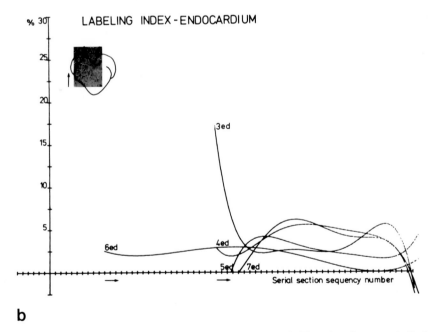

FIG. 4. Graphic reconstruction of DNA synthesis localization. In Figs. 4 to 6, *arrows* indicate the proximo-distal progression in the sequence of serial sections. e.d. = embryonic days.

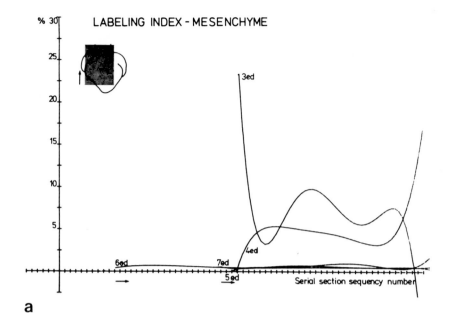

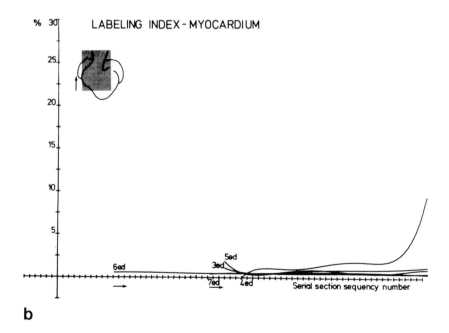

FIG. 5. Graphic reconstruction of DNA synthesis localizations.

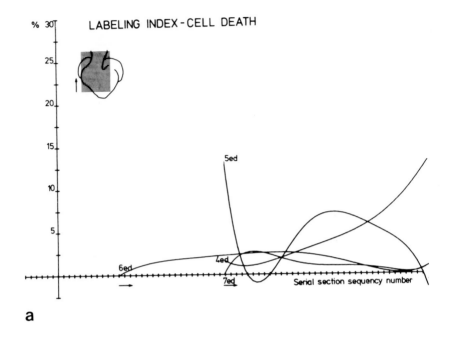

a

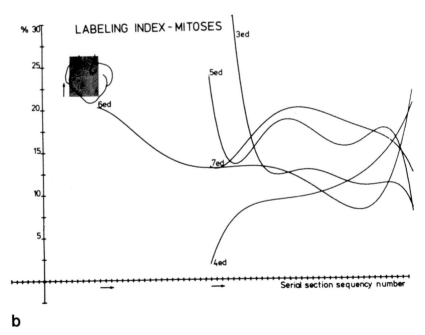

b

FIG. 6. Graphic reconstruction of the distribution of ³H-thymidine incorporation in dying and dividing cells.

outflow tract, corresponding to the formation of distal bulbar (truncus) cushions. On the 4th e.d. this index illustrates the appearance of the proximal (conus) cushions and continuing incorporation in the distal (truncus) cushions. All activity concentrates in the proximal bulbar (conus) cushion at 5th e.d. On 6th e.d. the endocardial labeling levels off. Seventh e.d. presents with a new proximal center.

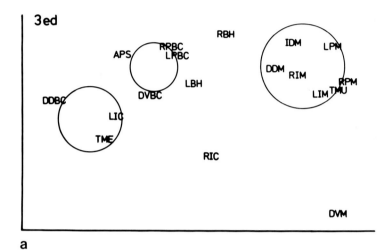

a

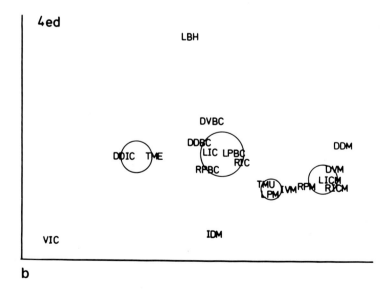

b

FIG. 7. Cluster analysis of proliferation compartments in the outflow tract of the chick embryonic heart. For abbreviations, see Table I. e.d. = embryonic days.

E. Labeling index of mesenchyme (Fig. 5A)

This index presents easily distinguishable trends. On the 3rd e.d. there are two peaks approximating the localization of two sets of cushions. On the 4th e.d. DNA synthesis is essentially localized in the area of proximal bulbar (conus) cushions. Fifth, 6th and 7th e.d. are characterized by an almost complete disappearance of thymidine incorporation into the cardiac mesenchyme.

F. Labeling index of myocardium (Fig. 5B)

With the exception of the 4th e.d., with a disto-proximal gradient of DNA synthesis, there was no local variation in this parameter.

IV. Search for proliferation foci along the outflow tract (Fig. 7, 8, 9)

Using thymidine incorporation as a principal criterion cluster analysis distinguished on the 3rd e.d. (Fig. 7A) three sets of localizations. The first grouped the mesenchyme of the truncus arteriosus, the distal dorsal bulbar cushion, and the mesenchyme between the cushions on the left side of the bulbus. The second set consisted of remaining bulbar cushions and of the aorticopulmonary septum. Finally, the third set was comprised of localizations involving important proportions of the myocardium.

The number of clusters increases by one on the 4th e.d. (Fig. 7B). The first of the four clusters identified was formed by mesenchymal localizations of the distal part of the outflow tract. The second cluster contains proximal bulbar cushions, whereas the third groups myocardium from the most extreme proximal and distal poles of the outflow tract. The last cluster is formed by myocardial localizations situated between these two poles.

On the 5th e.d. (Fig. 8A) there are again four clusters. The first groups future aortic and pulmonary valves with the distal ventral bulbar cushion. The second cluster contains the other bulbar cushions and the aorticopulmonary septum. The two remaining clusters group the distal and the ventral musculature containing localizations.

The distal cushions segregate in a separate cluster on the 6th e.d. (Fig. 8B). Proximal cushions, the aorticopulmonary septum, and presumptive cardiac valves form the second cluster. Surprisingly, the third cluster is formed by mesenchyme from the distal part of the outflow tract. The last cluster groups the myocardial localizations.

There have been only two clusters remaining on the 7th e.d. (Fig. 9). The first one represents the developing aortic and pulmonary valves. The second contains all of the localizations with important amounts of myocardium.

DISCUSSION

Our studies document the existence of interstage variations of thymidine incorporation in individual localizations. At the same time, they illustrate the important local differences in proliferation activity at one and the same developmental stage. The study was initially designed with the aim of discovering variations of proliferation activity which would underly morphogenetic changes in the

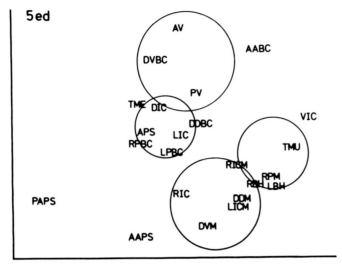

a

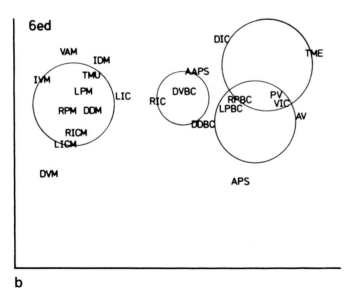

b

FIG. 8. Cluster analysis of proliferation compartments in the outflow tract of the chick embryonic heart. For abbreviations, see Table I.

heart at the organ level. We were unable to proceed further in this difficult task primarily because of a lack of quantitative data describing heart organogenesis for correlation. This is a situation very similar to that which we experienced at the end of our cell death studies (11). In the cell death studies, we were partially able to overcome this handicap by supravital staining and microdissec-

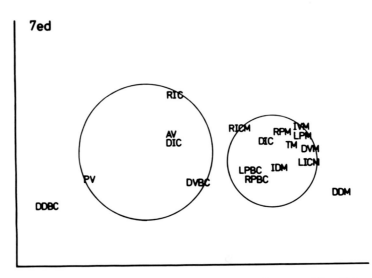

FIG. 9. Cluster analysis of proliferation compartments in the outflow tract of the chick embryonic heart. For abbreviations see Table I.

tion studies. Unfortunately, a selective supravital stain for mitotic cells has not yet been devised.

Interestingly, the two-phase behavior of the percentage of labeled mitoses (Fig. 1) can be correlated with the culmination of cell death in the outflow tract, situated between the 4th and 5th e.d. The steady increase of the total labeling index can be related to the concept of a continuing general growth of the embryonic heart. Constant and high percentages of thymidine incorporation into endocardial cells fit well with the endocardial seeding theory (5) of cellular colonization of the cardiac jelly. Our data are also in good agreement with the most recent observations of Thompson and Fitzharris (17), which are based, however, on simple mitotic counts. In contrast to the ventricles (2,3), the myocardial proliferation in the outflow tract morphogenesis is of lesser importance.

The two-dimensional graphic reconstructions (Figs. 4, 5, and 6) can be interpreted in at least two different ways. The first admits the premise of structure-related proliferation peaks, e.g., proliferation foci localized at specific bulbar cushions and/or valvular anlagen. If this is true, it might be interesting to speculate about the fact that on 3rd e.d. the proximal proliferation peak precedes the appearance of proximal bulbus cushions. The second interpretation extends to later stages of heart organogenesis the observation of Stalsberg (16) regarding mitotic waves traveling in the disto-proximal direction along the longitudinal axis of the outflow tract. Further cell kinetic studies will be necessary to analyze the possible effects of variations in cell cycle duration. It is interesting to note the role of the proximal part of the bulbus as a main proliferation center on 4 e.d. in relation to our recent work (14) on mechanisms of the midline bulbus shift. The presence of dead cells which have incorporated ^{3}H-thymidine illustrates the speed of the degeneration (30 minutes). However, it can be also interpreted as a sign of persistence of erratic DNA synthesis, even in advanced stages of cell degeneration.

Cluster analysis has shown that the initial subdivision into 28 localizations was not very meaningful either from the biological or the mathematical point of view. We would like to emphasize the stability and the restricted number of clusters formed. In other words, proliferative activity in the developing outflow tract of the embryonic heart seems to be resumed in a maximum of four categories. The proliferation structure of the outflow tract is homogenous at the beginning of organogenesis (3rd e.d.). Diversification of proliferation patterns on 4th, 5th and 6th e.d. is followed by the progressive disappearance of the proliferation gradients on 7th e.d. The analysis of formed clusters did not indicate any right–left DNA synthesis or proliferation asymmetry. Of interest was the singular behavior of the distal ventral bulbar cushion, which did not belong to the same cluster as all of the other bulbar cushions. Finally, the myocardium on the 4th and 5th e.d. does not seem to be homogenous as far as proliferation is concerned, being split into two different subsets.

Variations in mitotic activity, together with cell migration and cell death, are principal sources of tissue composition changes. These changes characterize the less immediate aspects of the growth of the heart and will be analyzed separately (7).

We must leave the reader for the moment with data that are difficult to interpret, in the hope that further studies will improve our understanding of the role cell division plays in organogenesis of the heart. Such studies should involve the quantitative description of shape changes accompanying morphogenesis of the heart, shortening of the sampling periods between the stages under study, and evaluation of cell cycle length variations at different stages.

ACKNOWLEDGMENT

This research was supported by Grants No. 3.844.0.72 and 3.465.0.75 from the Swiss National Science Foundation.

REFERENCES

1. De Haan, R. L., and O'Rahilly, R. (1978): Embryology of the heart. In: *The Heart,* 4th ed., edited by J. W. Hurst, R. B. Logue, R. C. Schlant, and N. K. Wenger, pp. 6-18. McGraw-Hill Book Co., New York.
2. Goerttler, K. (1956): Die Stoffwechseltopographie des embryonalen Hühnerherzens und ihre Bedeutung für die Entstehung angeborener Herzfehler. *Verh. Dtsch. Ges. Path.,* 40:181-185.
3. Grohmann, D. (1961): Mitotische Wachstumsintensität des embryonalen und fetalen Hühnchenherzens und ihre Bedeutung für die Entstehung von Herzmissbildungen. *Z. Zellforsch.,* 55:104-122.
4. Manasek, F. J. (1979): Organization, interactions, and environment of heart cells during myocardial ontogeny. In: *Handbook of Physiology, Section 2: The Cardiovascular System, Vol. 1: The Heart,* edited by R. M. Berne, pp. 29-42. *Am. Physiol. Soc., Bethesda.*

5. Markwald, R., Fitzharris, T. P., and Manasek, F. J. (1977): Structural development of endocardial cushions. *Am. J. Anat.,* 148:85-121.
6. Nie, N. H., Hull, C. H., Jenkins, J. G., Steinbrenner, K., and Bent, D. H. (1975): *SPSS— Statistical Package for the Social Sciences.* McGraw-Hill Book Co., New York.
7. Paschoud, N. (1980): *Cinétique des populations cellulaires lors du développement du coeur.* Thèse, Université de Lausanne.
8. Paschoud, N., and Pexieder, T. (1977): Development, topography and sizes of proliferative compartments in organogenesis of the heart. *Exc. Med. Int. Congr. Ser.,* 426:50.
9. Pexieder, T. (1973): The tissue dynamics of heart morphogenesis. II. Quantitative investigations. A. Method and values from areas without cell death foci. *Ann. Embryol. Morph.,* 6:325-334.
10. Pexieder, T. (1975a): Cell death in the morphogenesis and teratogenesis of the heart. *Adv. Anat. Embryol. Cell. Biol.,* 51/3:1-100.
11. Pexieder, T. (1975b): Teratogenic mechanisms in congenital cardiac anomalies. *Acta Anat. Neerl. Scand.,* 13:311-313.
12. Pexieder, T. (1978): Development of the outflow tract of the embryonic heart. In: *Morphogenesis and Malformation of the Cardiovascular System,* edited by G. C. Rosenquist and D. Bergsma, pp. 29-68. *Birth Defects:* Orig. Art. Ser., Vol. XIV, No. 7. Alan R. Liss, New York.
13. Pexieder, T. (1980): Cellular mechanisms underlying the normal and abnormal development of the heart. In: *Etiology and Morphogenesis of Congenital Heart Disease,* edited by R. Van Praagh and A. Takao, pp. 127-153. Futura Publ. Co., New York.
14. Pexieder, T., and Christen, Y. (1980): Quantitative analysis of the shape development in the chick embryo heart. In: *Mechanisms of Cardiac Morphogenesis and Teratogenesis,* edited by T. Pexieder, pp. 49-67. Raven Press, New York.
15. Sissman, N. J. (1966): Cell multiplication rates during development of the primitive cardiac tube in the chick embryo. *Nature (Lond.),* 210:504-507.
16. Stalsberg, H. (1969): Regional mitotic activity in the precardiac mesoderm and differentiating heart tube in the chick embryo. *Dev. Biol.,* 20:18-45.
17. Thompson, R. P., and Fitzharris, T. P. (1979): Morphogenesis of the truncus arteriosus of the chick embryo heart: The formation and migration of mesenchymal tissue. *Am. J. Anat.,* 154:545-556.
18. Wishart, D. (1975): *CLUSTAN User Manual.* University College, London.

DISCUSSION

Satow: You have mentioned the cell death labelling index. Does this mean that dying or dead cells can take up tritiated thymidine?

Paschoud: Yes, some dying cells can incorporate tritiated thymidine. These are either aberrant mitotic cells or cells proceeding to degenerate very rapidly. But the aberrant mitosis cannot be responsible for all of the cell death seen. When you compare the distributions of cell death and proliferation activity on 5th e.d., they are discordant.

Perspectives in Cardiovascular Research, Vol. 5,
Mechanisms of Cardiac Morphogenesis and Teratogenesis,
edited by Tomas Pexieder. Raven Press, New York © 1981

DNA Synthesis and Polyploidization of Chicken Heart Muscle Cells in Mass Culture*

E. Bogenmann and H. M. Eppenberger

Institut für Zellbiologie, Eidgenössische Technische Hochschule, Zürich, Switzerland

Heart muscle cells from 9-day-old chick embryos were grown *in vitro* in three different media. We investigated DNA synthesis and proliferation and the periodic acid Schiff reaction (PAS) for identification of cardiac muscle cells (myocytes). No increase in the number of myocytes was observed, whereas nonmuscle cells showed substantial proliferation. However, autoradiographic studies of cultures incubated for up to 5 days in methyl ^{3}H-thymidine revealed that an average of more than 50% of the myocytes synthesized DNA. Pulse labeling studies (2 h with ^{3}H-thymidine) demonstrated a maximum of DNA-synthesizing muscle cells (ca 40%) at day 2 of incubation.

The DNA content of mononucleated myocytes measured by cytofluorometry showed a shift from a diploid to a tetraploid state, whereas the nonmuscle cells behaved like a proliferating population. By comparison, heart cells from 5-day-old embryos showed a slight increase in the number of myocytes (ca 20%); however, tetraploidization was also regularly observed.

DISCUSSION

Gross: How can you be certain that the PAS-positive cells are all muscle cells? Using phase contrast microscopy, we have seen a gradual decrease of glycogen content in cultured heart muscle cells.

Bogenmann: I agree that PAS staining may not be a very good marker for muscle cells, but at present it is widely used for this purpose, especially in mass cultures.

De Haan: I would like to defend further the use of PAS staining to distinguish myocytes from fibroblasts. Polinger in my laboratory studied over five days the correlation between the decline of PAS-positive cells and the decline of beating cells. The number of PAS-positive cells can almost at will be influenced by the medium. If you use rich medium, containing embryo extract in addition to fetal calf serum, you will find that the number of PAS-positive cells and the number of beating cells remain constant.

Pexieder: What was the age of the embryos you used to set up your cultures? What do you know about the polyploidization of heart muscle cells *in vivo*?

Bogenmann: We have been analyzing heart muscle cells primarily from 9-day-old embryos. Some data obtained on 5-day-old embryos did not seem to be significantly

---

** Full text of this contribution has been published in *Journal of Molecular and Cellular Cardiology* (1980) 12:17-28.

different. Polyploidization has been well studied in human hearts of 8- and 12-year-old children, but no information is available on embryonic development.

Fischman: In vivo, as has been shown by Jeter and Cameron, all the cells of 9-day-old embryo synthesize DNA. Now, when you dissociate your cells and put them in a monolayer, almost all cells will show a 2–5 n DNA content. It seems that there is something wrong with our system. The cells are not duplicating what occurs *in vivo.* It may be that you lose cycling myocytes because they are very sensitive to trypsine.

De Haan: Your closing comment, "These results are an artifact of a culture condition" is true. We have to start looking at the effects of culture conditions. Also, the electrophysiological properties of cells in monolayer are different from those of an intact heart. The reaggregated cells will regain the electrophysiological properties of the intact heart.

Markwald: In tissue culture, fibroblasts as well as the myocytes continue to make glycoprotein, which adheres to the cell surface and should react with PAS just as well as glycogen reacts. How are you getting entire cell staining through an intact plasma membrane? You need to establish more critically which are muscle cells and which are not.

Fischmann: There is no question that this is not cell surface PAS-positive material. There is no problem about the cytoplasmic entry of the reactive in alcohol-fixed tissue. The cytoplasmic and cell surface PAS positivity can also be easily distinguished by diastase digestion.

De Haan: Dr. Fischmann has shown that a ratio of cell volume to DNA content remains constant from 3 or 4 e.d. up through hatching. Is it possible that under cell culture conditions we are holding cells back from undergoing cytokinesis and that what we see then is a kind of artificial polyploidization?

Bogenmann: We have tried to isolate nuclei from the heart to measure them, but we had a very low efficiency, about 2 to 3%, so that any measurements would hardly be significant. I would suggest trying to determine whether the tetraploid myocytes can be stimulated to re-enter the cycle.

Cell Death

Perspectives in Cardiovascular Research, Vol. 5,
Mechanisms of Cardiac Morphogenesis and Teratogenesis,
edited by Tomas Pexieder. Raven Press, New York © 1981

Introduction

Tomas Pexieder

Institut d'Histologie et d'Embryologie, Université, de Lausanne, Lausanne, Suisse

When looking at most normal and healthy tissues, especially those of the embryo, a good observer will note, in addition to the numerous mitotic figures, cells in various stages of degeneration. These cells are manifestations of "physiological cell death." The existence of physiological cell death was recognized as early as 1924 by Ernst (2). Its role as a general morphogenetic mechanism has been described by Glücksmann (5) and reviewed by Saunders (47), Wendler (49) and Pexieder (33). The concept of cell death as a mechanism of teratogenesis was introduced by Menkes (17). Physiological cell death has been described in almost every embryonic tissue. It has been most intensively studied in development of the limb, palatal shelves, urogenital tract, and central nervous system.

The history of physiological cell death studies of the embryonic heart began in 1957, when Goerttler (6) mentioned the necrotic cells. In 1965, Menkes and his coworkers (16) described the dying cells in the aorticopulmonary septum. Illies (12) was the first to report on the existence of degenerating cells in the human embryonic heart. Within the framework of his studies on histogenesis of heart tissues, Manasek (15) has seen myocardial cell death and associated phagocytosis in the embryonic chick ventricle.

My laboratory spent the years from 1968 to 1975 in extensive studies of the function of cell death in morphogenesis and teratogenesis of the heart. 1968 and 1969 saw our efforts concentrated on systematic studies of the localization and ultrastructure of cell death phenomena in the developing chick embryo heart (14,21,22,23,28,29). Quantitative investigations of the importance of cell death in the embryonic heart (24,25) enabled us to distinguish between background cell death, present overall, with dying and dead cells occupying less than 30 percent relative volume of a tissue, and cell death foci with 30 to 70 percent relative volume of degenerating cells. The simultaneous analysis of numbers of interphase, mitotic, and degenerating cells (24,25) and of their role in the cell turnover of the developing heart (31,32,50) permitted classification of cell death foci into morphogenetic, phylogenetic, and histogenetic categories, according to the principles devised by Glücksmann (5). We have also emphasized the possibility that individual foci can move from one category to the other during development, such as in the cell death observed in the aorticopulmonary septum (33).

In further studies of physiological cell death, we more or less restricted ourselves to the heart bulbus (conotruncus), because of its importance in formation of the outflow tracts and its accessibility to observation and experimental manipulation. There has been also a sufficient background of experimental embryological and teratological studies concerning this part of the heart.

In our ultrastructural studies (13,14,33), we have been able to identify three subpopulations of cells: pre-necrotic, necrotic, and phagocytic. In agreement with Forsberg and Abro (4), we could characterize the ultrastructural changes as a burst of autophagy followed by isogenic heterophagy. We have also discussed the difference between macrophages (blood-borne) and phagocytes (tissue-borne). The differentiation of phagocytes from neighboring healthy cushion tissue and myocardial cells is triggered when the intensity of autophagocytosis reaches a certain threshold level.

The pursuit of our investigations required a comprehensive technique allowing rapid topographic and quantitative assessment of cell death phenomena in large numbers of embryonic hearts. This technique took the form of microdissection of hearts stained supravitally with Nile blue sulphate. We have spent much time proving in cytological studies (33) that Nile blue sulphate stains both isolated dead cells and macrophages, as well as extra- and intracellulary localized cytolysomes and phagosomes. With these tools in hand, we approached (26) the problem of the morphogenetic role of physiological cell death in the conotruncus (heart bulbus). Correlating the specific localization and intensity of cell death with the form changes of selected bulbar (conotruncal) cushions, we concluded that cell death preceding the shape changes by 8 to 16 hours contributes to cushion molding. At that point, we stated for the first time the need for digital description of cardiac morphogenesis at the organ level.

Using the experimental pulmonary stenosis produced by clipping off both sixth aortic arches, we then decided to test two hypotheses in a common experimental situation (27). The first hypothesis concerned the causality of the relationship between cell death and morphogenesis of the bulbar (conotruncal) cushions. The second concerned the eventual causal relation between hemodynamic factors and variations in cell death intensity. Experimental intervention on the aortic arches was followed by the appearance of a new cell death focus in the space where future merging of the proximal right bulbus (dextroposterior conus) cushion and its distal ventral (dextrosuperior truncus) counterpart would normally occur. Here the increase in cell death intensity preceeded by 8 to 16 hr the signs of delayed merging of these cushions. Interestingly, as first noted by Rychter and Lemež (43), this hemodynamic intervention results in a 92% rate of ventricular septal defects (VSD). We therefore postulated either mechanical damage to subendocardial mesenchymal cells or the action on pre-necrotic cells as possible links among altered hemodynamics, the modulation of cell death intensity, and the pathogenesis of VSD.

In 1973 (30) we completed our investigations into the role of hemodynamics as an epigenetic regulating factor of cell death in the developing heart. This involved an inverse experiment using organ culturing of the bulbus (conotruncus) in a complete absence of blood flow. In contrast to the pattern of programmed cell death in chick embryonic limb explanted in organ culture by Fallon and Saunders (3), we found no signs of the existence of a "death clock." The intensity of cell death phenomena in explanted conotruncus (bulbus) was significantly reduced and completely lacked the pattern observed *in vivo*. Subsequent studies (1), however, have shown important differences in DNA and protein synthesis rates *in vivo* and *in vitro*, so that our conclusions based on the organ culture studies must now be reinvestigated.

In 1973 there appeared, in the form of an abstract, the first observation from the Hiroshima school on physiological cell death in the rat embryonic heart (45,46). Ojeda and Hurle (18) published, in a short form, their first paper on cell death during fusion of the endocardial tubes in the chick embryo.

To be sure that cell death related to the heart organogenesis is not a species-limited process, we proceeded to perform extensive comparative studies of rat and human embryos (33,42). These studies showed that the number of cell death foci decreases in the course of phylogenesis, passing from 31 in the chick to 21 in the rat and 16 in the human. However, the lesser availability of human embryonic material has to be taken into consideration. Cell death has been found in the following structures of all three species studied: atrioventricular cushions, zone of fusion of the atrioventricular cushions, conotruncal (bulbus) cushions, zone of fusion of the conotruncal (bulbus) cushions, walls of the aorta and the pulmonary artery, and semilunar valves of the aorta and the pulmonary artery.

Even in 1972 (27), we envisaged the possibility that physiological cell death zones in the heart represent a common target for both hemodynamic and chemical teratogens. To prove the interaction of chemical teratogens with physiological cell death, we have looked for chemical substances already known to produce specific heart anomalies in the chick embryo, which would act at the conotruncus. We expected these substances to be capable of interaction with either pre-necrotic cells or phagocytes. We selected cyclophosphamide, supposed to amplify cell death phenomena through alkylation of DNA, and dexamethasone, known to inhibit phagocytes. Cyclophosphamide injected into the amniotic fluid on 4th e.d. produced a 75% rate of cardiovascular defects, 75% of these being VSD. Dexamethasone treatment resulted in a 40% rate of cardiovascular defects, of which 31% were isolated VSD and 45% VSD combined with overriding aorta. The quantification of cell death intensity in the various structures of the embryonic hearts with a check for differences in phagocyte density (33) showed that chemical teratogens can modulate cell death phenomena. However, their effects on cell death were less pronounced than those of hemodynamics. When we discussed the mechanisms of cyclophosphamide and dexamethasone action, particularly their potential interaction with cell division (33), we were confronted with the very wide and rather unspecific effects of the majority of chemical teratogens and inhibitors. In this experimental set-up the bulbar (conotruncal) and atrioventricular cushions appeared as *loci minoris resistentiae* with regard to heart teratogenesis.

In 1975, the year of appearance of our monograph (33) on cell death in morphogenesis and teratogenesis of the heart, Ojeda and Hurle (19) published their full paper on cell death during formation of tubular heart of the chick embryo. At that time, they presented the unusual suggestion that cellular debris located between the double endocardial layers of the sagittal septum can participate in the elaboration of cardiac jelly. This idea, which does not seem to be quite plausible, still awaits experimental proof.

1975 also saw our preliminary report (34) on the first SEM studies of cell death. With the SEM, we were able to observe the exocytosis of cytolysomes and the presence of intercellular clefts between endocardial cells, and the phagocytes adhering to the luminal surface of the endocardium (35). Exploiting the advantages of SEM technology, we studied (36,37,40) the modifications of endocardial surface morphology following experimental elimination of both sixth aortic arches. Redistribution of laminar blood streams (39) following this experimental intervention induced rapid, precisely localized and unspecific damage to the endocardium. Later, giant intercellular clefts appeared at specific localizations as a sign of the amplified wash-out of phagocytes. In other regions, transendocardial passage of phagocytes was observed. This observation was interpreted as either an increase in the number of traversing phagocytes or a decrease in their wash-out. Our SEM studies showed that not only the focalized subendocardial intensification of cell death, but also the altered clearing of tissue from cell debris, is of importance in the pathogenesis of experimental VSD.

The years following 1976 have seen a refocusing of our interest from the problems of cell death to other developmental mechanisms (e.g., proliferation), to the integration of various developmental mechanisms, and to quantitative studies of heart organogenesis. More recently, we have discussed the importance of cell death in major papers on development of the outflow tract (38), on the effects of modifying the embryonic circulation (39), and on cellular mechanisms of cardiac morphogenesis and teratogenesis (41).

In 1976, Okamoto and Satow (20) from the Hiroshima group published a major paper concerning their observations of physiological cell death in the embryonic heart of normal and rapid-neutron-irradiated rats. From the greater length of cell death focus in the "inferior distal bulbar ridge" in radiation-produced double outlet right ventricle, they deduced its role in the shortening of this ridge. They also stated that "cell death found in the proximal inferior subaortic distal ridges suggests that the occurrence of cell death in the bulbus is *greatly related* to the migration of the aorta into the left ventricle." Still other rather unusual reasoning can be found in their statement, "It is reasonable to assume that the cell death masses in the distal bulbar ridge do not occur by chance, but by a *genetically* controlled program." Finally, they suggested that "the absorption of the bulbus . . . is caused by the cell death . . . ." Even if these are valuable hypotheses for further study, they have not yet been proved and lack sufficient experimental and descriptive support. Another problem with interpretation of observations obtained in Hiroshima results from the delay (several days) that separates irradiation from the observed modification of cell death. Furthermore (38), the abnormal looping seen as an early consequence of irradiation creates abnormal hemodynamic conditions. The most interesting part of the work done in Hiroshima is the observation that ionizing radiation delays the appearance of cell death and decreases its amplitude.

Hurle and his coworkers (8) published a paper confirming Manasek's (15) observations regarding phagocytosis by myocardial cells, and reported on the similar behavior of acid phosphatase, as we noted in 1973 and 1975 (13,14,33). They presented another strange reasoning, i.e., "the location of this area mainly in the *right* side of the wall of the bulbus could be a factor participating in the displacement of the bulbus towards the *left* side." The series of peculiar hypotheses issued by these authors was completed in the same year (10) by the statement that "cardiac jelly could participate in the fusion facilitating the endocardial cell death." The observations of phagocytosis by embryonic myocardial cells were developed by these authors (9) into another statement that "spontaneous degeneration of some of the cardiac muscle cells is related to the transformation into origins of the aorta and pulmonary artery." More realistic were the recent observations by Hurle (7) on the role played by physiological cell death in morphogenesis of semilunar valves.

In rather complete morphometric investigations, Satow and his collaborators (44) confirmed at the quantitative level the earlier idea of Schweichel and Merker (48) that there is no difference in the ultrastructure of physiological and teratogene-induced cell death. At the same time, these authors formulated supplementary hypotheses relating "positional changes in cell death focus to directional abnormalities of the invading myocardial cells," which would result in anomalies of the subpulmonary muscle bundles, leading to cardiac anomalies.

Finally, in 1979, instead of trying to test or otherwise verify some of their previous hypotheses, Hurle and Ojeda (11) had the audacity to state that "no comprehensive study has been made (on physiological cell death) which could serve as a basis for experimental studies." Ignoring our comparative studies on the use of various histological and supravital stains, they wondered, "we would not distinguish as many necrotic areas." Of course, when using Harris' instead of Meyer's hematoxylin, and neutral red instead of Nile blue sulphate. Stressing the importance of quantifying both dividing and dying cells, they seem to ignore the fact that we had already tackled this problem in 1973 (31, 32,33), including the question of cell death duration.

I would like to conclude by stating that there is now a whole host of hypotheses relating physiological cell death to various features of heart morphogenesis. The next useful step will be to select those which are both plausible and amenable to experimentation for serious testing and verification. Further research will be needed to analyze the integration of cell death with other developmental mechanisms. Wide horizons remain to be traversed as far as initiation and causation of physiological cell death at the level of cellular and molecular biology are concerned.

REFERENCES

1. Chavaz, P. (1977): *Synthèse des acides désoxyribonucléiques et des protéines dans les parties bulbaires des coeurs embryonnaires de poulet in vivo et in vitro.* Thèse, Université de Lausanne. Traitement du texte SA, Genève.

2. Ernst, M. (1926): Ueber Untergang von Zellen während der normalen Entwicklung bei Wirbeltieren. *Z. Anat. Entwickl.-Gesch.*, 79:228-262.

3. Fallon, J. F., and Saunders, J. W. Jr. (1968): *In vitro* analysis of the control of cell death in a zone of prospective necrosis from the chick wing bud. *Dev. Biol.*, 18:553-570.

4. Forsberg, J. G., and Abro, A. (1973): Ultrastructural studies on cell degeneration in the mouse uterovaginal anlage. *Acta Anat. (Basel)*, 85:353-367.

5. Glücksmann, A. (1951): Cell deaths in normal vertebrate ontogeny. *Biol. Rev.*, 26:59-86.

6. Goerttler, K. (1957): Ueber terminologische und begriffliche Fragen der Pathologie der Pränatalzeit. *Virchows Archiv.*, 330:35-84.

7. Hurle, J. M. (1979): Scanning and light microscope studies of the development of the chick embryo semilunar heart valves. *Anat. Embryol.*, 157:69-89.

8. Hurle, J. M., Lafarga, M., and Ojeda, J. L. (1977): Cytological and cytochemical studies of the necrotic area of the bulbus of the chick embryo heart: Phagocytosis by developing myocardial cells. *J. Embryol. Exp. Morph.*, 41:161-170.

9. Hurle, J. M., Lafarga, M., and Ojeda, J. L. (1978): *In vivo* phagocytosis by developing myocardial cells: An ultrastructural study. *J. Cell. Sci.*, 33:363-369.

10. Hurle, J. M., and Ojeda, J. L. (1977): Cardiac jelly arrangement during the formation of the tubular heart of the chick embryo. *Acta Anat. (Basel)*, 98:444-455.

11. Hurle, J. M., and Ojeda, J. L. (1979): Cell death during the development of the truncus and conus of the chick embryo heart. *J. Anat.*, 129:427-439.

12. Illies, A. (1967): La topographie et la dynamique des zones nécrotiques normales chez l'embryon humain. *Rev. Roum. Embryol. Cytol., Ser. Embryol.*, 4:51-85.

13. Krstić, R., and Pexieder, T. (1973): Ultrastructure of cell death in bulbar cushions of chick embryo heart. *Z. Anat. Entwickl.-Gesch.*, 140:337-350.

14. Krstić, R., and Pexieder, T. (1973): Elektronenmikroskopische Beobachtungen der Kulminationsphase des Zellunterganges in den Herzbulbuswülsten des Hühnerembryos. *Anat. Anz.*, 134, Erg.H., 613-618.

15. Manasek, F. J. (1969): Myocardial cell death in the embryonic chick ventricle. *J. Embryol. Exp. Morph.*, 21:271-284.

16. Menkes, B., Alexandru, C., Pavkov, A., and Mircova, O. (1965): Researches on the formation and the elastic structure of the aorto-pulmonary septum in the chick embryo. *Rev. Roum. Embryol. Cytol., Ser. Embryol.*, 2:79-91.

17. Menkes, B., Sandor, S., and Illies, A. (1970): Cell death in teratogenesis. In: *Advances in Teratogenesis, Vol. 4*, edited by D. H. M. Woollam, pp. 170-215. Logos Press, London.

18. Ojeda, J. L., and Hurle, J. M. (1973): Cell death during the fusion of the endocardial tubes in the chick embryo. *Int. Res. Comm. Syst.*, 73-5:1-4.

19. Ojeda, J. L., and Hurle, J. M. (1975): Cell death during the formation of tubular heart of the chick embryo. *J. Embryol. Exp. Morph.*, 33:523-534.

20. Okamoto, N., and Satow, Y. (1976): Cell death in bulbar cushion of normal and abnormal developing heart. In: *Developmental and Physiological Correlates of Cardiac Muscle*, edited by M. Lieberman and T. Sano, pp. 51-66. Perspectives in Cardiovascular Research, Vol. 1. Raven Press, New York.

21. Pexieder, T. (1969): Cell death in the development of the chick embryo heart. *Proc. XII. Congr. Czech. Morphol.*, Praha.

22. Pexieder, T. (1971): Zelltod als Faktor bei der Herzentwicklung des Hühnerembryos. *Acta Anat. (Basel)*, 78:150.

23. Pexieder, T. (1971): Zelluntergang im Herz von Hühnerembryonen zwischen dem 2. und 8. Tag der Entwicklung. *Acta Anat. (Basel)*, 78:159.

24. Pexieder, T. (1971): Die quantitative Karte des Zellunterganges in der Herzentwicklung der Hühnerembryonen zwischen dem 2. und 8. Tag der Inkubation. *Anat. Anz.*, 128, Erg. H., 295-300.

25. Pexieder, T. (1971): Zur quantitativen Auswertung der Gewebedynamik in der Herzorganogenese (mit besonderer Berücksichtigung des Zelltodes). *Acta Anat., (Basel)*, 79:156-157.

26. Pexieder, T. (1972): Beobachtungen über den lokalen Zelltod während der Herzbulbusseptierung des Hühnerembryos. *Anat. Anz.,* 130, Erg.H., 279-286.

27. Pexieder, T. (1972): Ueber die Wirkung der Hämodynamik auf den Zelluntergang in den Herz-bulbuswülsten des Hühnerembryos. *Acta Anat. (Basel),* 82:459-460.

28. Pexieder, T. (1972): The tissue dynamics of heart morphogenesis. I. Cell death phenomena. B. Topography. *Z. Anat. Entwickl.-Gesch.,* 138:241-253.

29. Pexieder, T. (1972): The tissue dynamics of heart morphogenesis. I. Cell death phenomena. A. Identification and morphology. *Z. Anat. Entwickl.-Gesch.,* 137:270-284.

30. Pexieder, T. (1973): Ueber die primären Ursachen des Zelltodes in den Herzbulbuswülsten des Hühnerembryos. *Anat. Anz.,* 134, Erg.H., 183-187.

31. Pexieder, T. (1973): The tissue dynamics of heart morphogenesis. II. Quantitative investigations. A. Method and values from areas without cell death foci. *Ann. Embryol. Morph.,* 6:325-334.

32. Pexieder, T. (1973): The tissue dynamics of heart morphogenesis. II. Quantitative investigations. B. Cell death foci. *Ann. Embryol. Morph.,* 6:335-346.

33. Pexieder, T. (1975): Cell death in the morphogenesis and teratogenesis of the heart. *Adv. Anat. Embryol. Cell Biol.,* 51/3:1-100.

34. Pexieder, T. (1975): SEM investigations on physiological cell death in the chick embryo heart. *Experientia,* 31:745.

35. Pexieder, T. (1976): Rasterelektronenmikroskopische Beobachtungen der Oberfläche der Herz-bulbuswülste der Hühnerembryonen. *Verh. Anat. Ges.,* 70:747-754.

36. Pexieder, T. (1976): Effets de l'hémodynamique sur la morphologie de l'endocarde embryonnaire. *Bull. Ass. Anat. (Nantes),* 60:399-406.

37. Pexieder, T. (1977): SEM observations of the embryonic endocardium under normal and experimental hemodynamic conditions. *Bibl. Anat.,* 15:531-534.

38. Pexieder, T. (1978): Development of the outflow tract of the embryonic heart. In: *Morphogenesis and Malformation of the Cardiovascular System,* edited by G. C. Rosenquist and D. Bergsma, pp. 29-68. *Birth Defects:* Orig. Art. Ser., Vol. XIV, No. 7. Alan R. Liss, New York.

39. Pexieder, T. (1978): Discussion of the topics: Effects of modifying the embryonic circulation. In: *Morphogenesis and Malformation of the Cardiovascular System,* edited by G. C. Rosenquist and D. Bergsma, pp. 449-455. *Birth Defects:* Orig. Art. Ser., Vol. XIV, No. 7. Alan R. Liss, New York.

40. Pexieder, T. (1979): Mechanisms of teratogenesis in hemodynamically induced ventricular septal defect. In: *Advances in the Detection of Congenital Malformation,* edited by E. B. Van Julsingha, J. M. Tesh, and G. M. Fara, pp. 264-268. Eur. Teratology Soc., Wethersfield.

41. Pexieder, T. (1980): Cellular mechanisms underlying the normal and abnormal development of the heart. In: *Etiology and Morphogenesis of Congenital Heart Disease,* edited by R. van Praagh and A. Takao, pp. 127-153. Futura Publ. Co., New York.

42. Pexieder, T., and Paschoud, N. (1973): La stabilité phylogénétique des zones de la mort cellulaire physiologique dans l'organogenèse du coeur. *Acta Anat. (Basel),* 86:321.

43. Rychter, Z., and Lemež, L. (1959): Vascular system of the chick embryo. IV. Descriptive morphology of experimentally produced ventricular septal defects. *Čs. Morfol.,* 7:21-32.

44. Satow, Y., Okamoto, N., Hidaka, N., Akimoto, N., and Miyabara, S. (1978): Intracellular mechanisms of teratogenesis of embryonic heart. In: *Morphogenesis and Malformation of the Cardiovascular System,* edited by G. C. Rosenquist and D. Bergsma, pp. 251-271. *Birth Defects:* Orig. Art. Ser., Vol. XIV, No. 7. Alan R. Liss, New York.

45. Satow, Y., Okamoto, N., Miyabara, S., Hidaka, N., and Akimoto, N. (1974): Cell death in the bulbar cushions in normal and abnormal development of rat embryonic hearts. *Teratology,* 10:96.

46. Satow, Y., Okamoto, N., Ueno, T., Miyabara, S., Hidaka, N., Akimoto, N., and Ikeda, T. (1973): Fine structural localization of the pyroantimonate precipitation in the cardiac jelly of the rat embryonic tubular heart after neutron irradiation. *Cong. Anom.,* 13:221-233.

47. Saunders, J. W. Jr. (1966): Death in embryonic systems. *Science,* 154:604-612.

48. Schweichel, J. U., and Merker, H. J. (1973): The morphology of various types of cell death in prenatal tissues. *Teratology,* 7:253-266.

49. Wendler, D. (1972): *Der embryo-fetale Zelltod während der Normogenese und im Experiment.* Acta Historica Leopoldina Nr. 8., J. A. Barth, Leipzig.

50. Wyss, P., and Pexieder, T. (1973): Quelques facteurs complémentaires dans l'évaluation quantitative de la dynamique tissulaire des bourrelets bulbaires chez l'embryon de poulet. *Acta Anat. (Basel),* 86:321.

Perspectives in Cardiovascular Research, Vol. 5,
Mechanisms of Cardiac Morphogenesis and Teratogenesis,
edited by Tomas Pexieder. Raven Press, New York © 1981

Establishment of the Tubular Heart. Role of Cell Death

J. L. Ojeda and J. M. Hurle

Department of Anatomy, Faculty of Medicine, University of Santander, Santander, Spain

Development of the embryonic organs involves several basic mechanisms, including cell differentiation, cell growth, cell migration, etc. The destruction of large numbers of cells at specific areas and specific times during development is also a mechanism involved in the morphogenesis of most embryonic organs (10,35). In the developing chick heart, several necrotic foci have been described (14,17,20,28,32,33). Most of these are observable only at advanced stages of development; their precise significance remains obscure, awaiting further experimental analysis.

In most vertebrates, the embryonic heart arises from two lateral primordia that fuse at the midline to form a single tubular structure (4,12,31,36). Some aspects of the fusion process have been analyzed in detail (29,30). On the basis of these analyses, it is now believed that structures extrinsic to the heart, such as the foregut endoderm, may be involved in the fusion process. However, the causes of the fusion process are far from being clarified.

In a previous paper (27), we have reported the presence of degenerating cells within the midline of the fusing endocardial tubes, suggesting that cell death might be a morphogenetic factor in the fusion process. However, several questions must be answered before this hypothesis can be demonstrated. For example, it must be determined whether fusion takes place in the absence of cell death. It must also be determined whether cell death is a consequence or a causal mechanism of the fusion process.

In the present work, we have studied, by use of several techniques, the occurrence of cell death during normal fusion of the heart primordia, as well as in embryos in which the process was prevented by a microsurgical procedure. In these experimental conditions, each primordium gives rise to an independently beating heart, resulting in a double-hearted embryo. Our results show that cell death takes place in the absence of fusion, thus suggesting that cell death is not a consequence of the fusion, but rather that is in some way previously programmed.

MATERIALS AND METHODS

White Leghorn chick embryos, staged according to Hamburger and Hamilton (13), were employed. Fusion of the heart primordia was studied by light, scanning, and transmission electron microscopy in normal embryos of stages 9 to 11 and in surgically induced double-hearted (cardia bifida) embryos of equivalent stages.

For the microsurgical production of cardia bifida, stage 8 embryos were explanted to watch-glass cultures with the ventral side up, by the method of New (26). In addition to the albumin medium employed in New's method, some embryos were cultured in agar–yolk medium (1), to discard possible alterations produced by the culture medium. Fusion of the heart primordia was prevented in these embryos by making a midline cut through the tissue of the anterior intestinal portal with a tugsten microneedle, as described by DeHaan (5). Control unoperated embryos were also studied.

Light Microscopy

The embryos were fixed in 3% glutaraldehyde buffered in 0.1 M sodium cacodylate at pH 7.3 for 3 to 4 h, washed in buffer alone, then dehydrated in a series of acetones and embedded in araldite.

Transverse serial sections 1 to 2 μm thick were cut and stained with 0.1% toluidine blue in 0.1% sodium borate and observed under the light microscope.

Scanning Electron Microscopy

Chick embryos fixed in glutaraldehyde, as above, were rinsed in cacodylate buffer and transversely cut through the heart. The fragments were dehydrated with acetone, dried by the critical point method, and gold sputter coated. The specimens were viewed using a Philips scanning electron microscope (SEM) 501.

Transmission Electron Microscopy

Chick embryos fixed in glutaraldehyde as above were washed in buffer solution and postfixed in 1% osmium tetroxide. After dehydration and embedding in araldite, ultrathin sections were obtained with a LKB ultratome III. The sections were stained with aqueous uranyl acetate and lead citrate and observed with a Philips EM 201 transmission electron microscope (TEM).

RESULTS

Heart Fusion in Normal Embryos

The mechanism of fusion is identical in normal embryos and in the cultured control embryos. It takes place between stages 9 and 12, and can easily be followed by SEM. The early paired primordia are tubular structures formed by an inner endocardial tube which is surrounded ventrally by the precardiac splanchnic mesoderm and dorsally by the open endoderm. Between the endocardium and the surrounding tissues, there is a large space filled with extracellular matrix. At stage 9 or 9+, the infolding of the endoderm reaches the level of the heart. Both primordia approach the midline and fuse, forming the tubular heart. This fusion process follows a cephalo-caudal sequence, so that in stage 11 the two rudiments of the sinus venosus have not yet joined. At the end of this process, the heart is an unpaired tubular structure, with an inner endocardial tube and an outer myocardial layer separated by the extracellular matrix (cardiac jelly) (3). This process implies both fusion of the paired endocardial tubes and fusion of the precardiac splanchnic mesoderm, termed the premyocardial layer, after Manasek (23) and Ho and Shimada (15).

The premyocardial layer displays a crescent shape in transverse sections, and fusion takes place both at the ventral and dorsal edges. At the ventral side, fusion occurs very quickly and is therefore difficult to observe in sections. When the ventral side of the heart is observed under the SEM (Fig. 1), it shows a prominent groove which corresponds with the zone in which fusion has taken place. In some instances, rounded cell profiles showing a pitted surface are observed in this zone, but they are very rare (Fig. 2). Fusion of the dorsal zone takes place very late in the stages covered in this study. During the studied stages, the heart remains open at the dorsal side in contact with the ventral foregut endoderm. This open zone is usually termed the dorsal mesocardium.

After infolding of the endoderm, the endocardial tubes appear, located laterally to each other under the floor of the ventral foregut endoderm (Fig. 3). The wall of each tube is composed of flattened cells, with the long axis arranged in a circular fashion. In some instances, cords of endocardial cells can be observed crossing the lumen of the tubes. These cords are joined to the endocardial wall by thin cytoplasmic processes, suggesting that they will later become detached. Once the endocardial tubes meet at the midline, their medial opposing walls undergo progressive changes until they disappear. Initially, some perforations produced by loss of cells are observed in their most ventral zones (Fig. 3). The number and size of these perforations increases later, forming wide communications between the tubes. At this stage, the tubes take the appearance of a single tube, with an incomplete septum in its medio-dorsal portion (Fig. 4). This process progresses dorsally until the septum is eliminated. At higher magnifications, rounded cell profiles in the process of detachment into the lumen can be observed in the zone of fusion during all these stages. These cells often show a rough surface with occasional holes, contrasting with the smooth surface of the flattened endocardial cells (Fig. 5). Constrictions are also a common feature of these cells.

These SEM observations are in accordance with light and TEM studies previously published by us (27). By use of these techniques, it can be observed that some endocardial cells of the midline die during the process of fusion and are

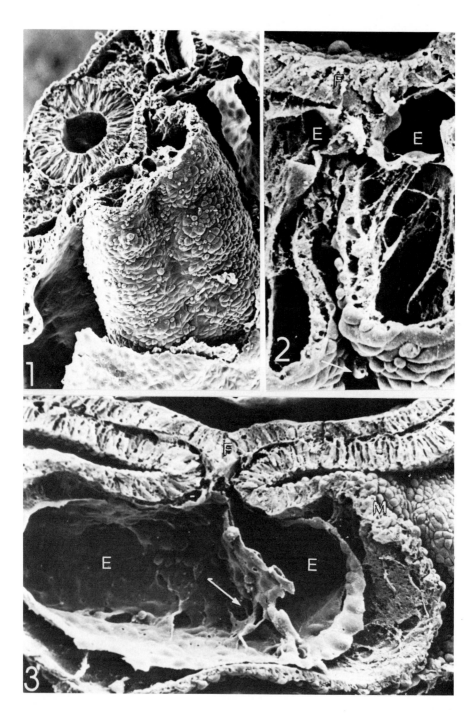

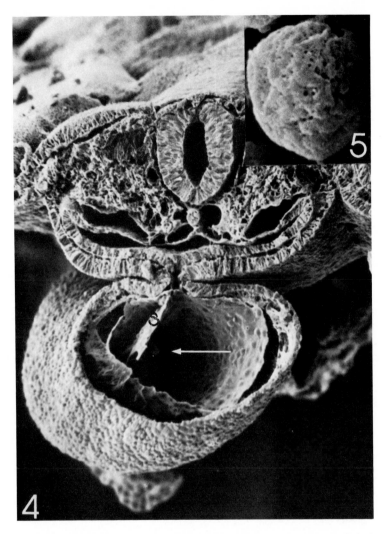

FIG. 4. Stage 10 chick embryo showing an intermediate stage of endocardial fusion. Both endocardial tubes are separated by an incomplete medio-dorsal septum (S). Note endocardial cells in process of detachment *(arrow)*. × 200.

FIG. 5. High-magnification SEM view of a detached endocardial cell displaying a rough and pitted surface. × 5,000.

FIG. 1. Ventral view of an embryo after fusion of the ventral mesocardium. The heart shows a prominent groove in the zone where the fusion has taken place. × 230.

FIG. 2. Transverse fracture of a stage 9+ embryo showing a rounded cell expelled towards the pericardial cavity *(arrow)*. F, foregut endoderm; E, endocardial tubes. × 900.

FIG. 3. Early stage of endocardial fusion. Some perforations are observed in the most ventral zone of the fusion *(arrow)*. Note some rounded endocardial cells protruding towards the lumen. E, endocardial tubes; F, foregut endoderm. M, premyocardial layer. × 500.

then detached either into the lumen of the heart or into the cardiac jelly (Fig. 6). However, it should be noted that, in addition to the degenerating cells, some apparently healthy endocardial cells can also be observed in the course of detachment. As can be seen in Fig. 7, these cells always show large cytoplasmic inclusions completely filled by extracellular matrix.

Double-Hearted Embryos

As shown in Fig. 8, the operated embryos develop two independent heart tubes, located in a ventro-lateral position. The structure of these hearts is similar to that of the paired primordia. They have an inner endocardial tube closely related to the unfolded endoderm and surrounded ventro-laterally by the myocardial layer. Cardiac jelly is also present between the different heart tissues. In these hearts, the zone of the endocardium related to the endoderm corresponds to the zone of fusion in the normal embryos; we shall call this area the "endocardial expected fusion zone" (EEFZ). The most medial zone of the myocardial layer is the "myocardial expected fusion zone" (MEFZ). When the hearts are observed at higher magnification, some rounded cells appear protruding or detached in the EEFZ (Fig. 9). These cells contact the endocardial wall and exhibit a rough and pitted surface. In other zones of the heart, cells with altered morphology are rare even in the MEFZ, and they never show a preferential location.

Both light microscopy and TEM show a good structural conservation of the heart tissues and also reveal pyknotic cells located in the EEFZ (Fig. 10). These cells usually protrude into the lumen, but they can also be observed detached into the cardiac jelly. Three different types of degenerating cells can be distinguished by their ultrastructural appearance. Some cells show only partial signs of degeneration. These are irregularly shaped endocardial cells still joined to the neighboring healthy cells. The most remarkable feature of these cells is the presence of abundant cytoplasmic vacuoles caused by swelling of the endoplasmic reticulum and mitochondria. In some instances, there are multinucleated

FIG. 6. Transverse semi-thin section of a heart at the same stage as that shown in Fig. 2. Arrows show dying cells in the endocardial septum. × 400.

FIG. 7. Viable endocardial cell in course of detachment from the zone of fusion. Note the large cytoplasmic inclusions containing extracellular material. × 9,000.

FIG. 8. Panoramic SEM view of a double-hearted embryo. C, unfused cardiac tubes. × 130.

FIG. 9. Higher magnification of the zone indicated by arrow in Fig. 8. Note several endocardial dead cells in the EEFZ *(arrow)*. × 900.

FIG. 10. Semi-thin section showing the EEFZ of a double-hearted embryo. Note dead cells being detached into the endocardial lumen *(large arrow)*. Small arrow shows a dead cell located in the cardiac jelly. F, unfolded endoderm; M, myocardial layer. × 450.

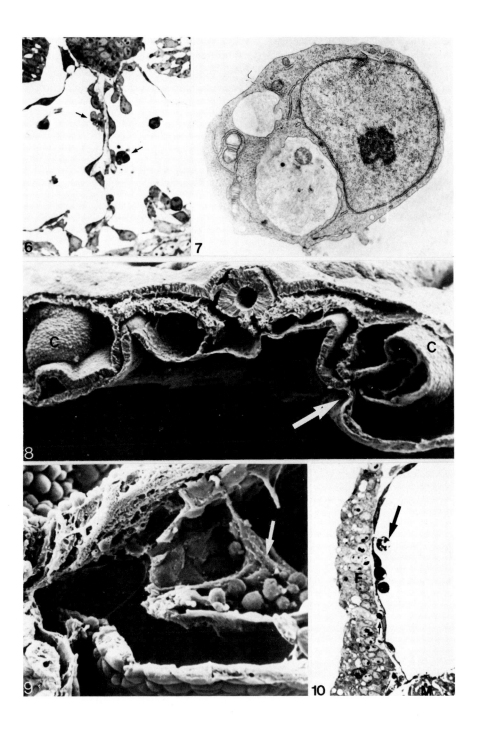

cells that show two or more rounded nuclei of different sizes (Fig. 11). Other cells appear as very dark rounded bodies. These degenerating cells are always detached from the endocardial wall, most often into the lumen and less frequently into the cardiac jelly. The nucleus always exhibits extensive chromatin condensation and frequently appears fragmented into several small pieces (Fig. 12). The cytoplasm is very electron-dense and shows widespread vacuolization of the organelles. The ribosomes very often appear to be aggregated, forming large crystalline structures (Fig. 13). The viable endocardial cells may show cytoplasmic processes contacting these dark cells. Cell fragments displaying a dramatic loss of matrix are a feature of the third type of degenerating cell. These degenerating cells appear as granular and membranous cell remnants surrounded by a membrane.

No differences were noted in histological and ultrastructural preservation of embryonic heart tissues grown in different culture media.

DISCUSSION

Our studies showed the occurrence of physiological cell death concomitant with fusion of the paired endocardial tubes, both *in ovo* and *in vitro*. Ultrastructural conservation of the heart tissues in the cultured embryos was very good, and no substantial modification in the pattern of cell death was observed under these conditions.

The presence of cell death in the EEFZ of the double-hearted embryos could possibly be interpreted as a technical artifact produced by the microsurgery, rather than as a physiologic process. However, the interval between the operation and the study of these embryos was long enough that this possibility can be discarded, since England and Cowper (6) have demonstrated by SEM that microsurgical wounds in the chick embryo endoderm are repaired within two hours. For this reason, our observations of the necrotic process occurring in the absence of fusion suggest that cell death is not dependent upon the contact between the endocardial tubes, but rather that it is programmed in earlier stages.

A pattern of programmed cell death, in some cases genetically dependent, has been clearly established for other necrotic areas (see 22 and 35 for reviews). These programmed necrotic processes may be triggered by locally diffusing materials. In the heart, it is possible that the endoderm and/or the cardiac jelly,

FIG. 11. Multinucleated degenerating endocardial cell of a double-hearted embryo. × 16,000.

FIG. 12. Dark endocardial dead cell of a double-hearted embryo showing the nucleus fragmented into several pieces. Note the good ultrastructural preservation of the healthy endocardial cells (E). × 6,000.

FIG. 13. Endocardial dead cell showing ribosome crystals *(arrow)*. × 16,000.

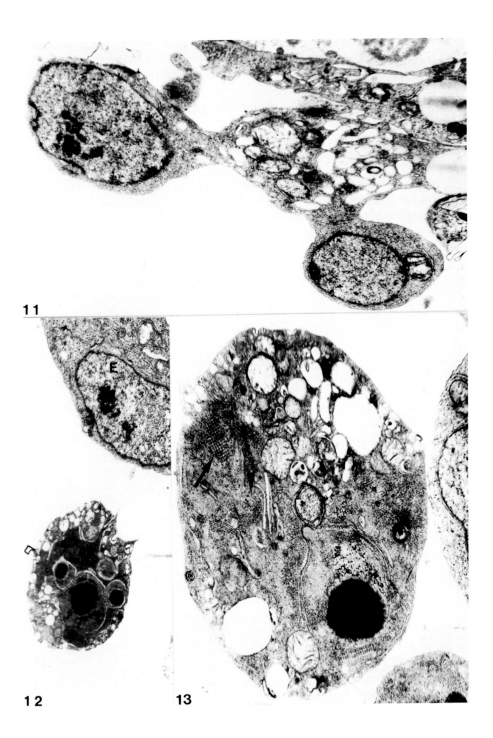

11

12

13

located between the fusing endocardial tubes, might trigger or control the necrotic process, since these are the only structures related to the necrotic zone. Orts Llorca (29,30) has demonstrated in previous experimental studies that fusion of the heart tubes requires the presence of the endoderm. On the other hand, we have also observed that the cardiac jelly associated with the zone of fusion displays morphologic features closely associated with the events of fusion, (19), and Manasek (24) has demonstrated that some of the components of this zone of the cardiac jelly are synthesized by the endoderm.

The mechanism of cell death is a controversial question. Most of the ultrastructural and surface characteristics of the dead endocardial cells observed here are similar to those reported in other necrotic areas (14,16,17,21). The presence of multiple nuclei is not a usual feature in degenerating cells, but it has been previously observed in the lens necrotic area of the chick embryo (8). This feature is consistent with the hypothesis that cell death is a consequence of aberrant mitotic divisions (7). The formation of ribosome crystals during physiological cell death, as described here, has been reported in other necrotic tissues (25). This observation also supports the altered-mitosis hypothesis for cell death, since ribosome crystallization is easier to induce by experimental procedures in mitotic cells than during interphase (2). However, the techniques employed here do not allow us to rule out other possible mechanisms of cell death, such as the involvement of lysosomes.

In most of the necrotic areas studied, the degenerating cells are rapidly removed by phagocytic activity by neighboring cells or by immigrating macrophages (9,18,21). However, in some instances they are expelled from the normal tissues into the extracellular space, where they disintegrate (11). In this study, we found that most of the dead cells were detached into the lumen of the heart and some into the cardiac jelly, and we presume that they might play an embryonic role. Recent experimental studies by Rajala et al. (34) suggest that initiation of the heartbeat is stimulated by a mechanical stretching of the heart wall, presumably caused by a temporary increase in intraluminal plasma volume and pressure. Since initiation of the heartbeat takes place at the same time as the degenerative process (stage 10), it can be suggested that the increase in intraluminal plasma pressure is caused by an osmotic effect of the detached cell detritus. On the other hand, we have previously suggested a possible involvement of the cell detritus detached into the cardiac jelly in production or modification of the extracellular components of the cardiac jelly (27).

We conclude from this study that elimination of most of the endocardial cells in the midline of the paired endocardial tubes is the result of a programmed necrotic process. However, it should be noted that, in addition to the degenerating cells, some healthy endocardial cells containing abundant extracellular material within cytoplasmic inclusions are also detached during the process. It is possible that these cells play a role in elimination of the extracellular matrix located between the fusing tubes.

ACKNOWLEDGMENTS

This work was supported by a grant from the *Fondo Nacional para el Desarrollo de la Investigación Científica* from the Spanish government.

REFERENCES

1. Britt, L. G., and Hermann, H. (1959): Protein accumulation in early chick embryos grown under different conditions of explantation. *J. Embryol. Exp. Morph.,* 7:66-78.
2. Byers, B. (1967): Structure and formation of ribosome crystals in hypothermic chick embryo cells. *J. Mol. Biol.,* 26:155-167.
3. Davis, C. L. (1924): The cardiac jelly of the chick embryo. *Anat. Rec.,* 27:201-202.
4. Davis, C. L. (1927): Development of the human heart from its first appearance to the stage found in embryos of twenty paired somites. *Carnegie Contribs. to Embryol.,* 19:245-284.
5. DeHaan, R. L. (1959): Cardia bifida and the development of pacemaker function in the early chick heart. *Dev. Biol.,* 1:586-602.
6. England, M. A., and Cowper, S. V. (1977): Wound healing in the early chick embryo studied by scanning electron microscopy. *Anat. Embryol.,* 152:1-14.
7. Forsberg, J. G., and Källén, B. (1968): Cell death during embryogenesis. *Rev. Roumaine Embryol. Cytol.,* 5:91-102.
8. Garcia-Porrero, J. A., Collado, J. A., and Ojeda, J. L. (1979): Cell death during detachment of the lens rudiment from ectoderm in the chick embryo. *Anat. Rec.,* 193:791-803.
9. Garcia-Porrero, J. A., and Ojeda, J. L. (1979): Cell death and phagocytosis in the neuroepithelium of the developing retina. A TEM and SEM study. *Experientia,* 35:375-376.
10. Glücksmann, A. (1951): Cell death in normal vertebrate ontogeny. *Biol. Rev.,* 26:59-86.
11. Glücksmann, A. (1965): Cell death in normal development. *Arch. Biol. (Liège),* 76:419-437.
12. Goss, C. M. (1952): Development of the median coordinated ventricle from the lateral hearts in rat embryos with three to six somites. *Anat. Rec.,* 112:761-796.
13. Hamburger, V., and Hamilton, H. L. (1951): A series of normal stages in the development of the chick embryo. *J. Morph.,* 88:49-92.
14. Hendrix, M. J., and Morse, D. E. (1977): Atrial septation. I. Scanning electron microscopy in the chick. *Dev. Biol.,* 57:345-363.
15. Ho, E., and Shimada, Y. (1978): Formation of the epicardium studied with the scanning electron microscope. *Dev. Biol.,* 66:579-585.
16. Hurle, J., and Hinchliffe, J. R. (1978): Cell death in the posterior necrotic zone (PNZ) of the chick wing-bud: A stereoscan and ultrastructural survey of autolysis and cell fragmentation. *J. Embryol. Exp. Morph.,* 43:123-136.
17. Hurle, J. M., Lafarga, M., and Ojeda, J. L. (1977): Cytological and cytochemical studies of the necrotic area of the bulbus of the chick embryo heart: phagocytosis by developing myocardial cells. *J. Embryol. Exp. Morph.,* 41:161-173.
18. Hurle, J. M., Lafarga, M., and Ojeda, J. L. (1978): In vivo phagocytosis by developing myocardial cells: An ultrastructural study. *J. Cell Sci.,* 33:363-369.
19. Hurle, J. M., and Ojeda, J. L. (1977): Cardiac jelly arrangement during the formation of the tubular heart of the chick embryo. *Acta Anat. (Basel),* 98:444-455.
20. Hurle, J. M., and Ojeda, J. L. (1979): Cell death during the development of the truncus and conus of the chick embryo heart. *J. Anat.,* 129:427-439.
21. Krstić, R., and Pexieder, T. (1973): Ultrastructure of cell death in bulbar cushions of chick embryo heart. *Z. Anat. Entwickl.-Gesch.,* 140:337-350.
22. Lockshin, R. A., and Beaulaton, J. (1974): Programmed cell death. *Life Sci.,* 15:1549-1566.
23. Manasek, F. J. (1969): Embryonic development of the heart. II. Formation of the epicardium. *J. Embryol. Exp. Morph.,* 22:333-348.
24. Manasek, F. J. (1976): Glycoprotein synthesis and tissue interactions during establishment of the functional embryonic chick heart. *J. Mol. Cell. Cardiol.,* 8:389-402.
25. Mottet, N. K., and Hammar, S. P. (1972): Ribosome crystals in necrotizing cells from the posterior necrotic zone of developing chick limb. *J. Cell Sci.,* 11:403-414.

26. New, D. A. T. (1955): A new technique for the cultivation of the chick embryo *in vitro. J. Embryol. Exp. Morph.,* 3:326-331.
27. Ojeda, J. L., and Hurle, J. M. (1975): Cell death during the formation of the tubular heart of the chick embryo. *J. Embryol. Exp. Morph.,* 33:523-534.
28. Okamoto, N., and Satow, Y. (1976): Cell death in bulbar cushion of normal and abnormal developing heart. In: *Developmental and Physiological Correlates of Cardiac Muscle,* edited by M. Lieberman and T. Sano, pp. 51-66. Raven Press, New York.
29. Orts Llorca, F. (1964): What are the factors which lead to the fusion of the two heart primordia? An experimental analysis. *W. Roux' Arch.,* 155:437-450.
30. Orts Llorca, F. (1964): Les facteurs déterminants de la morphogénèse et de la differentiation cardiaque. *Bull. Ass. Anat. (Nantes),* 122b:1-124.
31. Patten, B. M. (1949): Initiation and early changes in the character of the heartbeat in vertebrate embryos. *Physiol. Rev.,* 29:31-47.
32. Pexieder, T. (1972): The tissue dynamics of heart morphogenesis. I. The phenomena of cell death. B. Topography. *Z. Anat. Entwickl.-Gesch.,* 138:241-254.
33. Pexieder, T. (1975): Cell death in the morphogenesis and teratogenesis of the heart. *Adv. Anat. Embryol. Cell. Biol.,* 51:1-100.
34. Rajala, G. M., Pinter, M. J., and Kaplan, S. (1977): Response of the quiescent heart tube to mechanical stretch in the intact chick embryo. *Dev. Biol.,* 61:330-337.
35. Saunders, J. W. Jr. (1966): Death in embryonic systems. *Science,* 154:604-612.
36. Yoshinaga, T. (1921): A contribution to the early development of the heart in mammalia. *Anat. Rec.,* 21:239-308.

DISCUSSION

Fitzharris: How far back in development do you think those cells might be genetically programmed to die? Where would you, in terms of the programming, envision the program to be initiated?

Hurle: We really do not know. We see only that the cells die when fusion is prevented.

Fitzharris: Do the cells move in concert to the particular region, or is there a heterogenous population of cells that arrives at a certain point and then initiates the program?

De Haan: Using the tritiated thymidine labeling method, we were able to localize at stage 5 cells which will be in a prospective fusion region at stage 10. But we could not tell you whether at stage 5 they are already programmed to die. You could remove that little region at stage 5 and see if the prospective endocardial cells will die on time. I was intrigued by the presence of those little pores in the area of fusion. Do they represent an actual linkage point in the membrane, or are they true pores going all the way through a cell?

Hurle: The condensation in endocardial cells may be a way of providing nutrition to endocardial cells.

Pexieder: You will normally find these holes only in damaged or dying cells. In thousands of SEM pictures, we have seen they were never present on healthy living cells.

Fischman: Where might the macrophages have come from at the stage when there is nothing circulating?

Hurle: In fact, all the cells in the embryo are capable of phagocytosis. I have seen even clearly differentiated myocardial cells containing phagocytized dying cells.

Hay: It is interesting that rounded cells can be found in the heart lumen, particularly in regions where there is a minimum of cardiac jelly and many mesenchymal cells. I have found them in fusing AV cushions. I would expect the reason for this to be the ample phagocytosis by neighboring mesenchymal cells.

Pexieder: Not all of the fusion processes in the heart are accompanied by visible cell death. This may be a question of debris removal from the tissue. I guess that this removal is very rapid in the bulbar cushions, whereas in the aorticopulmonary septum the dead cells stay there for a while and can be observed more easily. I would suggest not using the term "macrophage," which is generally reserved for blood-borne cells or the monocyte line, in connection with embryonic cell death. Let us call just them phagocytes.

Langemeijer: I have seen in your SEM pictures only the fusion of endocardium. What happens when the myocardial mantles fuse? Is there any cell death?

Hurle: As fusion of the ventral myocardium is very rapid, observation is more difficult. Except for isolated dead cells, I did not see a true necrotic area there. Moreover, the morphology of fusion of endocardial and myocardial tubes is different.

Clark: The shedding of dead and dying cells seems to be a very common phenomenon even after completion of cardiac morphogenesis. For example, we can observe it in subacute bacterial endocarditis.

De Haan: Since Dr. Pexieder has some estimates on total necrotic cells, and since potassium is the most osmotically active component of the cellular detritus, it might be interesting to calculate whether or not there is a substantial increase of osmotic pressure in the fluid enclosed in the primitive heart.

Rychter: Many years ago, we used to speak about determination of embryological processes. Actually, we speak about genetic programming of these processes. This change seems to me to decrease our chance of conceiving a simple experiment, and requires new experimental designs. We made an interesting observation about the neural tissue. Its cells can only ingest the dying cells and transport them across the neuroepithelium, but are unable to digest them *in situ.* Perhaps the enzymatic apparatus is not adequate for this task.

Hurle: The myocardial cells I have seen were able to digest the phagocytized material. In fact, Arnold et al. have recently categorized two kinds of phagocytes—professional and amateur—according to the degree of involvement of pseudopods and according to the intracellular localization of ingested particles.

Perspectives in Cardiovascular Research, Vol. 5,
Mechanisms of Cardiac Morphogenesis and Teratogenesis,
edited by Tomas Pexieder. Raven Press, New York © 1981

Comparative and Morphometric Study on Genetically Programmed Cell Death in Rat and Chick Embryonic Heart

Yukio Satow, Naomasa Okamoto, Naotaka Akimoto, Nobuto Hidaka, Shinichi Miyabara, and *Tomas Pexieder

*Research Institute for Nuclear Medicine and Biology, Hiroshima University, Hiroshima, Japan; *Institute of Histology and Embryology, University of Lausanne, Lausanne, Switzerland*

For more than two centuries, many researchers have studied normal and abnormal morphogenesis of embryonic hearts in various species (9). Chick embryonic hearts have been studied more frequently than rat or human hearts. Since Ernst (3) reported on cell death during the embryogenesis of various organs in a variety of species, many investigators have emphasized the importance of cell death during embryonic development. However, there are few reports on cell death in developing cardiovascular systems. In the chick embryo, the occurrence of cell death during remodeling of the dorsal aorta, involution of the ductus arteriosus, formation of the aorticopulmonary septum, and absorption of the cardiac bulb has been described by Hughes (5) and Menkes et al. (13). Ilies (6) reports on a constant zone of cell death in the pericardial region of human embryonic heart. Menkes et al. (14) also point out that the occurrence of cell death in abnormal areas may lead to abnormal cardiac development. Recently, Pexieder (21,22,23) and Krstić and Pexieder (8) have systematically studied cell death in the chick embryonic heart. They have described the presence of many dying cells in the heart bulbar cushions, suggesting that the physiological cell death zone is a common target for teratogens (23). We have pointed out that physiological cell death in the conal ridges of rat embryonic heart plays an important role in normal and abnormal morphogenesis (18,20,25). We believe that comparative study of the embryonic hearts in different species is necessary, since it is known that the types and frequencies of experimentally induced heart anomalies vary among species (16,17,20). This may be due to methodologic differences or to differences in the genetic and environmental background of each species. The present study attempts to compare the initial steps of physiological cell death in rat and chick embryonic hearts. Its aim is to determine the relationship between morphogenesis of the heart and physiological cell death in the conal ridge.

MATERIALS AND METHODS

Chick Embryonic Heart

White Leghorn chick embryos were incubated at 38.5°C and 60 to 70% relative humidity. The embryos on 3rd, 3⅓, 3⅔, and from 4th to 18th day of incubation were sampled in the laboratories of Lausanne and Hiroshima Universities. At each stage, 5 to 6 embryonic hearts were perfused with 2% glutaraldehyde with 1% formaldehyde in a 0.1M cacodylate buffer adjusted with NaCl to 290 mOsm/l, pH 7.2. After prefixation for 30 minutes, postfixation was performed for 2 hours in cacodylate-buffered 1% osmium tetroxide with 5% saccharose. After dehydration by a series of graded alcohols and propylene oxide, the bulbi were embedded in Epon. The regions for ultra-thin sectioning were selected from semi-thin sections stained by toluidine blue or Richardson's solution. Sections contrasted by uranyl acetate and lead acetate were viewed with the electron microscope.

Rat Embryonic Heart

Rat embryos of the Donryu strain, from 13 to 17 days after conception, were used. The hearts were prepared in the same way as those of the chick embryos. Details of this method have been reported previously (25). The osmotic pressure of the buffer solution was adjusted from 290 to 310 mOsm/l, pH 7.2. For quantification of the cellular components of the dying cells in the conal ridges, the Semiautomatic Manual Optical Picture Analyzing System M.O.P. AM/0l was used. The fundamental principle of calculation is similar to that of a point-counting method (28).

RESULTS AND DISCUSSION

External Configuration of Chick and Rat Embryonic Hearts

In the chick embryo at stages 15 to 18 of Hamburger and Hamilton (4), (2.5 to 3rd day of incubation), the truncus arteriosus occupies a ventral and right-sided position to the atrium (Fig. 1-1) and at stage 25 (4.5 to 5th day) its proximal end is continuous with the bulbus cordis (Fig. 1-2). On about the 5th day of incubation (stage 28), displacement of the truncus arteriosus to the middle part of the heart is observed (Fig. 1-3). At approximately stages 29 to 32 (6 to 7.5th day), external separation between the aorta and the pulmonary artery is evident (Fig. 1-4). Chick embryonic heart up to this stage corresponds to rat embryonic heart about 14 to 15 days after conception, showing almost the same external configuration (Fig. 1-1—4). From stages 25 to 36 (Fig. 1-2—6), shortening of the bulbus cordis is observed. After stage 35 (about 8.5th day), the great arterial vessels have almost definitive shapes (2). The primary difference between the external aspect of definitive chick heart and that of rat

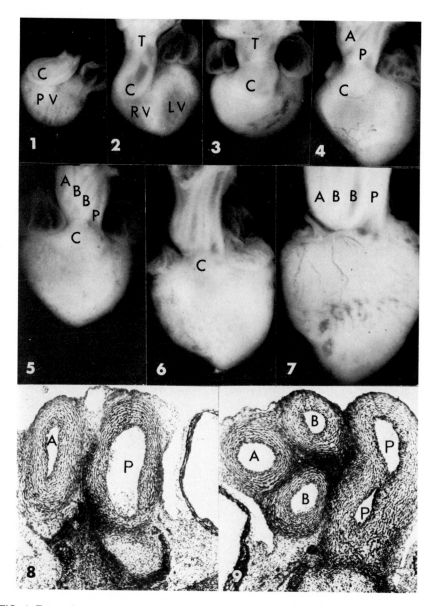

FIG. 1. External aspects of chick embryonic hearts at stages 15 to 18 (1), 25 (2), 28 (3), 29 (4), 35 (5), 36 (6) and 40 (7). Truncus arteriosus (T) separates into aortic (A) and pulmonary (P) tracts (2,3,4,8) before the two brachiocephalic arteries (B) (5,6,7,9) ramify from the aorta. C = bulbus cordis; PV = primitive ventricle; RV, LV = right and left ventricle.

is that chick heart has a right-sided aortic arch and two brachiocephalic arteries that arise from the aortic root (Fig. 1-5—7). There may be no direct relationship between the conotruncal ridges and formation of the two brachiocephalic arteries, since these two arteries ramify in stages 32 to 35 (7 to 8.5th day) (Fig.

1-5,9) after septation of the truncus arteriosus and formation of the presumptive aortic and pulmonary valves (Fig. 1-4,8).

Internal Aspect of the Truncus Arteriosus

In rat embryonic heart 13 days after conception, two swellings are formed, probably through proliferation of mesenchymal cells, in the truncal lumen, facing each other (Fig. 2-7,8). These subsequently fuse together 14 to 15 days after conception (Fig. 3-4—6). One truncal swelling is called the dextro-superior, and the other is the sinistro-inferior (12,15,27). The conal ridges appear at almost the same stage as the truncal swellings, and this is followed by rapid growth after completion of the truncal septum. One is the sinistro-ventral conal ridge connected with the sinistro-inferior truncal swelling through its distal end. The other is the dextro-dorsal conal ridge connected with the dextro-superior truncal swelling by its distal end. In chick embryonic heart on 4th to 5th day of incubation, the cono-truncal ridges are readily visible in a microdissection or serial sections of the heart (Fig. 2-3—6).[1] At stage 28 (5.5th day), the ventral-distal and dorsal-distal bulbar cushions begin to fuse (Fig. 3-1). These bulbar cushions (23,24,26) (Fig. 2-5,6) correspond to the sinistro-superior and dextro-posterior truncal swellings (7,11). The right-proximal and left-proximal bulbar cushions, which correspond to the dextro-dorsal and sinistro-inferior conal ridges, fuse to form the conal septum (Fig. 3-2,3). In stage 29 (6th to 6.5th day), the septation process is almost complete (Fig. 3-2,3). In this stage, the primordia of the cusps of the aortic and pulmonary semilunar valves are already visible (Fig. 2-1).[2] In chick embryonic heart, the distal-ventral and distal-dorsal ridges (Fig. 2-4) separate from the left-proximal ridge in stage 25 (4th to 5th day). Although in the chick the shape of the mesenchymal swellings of the above-mentioned cono-truncal ridges is somewhat different from that of rat, no fundamental differences regarding the formation of the aortic and the pulmonary tracts or conal septum are observed (Fig. 1-8,2-1—4) between the two species on serial sections. In the horizontal plane of the sections of the cono-truncal ridges on 4th to 5th day of incubation (Fig. 2-1—3), two dense mesenchymal cell masses are observed. One of these cell masses is found in the dorsal-right conal ridge (Fig. 2-2,3) and the other in the ventral or left-dorsal conal ridge (Fig. 2-2). Laane (10) points out that the aorticopulmonary septum in the chick extends two limbs of dense mesenchymal cell accumulation into the cono-truncal ridges (Fig. 2-1—4). In the rat, only one cell mass is seen, almost in the middle part of the mesenchyme in the truncus arteriosus, suggesting that no limbs are separated from the descending aorticopulmonary septum (1).

---

[1] They are called proximal and distal bulbar cushions by Rychter (24).

[2] According to Laane (10), using another nomenclature.

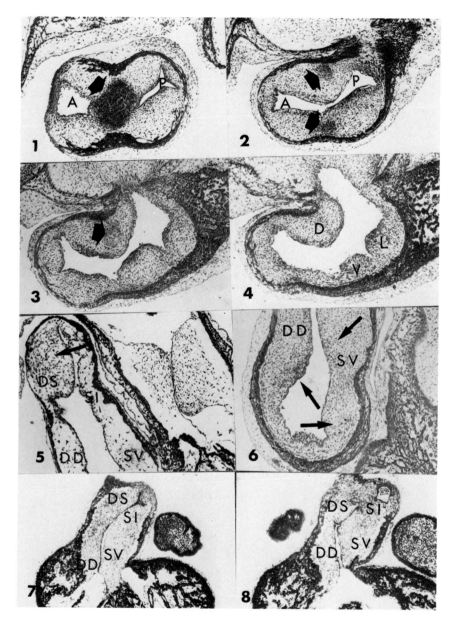

FIG. 2. Transverse sections (1,2,3,4) and sagittal sections (5,6) of chick embryonic heart at stage 25. Mesenchymal cell columns (†) are seen showing two limbs of aorticopulmonary septum. A = aorta; P = pulmonary artery; D = dorsal-right ridge; V = ventral ridge; L = dorsal left-ridge; DS = dextro-superior truncus swelling; SI = sinistro-inferior truncus swelling; DD = dextro-dorsal conal ridge; SV = sinistro-ventral conal ridge. Arrows indicate some dying cells. Fig. 2-7,8 show sagittal conotruncal ridges of rat 13 days after conception.

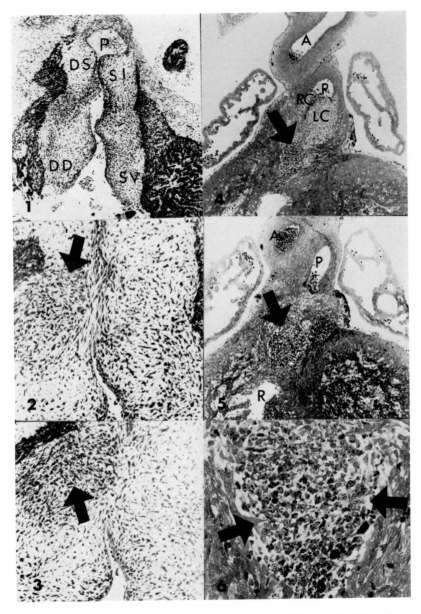

FIG. 3. Sagittal sections of chick embryonic heart at stage 28 (1) and 29 (2,3). In the conal septum some dying cells are seen (2,3) (↑). In rat heart at 15 days after conception (4,5,6), cell death focus (↑) is seen under the right (RC) and left cusps (LC) of the pulmonary valves. R = right ventricle.

Cell Death Foci in the Conal Ridges

The term "cell death" used in this study refers to cells that die spontaneously in a process which is called, with some ambiguity, physiological or spontaneous cell death. These cells die under normal conditions in healthy subjects as a result of normal genetic or epigenetic regulation (23). In rat embryonic heart, a cell death focus begins to appear 13 days after conception in the mesenchymal cells of the dextro-dorsal and the sinistro-ventral conal ridges. This focus gradually increases in size and becomes very dense 15 to 16 days after conception (Fig. 3-4—6,4-6), decreasing rapidly after 17 and 18 days (18,19,25). Cell death that occurs in the normal process of cardiac development is almost always found at the proximal part of the conal ridge under the presumptive pulmonary right and left semilunar valves (Fig. 3-4). This cell death focus appears and disappears in the same place and at the same stage of development, and its extent is almost always constant. It may be reasonable to assume that cell death focus in the conal ridge does not occur by chance, but is genetically or epigenetically programmed (18,19,25). In rat embryonic heart 13 days after conception, round or irregularly shaped amorphous materials, 2 to 3 μm in size, begin to appear in the cytoplasm of the mesenchymal cells of the conal ridges (Fig. 4-3,4). Most of these amorphous materials, which increase in size to 5 to 8 μm and in number with development, may develop into autophagic lysosomes and residual bodies that occupy the greater part of the cytoplasm (Fig. 4-6). Fifteen to 16 days after conception, many large vacuoles are observed in the cytoplasm, and cell lysis or rupture is also seen (Fig. 4-6). The nuclei are deformed by residual bodies, but no remarkable changes are observed in the nucleoplasm. Developing myocardial cells are visible around the cell death focus, especially adjacent to the pulmonic valve. This suggests gradual replacement by myocardial cells which invade the cell death focus from its circumference (Fig. 3-6). Serial sections of hearts from 14 to 16 days after conception reveal that the presumptive right and left semilunar valves of the pulmonary trunk are connected with the right and left conal ridges, respectively. Since cell death foci are seen at the proximal part of the right and left presumptive semilunar valves in the conal septum, the invading muscle cells may contact these two semilunar valves. The myocardial cells may therefore form the parietal portion of the definitive right ventricular cavity, while the pulmonary anterior semilunar valve, which originates from the pulmonary intercalated valve swelling, directly communicates with the myocardial cells of the right ventricle. These myocardial cells form the septal portion of the definitive heart in the right ventricular cavity (1,18,19,25). In chick embryonic heart on 4th day of incubation, cell death occurs in the left-proximal and the ventral-distal bulbar cushions (sinistro-ventral conal ridge and dextro-superior truncal swelling), as well as in the right-proximal and dorsal-distal bulbar cushions (dextro-dorsal conal ridge and sinistro-inferior truncal swelling) (21,22,23). Although many cell death foci are seen in chick embryonic heart, there are at this stage fewer dying cells in the foci

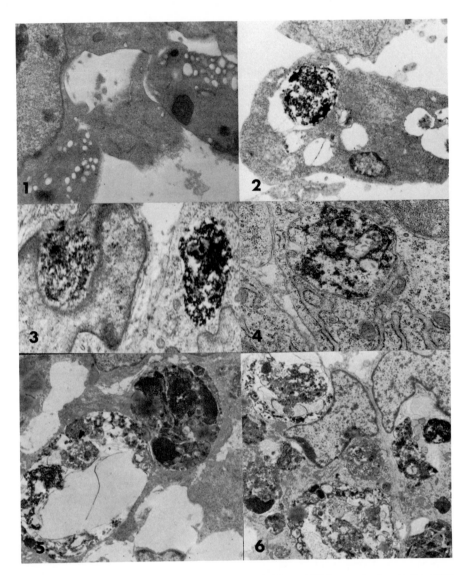

FIG. 4. Electron micrographs of dying cells in conal ridges. Initial vacuolization in the chick outflow tract on 3rd day of incubation (1,2). Amorphous materials in rat outflow tract 13 days after conception (3,4). Final phases of cell death in chick (5) and rat (6).

as compared to rat embryo. These cell death foci may have a net morphogenetic significance, although it would be an oversimplification to consider cell death as the sole active agent in heart morphogenesis (23). The most characteristic finding of the initial change of the dying cell in chick, in comparison with that of rat, is the earlier occurrence of vacuolization in the cytoplasm. The amorphous materials appear later. Formation of the vacuoles seems to be initiated in the Golgi region by the appearance of a single, smooth membrane-bound structure with a diameter of about 0.3 μm and no distinguishable contents (Fig. 4-1). Since osmotic pressure of the fixative solution is adjusted to that of the serum of the embryo, they do not represent fixation artifacts. These vacuoles later contain condensed cytoplasmic matrix (Fig. 4-2). Subsequently, the number of dying cells that contain vacuoles or amorphous or dense materials in the cytoplasm increases.

Quantification of Intracellular Organelles of Cell Death Foci

Quantitative analysis of such cell components as the nucleus, mitochondria, rough endoplasmic reticulum (R-ER), lipid droplets, dense bodies, amorphous material, and vacuoles was carried out to investigate the relationship between the intracellular organelles and the initial phases of physiological cell death. Rat embryonic conal ridge on 13, 13.5, and 14 days after conception and its homologue in the chick on 3rd, $3\frac{1}{3}$, and $3\frac{2}{3}$ day of incubation were studied. The cell components are represented as percentages of the whole cytoplasm. The dying cell is defined as the cell that contains some dense bodies, amorphous materials, and/or vacuoles. In each stage, about 30 to 40 electron micrographs were measured. The ratio of the organelles to cytoplasmic volume in rat embryo is similar to that of chick, except for dense bodies, amorphous materials, and vacuoles (Fig. 5). In rat, the ratio of amorphous material to cytoplasm is higher than that of dense bodies or vacuoles. In chick embryo, the ratio of dense and amorphous materials to cytoplasm is low, and the ratio of vacuoles is high (Fig. 5). In the final stages of cell death in bulbar cushion, the ratio of vacuoles and amorphous materials to the cytoplasm is high both in rat and chick embryos (Fig. 5). The difference in number and amount of cell death foci in the conal ridges may indicate that the mechanism of morphogenesis of the outflow tract of the right ventricle is different in the two species. The difference in ultrastructure of the initial stages of cell death in conal ridges in the chick and rat may also suggest some differences in genetic or epigenetic background of this phenomenon in the two species.[1]

CONCLUSIONS

Comparative study of rat and chick embryonic hearts was carried out to determine the relationship between cardiac morphogenesis and physiological cell death in the conal ridges. The results reveal that in rat embryonic heart, the cell death focus which is seen mostly in the conal septum may play an important role in formation of the right ventricular outflow tract. In chick

---

[1] The necessary prerequisite for further analysis must be the determination of corresponding developmental stages, to see if the 3rd day of incubation in chick is comparable with the 13th day after conception in rat.

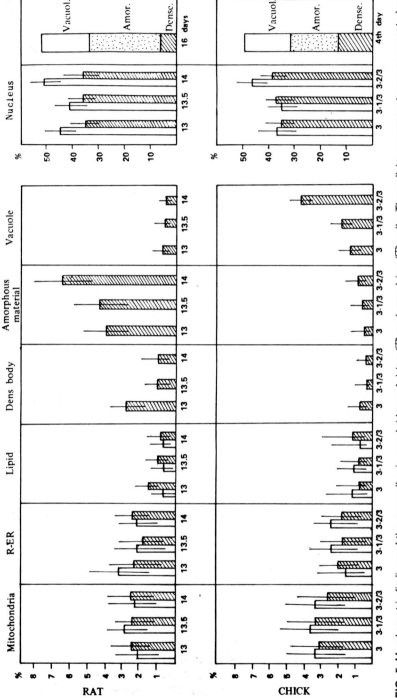

FIG. 5. Morphometric findings of the organelles in conal ridges of dying (▨) and non-dying (▥) cells. The cellular components are represented as percentages of the whole cytoplasm. The high ratio of amorphous materials in the rat and vacuoles in the chick is remarkable. The right side graphs show final phases of cell death indicating the ratio of vacuoles, amorphous, and dense materials. (Mean ± standard deviation).

embryo, cell death is less intensive than in rat. Observations of the initial stage of cell death shows that vacuolization appears as the first sign of cell death in chick, and that amorphous materials are visible in the case of rat. These results may suggest some differences in physiological cell death in the two species.

REFERENCES

1. Akimoto, N. (1979): Study on the septation of the truncus arteriosus and conus cordis. *Med. J. Hiroshima Univ.*, 27:103-129 (in Japanese with English abstract).
2. de la Cruz, M. V., Muñoz-Armas, S., and Muñoz-Castellanos, L. (1972): *Development of the Chick Heart.* Johns Hopkins University Press, Baltimore and London.
3. Ernst, M. (1926): Über Untergang von Zellen während der normalen Entwicklung bei Wirbel-tieren. *Z. Anat. Entwickl. Gesch.*, 79:228-262.
4. Hamburger, V., and Hamilton, H. L. (1951): A series of normal stages in the development of the chick embryo. *J. Morph.*, 88:49-92.
5. Hughes, A. F. W. (1948): The histogenesis of arteries in the chick embryo. *J. Anat.*, 77:266-287.
6. Ilies, A. (1967): La topographie et la dynamique des zones nécrotiques normales chez l'embryon humain. *Rev. Roum. Embryol. Cytol.*, 4:51-84.
7. Kramer, T. C. (1942): The partitioning of the truncus and conus and formation of the membra-nous portion of the interventricular septum in the human heart. *Am. J. Anat.*, 71:343-370.
8. Krstić, R., and Pexieder, T. (1973): Ultrastructure of cell death in bulbar cushions of chick embryo heart. *Z. Anat. Entwickl. Gesch.*, 140:337-350.
9. Laane, H. M. (1974): The nomenclature of the arterial pole of the embryonic heart II. Review of the literature from 1750-1890. *Acta. Morphol. Neerl.-Scand.*, 12:177-184.
10. Laane, H. M. (1978): The septation of the arterial pole of the heart in the chick embryo II. Development of the truncus arteriosus of the heart of chick embryos from 4 to 5 days of incubation. *Acta. Morphol. Neerl.-Scand.*, 16:29-53.
11. Langman, J., and Van Mierop, L. H. S. (1968): Development of the cardiovascular system. In: *Heart Disease in Infants, Children and Adolescents,* edited by A. J. Moss and F. H. Adams, pp. 3-25. Williams and Wilkins, Baltimore.
12. Los, J. A. (1968): Embryology. In: *Pediatric Cardiology,* edited by H. Watson, pp. 1-28. Lloyd-Luke, London.
13. Menkes, B., Alexandru, C., Pavkov, A., and Mircova, O. (1965): Researches on the formation and the elastic structure of the aortopulmonary septum in the chick embryo. *Rev. Roum. Embryol. Cytol.*, 2:79-91.
14. Menkes, B., Sandor, S., and Ilies, A. (1970): Cell death in teratogenesis. *Adv. Teratol.*, 4:170-215.
15. Netter, F. H., and Van Mierop, L. H. S. (1969): Embryology. In: *CIBA Collection of Medical Illustrations. Heart,* edited by F. H. Netter, pp. 115-130. Ciba Pharmaceutical Co., New Jersey.
16. Okamoto, N. (1969): Experimental production of congenital cardiovascular anomalies. *Cong. Anom.*, 9:45-59 (in Japanese with English abstract and literature).
17. Okamoto, N. (1969): Experimental production of congenital cardiovascular anomalies (con-cluded). *Cong. Anom.*, 9:117-132 (in Japanese with English abstract and literature).
18. Okamoto, N., and Satow, Y. (1975): Cell death in bulbar cushion of normal and abnormal developing heart. In: *Developmental and Physiological Correlates of Cardiac Muscle,* edited by M. Lieberman and T. Sano, pp. 51-65. Raven Press, New York.
19. Okamoto, N., Satow, Y., Hidaka, N., Akimoto, N., and Miyabara, S. (1978): Morphogenesis of congenital heart anomaly—Bulboventricular malformations, *Jpn. Circ. J.*, 42:1105-1120.
20. Okamoto, N. (1979): *Congenital Anomalies of the Arterial End of the Heart—Embryologic, Morphologic and Experimental Teratologic Consideration.* Igaku Shoin, Tokyo.
21. Pexieder, T. (1972): The tissue dynamics of heart morphogenesis. 1. The phenomena of cell death. A. Identification and morphology. *Z. Anat. Entwicklungsgesch.*, 137:270-284.
22. Pexieder, T. (1972): The tissue dynamics of heart morphogenesis. 1. The phenomena of cell death. B. Topography. *Z. Anat. Entwickl. Gesch.*, 138:241-253.
23. Pexieder, T. (1975): *Cell death in the morphogenesis and teratogenesis of the heart: Adv. anat. embryol. cell biol.* 53:1-100. Springer-Verlag, Berlin, Heidelberg, New York.

24. Rychter, Z. (1959): Vascular system of the chick embryo. III. To the problem of heart bulb and trunk septation in the chick embryo. *Čs. Morphol.,* 8:1-20.

25. Satow, Y., Okamoto, N., Hidaka, N., Akimoto, N., and Miyabara, S. (1978): Intracellular mechanism of teratogenesis of embryonic heart. In: *Morphogenesis and Malformation of the Cardiovascular System,* edited by G. C. Rosenquist and D. Bergsma, pp. 251-271. Alan R. Liss. Inc., New York.

26. Tandler, J. (1912): The development of the heart. In: *Manual of Embryology,* edited by K. Mall, pp. 534-570.

27. Van Mierop, L. H. S., Alley, R. D., Kausel, H. W., and Stranahan, A. (1963): Pathogenesis of transposition complexes. 1. Embryology of the ventricles and great arteries. *Am. J. Cardiol.,* 12:216-225.

28. Weibel, E. R. (1969): Stereological principles for morphometry in electron microscopic cytology. *Int. Rev. Cytol.,* 26:235-300.

DISCUSSION

Laane: Did I understand correctly that the truncus, in your interpretation, is that part of the outflow tract at which the semilunar valves will later be situated?

Pexieder: I am not very enthusiastic about discussing the terminology. I think, however, that we can agree that in the majority of embryonic hearts there are two structures (cushions or ridges) at the level of what you may call conus or bulbus or proximal bulbus. Then there are another two structures (cushions or ridges) at the level of what you may call truncus or distal bulbus. Finally, there are the two anlagen of the aorticopulmonary septum and their invasion in the proximal direction. I believe that if we can keep these structural principles in mind and translate the terminology the other people are using, we can understand each other. Unfortunately, there is at present no way to unify the terminology. Does it clarify your question?

Laane: No, because I do not understand the truncus nomenclature. I thought it was not the vascular part.

Pexieder: "Amsterdam's" truncus is everything which is not ventricle. Dr. Satow was confronted with our nomenclature of the chick embryonic heart in contrast to the rat nomenclature used in Hiroshima. This study reflects this controversial situation.

Oppenheimer-Dekker: Did you find any difference in the region of cushion fusion between the chick and the rat?

Satow: We did not study the fusion process; we limited our investigations to the cell death foci occurring in cono-truncal ridges.

Oppenheimer-Dekker: Dr. Pexieder warned in his introduction against use of the term "programmed cell death." Can you explain to me the reason for this warning?

Pexieder: With the advent of molecular biology and the discovery of the role of DNA, everything in embryology was conceived of as genetically programmed. I would like to stress that, generally speaking, some cells have the potential to die or to live. This potential is probably genetically programmed, but the actual decision that this or another particular cell will live or die may quite well be under the control of epigenetic factors.

De Haan: I think that when something is programmed, this implies that there is a certain amount of flexibility, whereas "determined" has a more rigid quality. I do not think that we know enough to speak about genetic programs.

Perspectives in Cardiovascular Research, Vol. 5,
Mechanisms of Cardiac Morphogenesis and Teratogenesis,
edited by Tomas Pexieder. Raven Press, New York © 1981

Role of Cell Death in Conal Ridges of Developing Human Heart

Naomasa Okamoto, Naotaka Akimoto, Yukio Satow, Nobuto Hidaka, and Shinichi Miyabara

Research Institute for Nuclear Medicine and Biology, Hiroshima University, Hiroshima, Japan

Embryological studies of the partitioning of the conotruncal and ventricular regions of the human embryonic heart have been reported by many investigators (2,4,15,18,19,27-29). However, understanding of the developmental process in the subpulmonary conus and aortic–mitral continuity (formation of the ventricular outflow tract) remains unsatisfactory.

Pexieder (21,22) has emphasized the importance of physiological cell death in the proximal left bulbar cushion, which is located in the vicinity of the bulboventricular ledge. He suggests that this localization of physiological cell death effects the regression of the bulboventricular ledge. Okamoto and his colleagues (17-19) stress the role of physiological cell death in the conal ridges during morphogenesis of the ventricular outflow tract of the heart in both normal and abnormal conditions. The relationship between physiological cell death and the invasion by muscle cells of the conal ridge of rat heart was described by Akimoto (1) and Sicking (23).

In the human embryo, the occurrence of physiological cell death in the pericardio-cardinal zone of embryos 8 to 10 mm crown–rump length was described by Ilies (10). Pexieder (21) has studied physiological cell death in human embryonic hearts of 4 to 14 mm crown–rump length, and discovered 16 foci of cell death in these hearts. He suggests that the intensity of cell death foci in human embryo is lower than that in chick or rat heart. Wendler (30), however, was unable to find such cell death foci in human embryos.

DEFINITION AND TERMINOLOGY

The term "cell death" as we use it here refers to the physiological or programmed cell death that occurs during normal embryogenesis. The time of appearance and disappearance of cell death foci parallels the most important stage of morphogenesis of the heart and great vessels. This type of cell death should be distinguished from necrosis in a pathological sense (17,19,21).

The first description of the foci of accumulations of cell nuclei located in the center of the dorsal ridge and an eccentric position of the ventral ridge in the conus of chick embryonic hearts was reported by Langer (14). The existence of sheets or areas of dense tissue in the condensing reticulum of the human embryonic heart at stage 18 is illustrated by Streeter (24, Fig. 3., p. 193). Krammer (13) also showed such condensed areas in conal ridges of a 13 mm human embryonic heart (Fig. 4A, B, p. 356). Judging from those figures showing the site and stage of appearance of sheets (areas) of condensed tissue in the conal ridges, it seems likely to us that these observations coincide with the description of cell death foci which will be discussed here.

Embryological studies of the role of cell death in the conal ridges and truncal swellings accompanying the formation of the muscle band of the outflow tract of the human embryonic heart and of abnormal hearts induced by experiment have recently been published (18,19). Details of the materials and methods are described in one of these reports (18). These specimens were recently restudied, and we can now discuss this phenomenon with some new information.

NORMAL DEVELOPMENT OF THE VENTRICULAR OUTFLOW TRACTS

Development of the Truncal and Conal Ridges

Externally, the truncus arteriosus and distal portion of the conus gradually become bulky as the result of growth of the two truncal swellings that appear facing each other on two sides in the truncal cavity. Great arteries become externally recognizable in embryos of stage 17. The aortic channel is located to the right of the pulmonary channel. With further development, the length of the great arteries increases and relative shortening of the conus cordis, accompanied by the descent of arterial valves, becomes apparent (Fig. 1A; Fig. 3A, B).

Internally, early in stages 11 to 14, the space between the endocardial layer and epimyocardial layer becomes filled with a gelatinous material, called cardiac jelly. This also happens in other segments of the cardiac tube (Fig. 4). The dextro-superior and sinistro-inferior truncal swellings are formed on the walls of the truncal lumen facing each other by subendothelial proliferation of mesenchymal cells. In stages 16 to 17, each of these swellings increases in volume asymmetrically, forming a large group of mesenchymal cells, and fusing.

The dextro-superior and sinistro-inferior truncal swellings are proximally aligned with the dextro-dorsal and sinistro-ventral conal ridges. These ridges twist at the site of the truncobulbar sulcus (Fig. 3A, A1, and B, B1). At stage 17, fusion of the conal ridges is not yet seen. After fusion of the truncal swellings and aorticopulmonary septum has been completed, both the aortic and pulmonary channels are formed. Part of the truncal mesenchymal tissue is differentiated into valvular tissue to form the right and left semilunar valves of the pulmonary artery and aorta. The mesenchymal primordia which are located opposite the

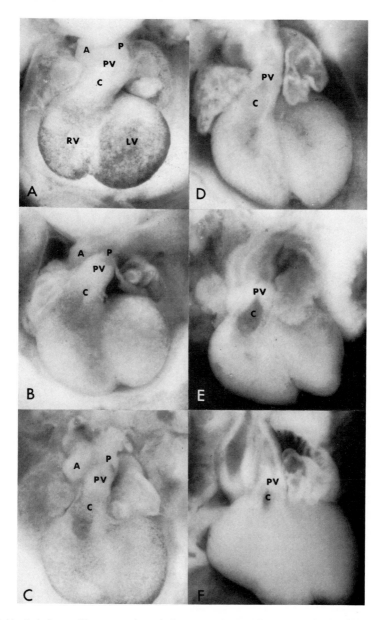

FIG. 1. Ventral views of human embryonic heart at stage 17 (A and B), 18 (C and D), 19 (E), and over 20 (F). **A:** Histologically (Fig. 3A, A1), septation of the truncus arteriosus and aortic sac is completed, but conal ridges are not yet fused. Note the bulky truncus arteriosus (X 21). **B:** Histologically (Fig. 3B, B1), septation of the truncus arteriosus and distal part of the conal ridges is completed and there is no fusion of the proximal parts of the conal ridges (x 21). **C:** The same heart as Fig. 5 (x 21). Septation of the conus is completed and cell death foci in the conal ridge are seen histologically (Fig. 5C, D, E and F) (x 18). **E:** Septation of the truncus arteriosus, the conus, and the ventricular septum is completed, and cell death foci have disappeared. Note the elongation of the aortic (A) and pulmonary channels (P), the downwards shift of the pulmonary valve (PV) with shortening of the conus (C), and the development of the right ventricle (RV) (x 18). LV: left ventricle. **F:** Heart at stage older than 20 (x 15).

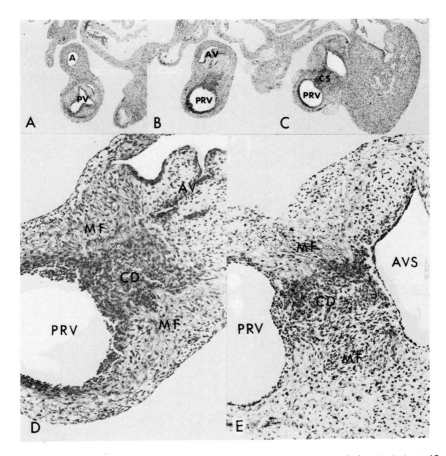

FIG. 2. Photomicrographs of the transverse sections of human embryonic heart at stage 18. **A:** Section at the level of the pulmonary semilunar valves (PV) (x 25). **B:** Section at the level of the aortic semilunar valves (AV) (x 25). **C:** Section at the level of the conus septum (CS) (x 25). **D:** High-power view of the same section as Fig. 2B showing invasion of muscle fibers (MF) into the cell death focus (CD). Note the site of the cell death focus directly facing the presumptive right ventricular cavity (PRV) (x 125). **E:** High-power view of the same section as Fig. 2C, showing the cell death focus and invasion of muscle fibers (x 125). A, aorta; AVS, aortic vestibulum; P, pulmonary artery.

fused truncal swellings, appear on the inner wall of the truncus to form both aortic and pulmonary channels. These form the non-coronary semilunar valve of the aorta and the anterior semilunar valve of the pulmonary artery. Neither of the semilunar valves is continuous with the conal ridge.

At the beginning of formation of arterial semilunar valves, the pulmonary semilunar valves are located distally and to the left of the aortic semilunar valves (Fig. 3A, A1 and B, B1). As involution of the conal septum proceeds, the former moves downwards to the presumptive right ventricle, which is formed by division of the primitive right ventricle. The latter becomes connected to

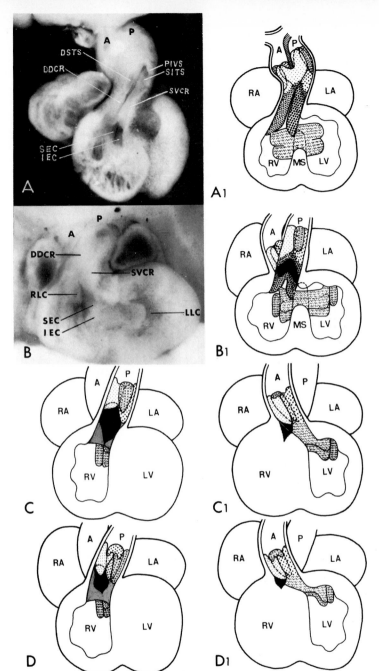

FIG. 3. Schematic diagrams showing development of the ventricular outflow tract. **A:** Internal view of the conus and right ventricle at stage 17. Note the non-fused conal ridges and fused bulky truncus swellings (x 24). **A1:** Schematic diagram of the same heart as **A. B:** Internal view of the conus and both ventricles at early stage 18. Note the non-fused proximal portion of the conal ridges (x 21). **B1:** Schematic diagram of the same stage of the heart as **B. C** and **C1:** The heart at stage 18 showing anterolateral (C) and posteromedial (C1) portions. Note the invasion of muscle fibers into the cell death focus. **D** and **D1:** The heart at early stage 19, showing anterolateral (D) and posteromedial (D1) portions.
▒▒▒, sinistroventral conal ridge (SVCR); ∷∷∷ , dextrodorsal conal ridge (DDCR); ⸪⸪⸪ , dextrosuperior truncal swelling (DSTS); ⸬⸬⸬ , sinistroinferior truncal swelling (SITS); ✕✕✕✕ , aortic (AIVS) and pulmonary (PIVS) intercalated valve swellings; ■■■ , cell death focus; ∿∿∿ , superior endocardial cushion (SEC); ≋≋≋ , inferior endocardial cushion (IEC); ⌇⌇⌇ , right (RLC) and left (LLC) lateral cushions; ▨▨▨ , aorticopulmonary septum; ▨▨▨ , muscle tissue of the right ventricle. A, aorta; P, pulmonary artery; RA and LA, right and left atrium; RV and LV, right and left ventricle; MS, muscular ventricular septum.

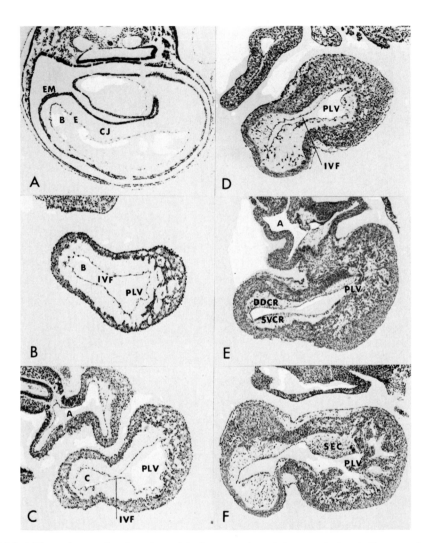

FIG. 4. Photomicrographs of sections of the human embryonic heart at the level of interventricular foramen. **A:** Heart at stage 11. Note the space between endocardium (E) and epimyocardium (EM) filled with cardiac jelly (x 120). **B:** Heart at stage 12. Increased thickness of myocardium (x 60). **C:** Heart at stage 13, showing beginning of colonization of cardiac jelly (CJ) by mesenchymal cells from endocardial epithelial side (x 60). **D:** Heart at stage 14. Note the increased number of mesenchymal cells in the cardiac jelly (x 60). **E:** Heart at stage 15. Sinistro-ventral (SVCR) and dextro-dorsal (DDCR) conal ridges are forming (x 40). **F:** Heart at stage 16. Superior endocardial cushion (SEC) can be seen (x 40). A, atrium; B, bulbus cordis; C, conus cordis; PLV, primitive left ventricle; IVF, interventricular foramen.

the primitive left ventricle through the aortic vestibulum (Fig. 3C, C1 and D, D1).

On the other hand, in stage 14, the conal ridges appear as a proliferation of mesenchymal cells at almost the same time as the truncal swellings. This is followed by rapid growth after the completion of the truncal septum (Fig. 4D, E). These are the sinistro-ventral and dextro-dorsal conal ridges. The former is connected with the sinistro-inferior truncal swelling via its distal end. Its proximal end connects with the inferior anterior edge of the bulboventricular foramen or the right anterior edge of the muscular portion of the interventricular septum (Fig. 3A, A1, B, B1, and C, C1; Fig. 4D, E, and F). The dextro-dorsal conal ridge is connected with the right side of the superior endocardial cushion and bulboventricular flange via its proximal end and with the dextro-superior truncal swelling via its distal end (Fig. 3A, A1 and B, B1; Fig. 4E, F). By the end of stage 16, the continuity between the sinistro-ventral conal ridge and subendocardial mesenchymal tissue of the left ventricle has disappeared (Fig. 4F; Fig. 5A). However, the continuity between the dextro-dorsal conal ridge and superior endocardial cushion remains until septation of the heart has been completed (Fig. 5B, C). From the end of stage 17 to the beginning of stage 18, both ridges fuse to form the conus septum, which is located at the superior part of the primitive right ventricular cavity. The posteromedial portion of the conus septum communicates with the proximal end of the right semilunar valve of the aorta, whereas the proximal end of the non-coronary and left semilunar cusps of the aorta is connected with the fused superior and inferior endocardial cushions through mesenchymal tissues (Fig. 3C1, D1; Fig. 5D, E, and F).

Involution of the Conus Septum

At about the beginning of fusion of the distal portions of the conal ridges (older members of stage 17), a focus of cell death appears in part of the mesenchymal cells of the dextro-dorsal conal ridge, followed by a similar process in the sinistro-ventral conal ridge. At the beginning of stage 18, cell death foci appearing independently on both ridges fuse to occupy the central area of the conus septum (Fig. 3C). Later, myocardial cells surrounding the foci of cell death invade each focus (Fig. 3D). At stages 19 and 20, the cell death zone gradually decreases in volume through progressive replacement by myocardial cells from the right ventricle. As the amount of muscle cells increases, the presumptive right ventricle, which was smaller than the left, grows rapidly. The left and right semilunar valve primordia of the pulmonary artery connect with the left and right conal ridges, so that the muscle fibers invading the cell death foci come into contact with pulmonary valves (Fig. 3B1, C, and D). These muscle fibers form the parietal portion of the right ventricular outflow tract. The anterior semilunar valve of the pulmonary artery communicates directly with the muscle cells of the right ventricle proper. These muscle fibers form the anterior or septal portion

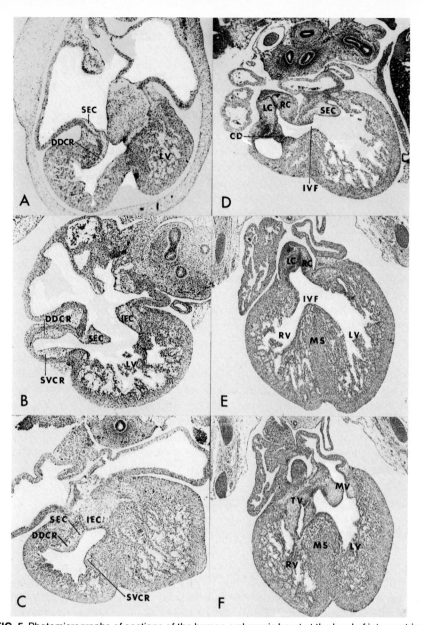

FIG. 5. Photomicrographs of sections of the human embryonic heart at the level of interventricular foramen. **A:** Heart at stage 16. The dextro-dorsal conal ridge (DDCR) is continuous with the superior endocardial cushion (SEC) via mesenchymal tissue (x 35). **B:** Heart at stage 17, showing the continuity of the dextro-dorsal conal ridge and the superior endocardial cushion tissue (x 25). **C:** Heart at early stage 18, showing the transition zone between the dextro-dorsal conal ridge and the superior endocardial cushion. The proximal portion of the conal ridges is not yet fused (x 25). **D** (the same heart as Fig. 1C): Heart at middle stage 18, showing cell death foci of the conal septum continuous with the right cusp of the aorta. The left cusp of the aorta is continuous with the right cusp of the aorta. The left cusp of the aorta is continuous with the superior endocardial cushion by way of fibrous tissue. Note the absence of cell death foci at the region beneath the left cusp of the aorta (x 25). **E** (the same heart as Fig. 1D): Heart at later stage 18, showing section at the level of aorta. Left cusp of the aorta (LC) is continuous with anterior leaflet of the mitral valve (MV, see Fig. 4F), (x 25). **F:** The same heart as **E,** showing the mitral and tricuspid valves (x 25). CD, cell death focus; AV, developing aortic valve leaflet; IVF, interventricular foramen II; RV, right ventricle; LV, left ventricle; SEC, superior endocardial cushion; IEC, inferior endocardial cushion; R(L)LC, right and left lateral cushion; TV, tricuspid valve; MV, mitral valve; MS, muscular ventricular septum.

of the right ventricular outflow tract. Consequently, the two muscle bundles grow in different directions.

The cell death zone is closely related to the right ventricular cavity through only one layer of endothelial cells (Fig. 2B, E). It is separated by many mesenchymal cells from the presumptive left ventricular cavity below the non-coronary and left semilunar valves of the aorta (Fig. 2C, E; Fig. 3C1, D1). The cell death focus on the pulmonary side is located beneath the pulmonary semilunar valves. On the aortic side it is only in slight contact with the lateral side of the aortic semilunar valve lying obliquely to the plane of the pulmonary valves (Fig. 2A, B; Fig. 5D). The cell death focus is continuous only with the proximal portion of the right semilunar valve of the aorta (Fig. 5E). Most of the invading muscle cells participate in formation of the muscle bundles of the right ventricular outflow tract. Only a small number of the invading muscle fibers take part in formation of the left ventricle. The high position of the pulmonary valves in normal adult heart may be explained by the localization of cell death focus.

The right semilunar valve of the aorta, on the other hand, is located somewhat inferior to those of the pulmonary artery, as the result of bending of the conotruncal region (Fig. 3A, A1 and B, B1). Since this infravalvular portion is located close to the cell death focus, muscle cells have invaded it to form muscle bundles. The left and non-coronary semilunar valves of the aorta are connected with the superior endocardial cushion via mesenchymal tissue; aortic–mitral continuity therefore is seen in the definitive heart.

Macroscopically, after the conus septum has been formed, muscle elements which grow from the right ventricle invade the conus (7,12,25,27). Recently, Asami (3) has demonstrated that the muscle elements of the right ventricle invade the bulbar cavity. Goor et al. (8) suggested that after formation of the septum membranaceum, the muscle elements that originated from the right ventricle invade the conus septum, especially the dextro-dorsal conal ridge, forming the characteristic morphology of the right ventricular outflow tract.

Migration of the Arterial Valves into the Ventricles

Orientation of the arterial semilunar valves changes during development. Before invasion of muscle cells into the conus septum, the aortic and pulmonary valve primordia are arranged side by side (Fig. 3A, A1). At the stage when semilunar valve primordia of the aorta and the pulmonary artery are being formed and cell death foci in the conal ridges are being replaced by muscle cells, the aortic valve becomes located vertically or somewhat obliquely and posterior to the pulmonary valve. The pulmonary valve primordia are then situated obliquely and to the left of the aortic valve primordia (Fig. 2A, B; Fig. 3B1). The aortic valve primordia are lying lower than that of the pulmonary artery. This situation might be brought about by the topographical relationships between the truncal swelling, the site of junction of the conus and truncus, and that of invasion of the muscle fibers into the conal ridges.

The shortening (absorption) of the conus which results in the migration of the conus septum towards the ventricle and aortic–mitral continuity has been described by many authors (2,3,5,8,11,18,20,26), but not all (6,9). With regard to the attenuation of the bulboventricular ledge, many investigators believe that this process leads to positioning of the aorta above the left ventricular cavity (2,6,16,20,25).

CONCLUSIONS

The hearts of human embryos ranging from Streeter's stage 11 to over stage 20 were studied. From the standpoint of differentiation, the truncal swellings are entirely distinct from the conal ridges. The truncal swellings differentiate into fibrous tissue to form the semilunar valves, while the conal ridges disappear and are replaced by muscle cells from the wall of the presumptive right ventricle. The final position of the arterial valves of the mature heart is due to the existence of cell death foci which are replaced by the muscle cells in the conal ridge during stages 17 to 18 (formation of subpulmonary conus) and to the persistence of the continuity between the dextro-dorsal conal ridge and superior endocardial cushion (aortic–mitral continuity).

REFERENCES

1. Akimoto, N. (1979): The study on the septation of the truncus arteriosus and conus cordis. *Hiroshima M. J.,* 27:103-129.
2. Anderson, R. H., Wilkinson, J. L., Arnold, R., and Lubkiewicz, K. (1974): Morphogenesis of bulboventricular malformations. I: Considerations of embryogenesis in the normal heart. *Brit. Heart J.,* 36:242-255.
3. Asami, I. (1969): Beitrag zur Entwicklung des Kammerseptums in menschlichen Herzen mit besonderer Berücksichtigung der sogenannten Bulbusdrehung. *Z. Anat. Entwickl. Gesch.,* 128:1-17.
4. Asami, I. (1978): Development of the heart. In: *Handbook of Internal Medicine, Circulation Disease Ia,* 30(A):3-38, Nakayama Shoten, Tokyo (Japanese).
5. Bersch, W. (1971): On the importance of the bulboauricular flange for the formal genesis of congenital heart defects with special regard to the ventricular septum defects. *Virchows Arch. Path. Anat.,* 354:252-267.
6. de la Cruz, M. V., and Da Rocha, J. P. (1956): An ontogenetic theory for the explanation of congenital malformations involving the truncus and conus. *Am. Heart J.,* 51:782-805.
7. Frazer, J. E. (1916): The formation of the pars membranacea septi. *J. Anat. Physiol.,* 51:19-29.
8. Goor, D. A., Dische, R., and Lillehei, C. W. (1972): The conotruncus. I. Its normal inversion and conus absorption. *Circulation,* 46:375-384.
9. Grant, R. P. (1962): The embryology of ventricular flow pathways in man. *Circulation,* 25:756-779.
10. Ilies, A. (1967): La topographie et la dynamique des zones nécrotiques normales chez l'embryon humain. *Rev. Roum. d'Embr. et Cyt., Séri. Embryol.,* 4:51-85.
11. Keith, A. (1909): The hunterian lectures on malformation of the heart. Lecture I. *Lancet,* 2:359-363.
12. Keith, A. (1924): Fate of the bulbus cordis in the human heart. *Lancet,* 20:1267-1273.
13. Kramer, T. C. (1942): The partitioning of the truncus and conus and the formation of the membranous portion of the interventricular septum in the human heart. *Am. J. Anat.,* 71:343-370.

14. Langer, A. (1894): Zur Entwicklungsgeschichte des Bulbus cordis bei Vögeln und Säugethieren. *Morph. Jb.,* 22:99-112.
15. Los, J. A. (1968): Embryology. In: *Paediatric Cardiology,* edited by H. Watson, pp. 1-28, Lloyd-Luke, London.
16. Moulaert, A. J., Bruins, C. C., and Oppenheimer-Dekker, A. (1976): Anomalies of the aortic arch and ventricular septal defects. *Circulation,* 53:1011-1015.
17. Okamoto, N., and Satow, Y. (1975): Cell death in bulbar cushion of normal and abnormal developing heart. In: *Developmental and Physiological Correlates of Cardiac Muscle,* edited by M. Lieberman and T. Sano, 1:51-65, Raven Press, New York.
18. Okamoto, N., Satow, Y., Hidaka, N., Akimoto, N., and Miyabara, S. (1978): Morphogenesis of congenital heart anomaly. Bulboventricular malformations. *Jap. Circulation J.,* 42:1105-1120.
19. Okamoto, N. (1980): *Congenital Anomalies of the Heart: Embryologic, Morphologic and Experimental Teratologic Considerations.* Igaku Shoin, Tokyo.
20. Pernkopf, E., und Wirtinger, W. (1933): Die Transposition der Herzostien—ein Versuch der Erklärung dieser Erscheinung. Die Phoronomie der Herzentwicklung als morphogenetische Grundlage der Erklärung. *Z. Anat. Etwickl.-Gesch.,* 100:563-711.
21. Pexieder, T. (1975): Cell death in the morphogenesis and teratogenesis of the heart. *Adv. Anat. Embryol. Cell Biol.,* 51:5-100, Springer-Verlag, Berlin.
22. Pexieder, T. (1978): Development of the outflow tract of the embryonic heart. In: *Morphogenesis and Malformation of the Cardiovascular System,* edited by G. C. Rosenquist and D. Bergsma, pp. 29-68. *Birth Defects:* Original Article Series 14 (7), The National Foundation, Alan R. Liss, Inc., New York.
23. Sicking: cited by Los, J. A. (1978): Cardiac septation and development of the aorta, pulmonary trunk, and pulmonary veins: Previous work in the light of recent observations. In: *Morphogenesis and Malformation of the Cardiovascular System,* edited by G. C. Rosenquist and D. Bergsma, pp. 127. *Birth Defects:* Original Article Series 14 (7), The National Foundation, Alan R. Liss, Inc., New York.
24. Streeter, G. L. (1958): Developmental horizons in human embryos. Description of age group XV, XVI, XVII, XVIII, being the third issue of a survey of the Carnegie Collection. *Contrib. Embryol.,* 32:113-203.
25. Tandler, J. (1912): The development of the heart. In: *Manual of Human Embryology,* edited by F. Keibel and E. P. Mall, pp. 534-570, 2. Lippincott, Philadelphia.
26. Thiene, G., Razzolini, B., and Della-Volta, S. (1976): Aorticopulmonary relationship, arterio-ventricular alignment, and ventricular septal defects in complete transposition of the great arteries. *Eur. J. Cardiol.,* 4:13-24.
27. Van Mierop, L. H. S., Alley, R. D., Kausel, H. W., and Stranahan, A. (1963): Pathogenesis of transposition complexes. I. Embryology of the ventricles and great arteries. *Am. J. Cardiol.,* 12:216-225.
28. Van Mierop, L. H. S. (1969): Section III: Embryology. In: *The Ciba Collection of Medical Illustrations, Volume V, Heart,* prepared by F. H. Netter and edited by F. H. Yonkman, pp. 112-130. Ciba Foundation, New York.
29. Van Mierop, L. H. S. (1974): Anatomy and embryology of the right ventricle. In: *The Heart,* edited by J. E. Edwards, M. Lev, and M. E. Abell, pp. 1-16. Williams & Wilkins, Baltimore.
30. Wendler, D. (1972): Der embryo-fetale Zelltod während der Normogenese und im Experiment. *Acta Historica Leopoldina,* 8:300, Leipzig., cited by 21.

DISCUSSION

De Vries: I have the same problem that Dr. Laane had. Where in the conus do these cells die? How do you define the conus in regard to the aortic and pulmonary truncus?

Los: In your diagram there was a continuity of distal ventral to distal dorsal truncus ridge and the upper atrioventricular cushion. Do you have histological evidence of this continuity?

Okamoto: Yes, I have.

Perspectives in Cardiovascular Research, Vol. 5,
Mechanisms of Cardiac Morphogenesis and Teratogenesis,
edited by Tomas Pexieder. Raven Press, New York © 1981

Formation of Foramina Secunda in the Chick

Dennis E. Morse

Department of Anatomy, Medical College of Ohio, Toledo, Ohio 43699

One of the unresolved questions regarding atrial septation concerns the mechanism involved in the formation of perforations in the septum primum that permit a right-to-left shunt of blood in the heart of the fetus. Collectively, these perforations are referred to as the foramen secundum. This system of perforations forms a vital bypass of the immature respiratory system, and its prenatal closure is incompatible with postnatal survival (13).

Heart development has been extensively studied in chick embryo, and the information thus gained forms the basis for much of our knowledge of cardiogenesis. In the chick, the foramen secundum is represented by multiple perforations (foramina) of varying sizes, each of which is bordered by thin endocardium-covered cords of tissue (3,5-8,11,12). Several theories have emerged with regard to formation of the foramina secunda. Chang (1) and Quiring (11) proposed that small focal areas of rupture develop as a result of increased pressure in the right atrium. Odgers' (7) work suggested that the foramen secundum is created as a result of incomplete growth of the various components of the septum primum. A third proposed contributing factor is programmed cell death, leading to a breakdown of precise regions of the septum (3,9).

Previous studies show that days 5 and 6 in chick embryo are the stages that best represent formation of foramina secunda (3,6). This study describes the ultrastructure of cell types found in the embryonic septum and defines some of their contributions to the formation of foramina secunda. The primary cell types to be considered are the endocardial cells, myocardial cells of the septal core, dead/dying cells, and associated phagocytes. Light and transmission electron microscopy were employed.

MATERIALS AND METHODS

Chick embryos of the White Leghorn strain were incubated to days 5 and 6 at constant temperature, humidity, and ventilation. Whole embryos were removed from the shell and immersed in cold aldehydes fixative buffered with 0.2 N cacodylate (4). Following staging according to the Hamilton–Hamburger series (2), the hearts were dissected free from the chicks and maintained in fixative for a minimum of one hour. Other techniques for preparing the tissue for electron microscopy were routine. Toluidine blue-stained thick sections of the epoxy-embedded tissue were used for orientation.

Whole embryos for light microscopy were immersion-fixed in ice-cold 80% ethanol:formalin (9:1). After staging and dissection, as above, the hearts were placed in vials of alcoholic formalin. These were maintained at 0°C for at least 24 hours. After fixation, the tissue was dehydrated (starting with 80% ethanol), cleared, and embedded in paraffin, according to routine procedures for light microscopy. Sectioned material was floated on 95% ethanol and mounted on glass slides. When dry, the sections were stained with Best's carmine stain for glycogen (10) and counterstained with Ehrlich's hematoxylin. Control slides were immersed in 5% diastase solution for 5 hours and washed for 15 minutes in running water before staining.

RESULTS

The atrial septum as it appears during day 6 of incubation is represented diagrammatically in Fig. 1. This drawing is based on scanning electron microscopic observations when viewed from the right atrial chamber. The foramen secundum complex is composed of several foramina of varying sizes. The smaller foramina tend to lie at the periphery of the complex. The entire system of foramina lies in the dorsal portion of the septum, and perforations were never observed to form in its ventral half. Each of the foramina is separated from adjacent ones by a thin endocardium-covered cord of septal tissue.

The atrial septum representing the period studied is shown in Fig. 2. This toluidine blue-stained light microscopic section is from the cranial portion of the septum, approaching the region of the foramen secundum. One interatrial communication exists in this field, and in several areas the septum is very thin. The endocardial cells of this region (future foramen secundum) are either flat and attenuated or notably rounded, and they project from the septal surface. The flat cells are typical of those found elsewhere on the atrial wall, whereas the rounded cells are concentrated in the regions of foramina formation. The projection of the rounded cells, together with what appear to be extensions of these cells into the septal core, tends to give the surface of the septum an irregular contour. The cells of the septal core are compact. Large areas of cytoplasm in these cells have very homogeneous staining characteristics.

FIG. 1. Diagrammatic representation of the right side of the atrial septum based on scanning electron microscopic evidence. The foramen secundum is represented by several perforations in the dorsal portion of the septum. Most of the foramina form between 4 and 8 days of incubation.

FIG. 2. A one-micrometer section through the portion of the atrial septum immediately cranial to the region of the foramen secundum. Note the presence of numerous rounded endocardial cells *(dot)* and endocardial cells extending processes into the septum *(arrows)*. The communication between the right (RA) and left (LA) atria represents one of the foramina (× 180).

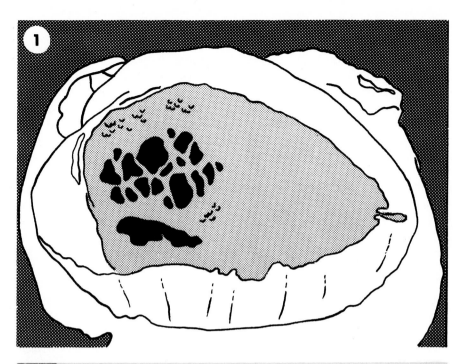

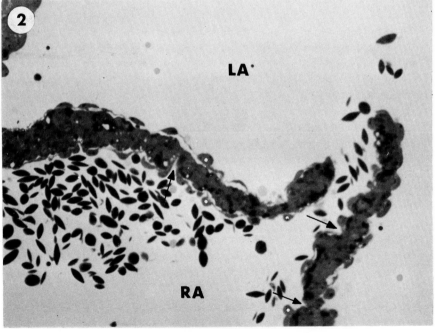

The structure of the cords of tissue that border individual foramina can be studied when the plane of section passes through the septum at the level of the foramina secunda (Figure 3). Numerous rounded endocardial cells are present. The structure of the core of each cord resembles that of the intact portion of the septum. The diameter of the cords is highly variable.

Rounded cells exist on both the right and left sides of the septum. Transmission electron microscopy of the developing foramen secundum region shows that the rounded cells possess multilobed nuclei, abundant Golgi zones, lipid droplets, and debris-filled vesicles. These cells also extend cytoplasmic processes toward the septal core (Fig. 4 and 5). The myocytes of the cord are separated as these processes traverse the thickness of the septum. At numerous points, the septum becomes very thin, and the endocardial cells of the two sides are separated by the cytoplasm of one myocyte (Fig. 6 and 7). Transseptal communication is eventually established by the cell processes. Separation of parallel, adjacent transseptal processes create new foramina secunda.

Subdivision of the septal tissue by the endocardial cells creates islands of endocardium-covered septal tissue (Figures 8 and 9). These islands represent the cords that separate the foramina at the light and scanning electron microscopic levels of observation (Fig. 1-3). Further subdivision of the cords is commonly seen (Figure 8). The mechanism is the same as that described above. The smaller cords created by this mechanism consist of one or two endocardial cells surrounding one to three myocytes (Fig. 9).

A well-defined subendocardial tissue space is commonly present. Cells are rarely found in this zone between the basal laminae of the endocardium and myocytes. Focal areas of fine extracellular connective tissue fibrils are characteristic (Fig. 4-9).

The cells of the core of the septum in the area studied all contain myofilaments which tend to have a random arrangement in the cytoplasm. Most characteristic of these cells in the electron micrograph is the presence of large areas of cytoplasm that appear void of organelles. These portions of the cytoplasm typically lie nearest the endocardium (Fig. 4-9). Best's carmine staining of paraffin-embedded sections reveals that these areas represent large depots of glycogen. Although the glycogen can be demonstrated throughout the atrial wall, its concentration is significantly higher in the septum (Fig. 10). This glycogen is apparently extracted during our electron microscopic preparations. Infrequently, the myocar-

FIG. 3. A one-micrometer section through the foramen secundum area. Numerous cords (C) border the foramina. There are many rounded endocardial cells *(dots)*. The core of each cord contains very little intercellular space, and many of the cells contain large areas of homogeneously staining cytoplasm ($\times$ 500).

FIG. 4. In thin section, the rounded endocardial cells (R) contain well-formed Golgi zones (G), lipid droplets (L), and other organelles characteristic of metabolically active cells. These cells extend processes (P) into the septal core. The myocytes (M) of the septal core are separated by invading rounded cell process ($\times$ 6,000).

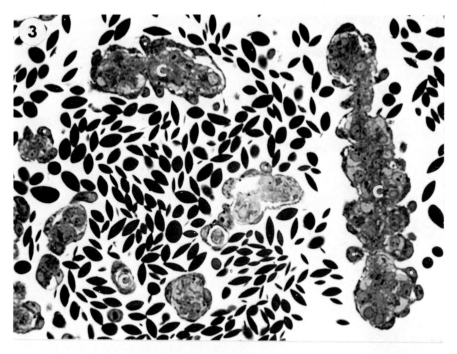

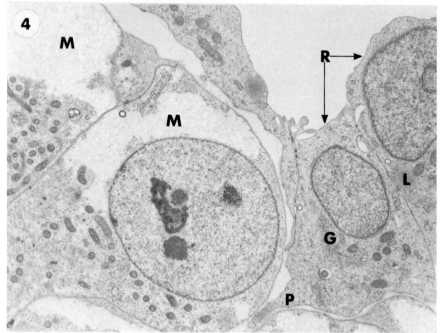

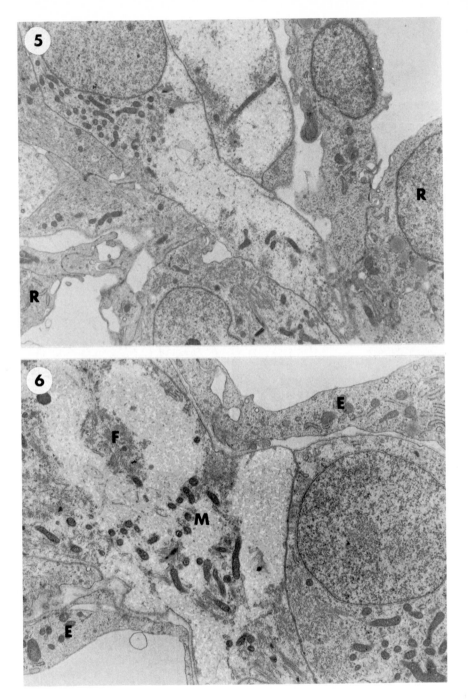

dial cells display evidence of degenerative phenomena in the form of debris-laden inclusions.

An additional cell type found in the region of the developing foramen secundum complex is the phagocytic cell of the septal core. These cells, although seldom observed, are conspicuous because of their large size and the abundance of cellular debris in various stages of degradation. Free, dead cells are rarely seen.

DISCUSSION

Precision in timing is of critical importance in formation of the atrial septal complex. As the septum approaches the endocardial cushions, the interatrial communication at the septum's lower edge (foramen primum) narrows. Fusion of the septum and cushions occludes this opening, making it necessary for blood entering the heart to be diverted away from the lungs by other means. Thus, as occlusion of foramen primum occurs, new interatrial communications form in the mid-dorsal portion of the septum. These are multiple in the chick, and are designated the foramina secunda. They first appear on day 4, and increase in number and size during the remainder of the first week of incubation (3,6).

Hendrix and Morse (3) demonstrated by scanning electron microscopy that the endocardium remains intact during formation of individual foramina. This observation suggests that the cells of the endocardium might be an important factor in foramina formation. Further support is given to this possibility by the fact that a conspicuous, rounded endocardial cell can be demonstrated at the time of foramen development.

The present report demonstrates in thin sections that the rounded endocardial cells possess characteristics of phagocytes (multilobed nuclei, lysosomal elements, lipid droplets). More important, these rounded cells extend cytoplasmic processes into the septum and probably serve to separate the cells of the septal core. The processes establish transseptal communication, and parallel processes separate to create new foramina. The effect is twofold: (1) the septum is subdivided to allow for development of additional foramina secunda; and (2) endocardial integrity is maintained.

The cells of the septal core all possess characteristics of myocytes. In addition, these cells contain amounts of glycogen exceeding that of other cells of the atrium. Although cell junctions between these cells are common, they appear

---

FIG. 5. The entire thickness of the atrial septum is shown in this field. The endocardial layers each contain rounded cells (R). The myocytes of the septal core contain large areas of cytoplasm which appear devoid of organelles (glycogen). The atrial chambers are at the extreme upper right and lower left of this field (× 4,500).

FIG. 6. In some instances, the thickness of the septum in the zone of foramina formation is restricted to the two endocardial cell layers (E) and one myocyte. Myofilaments (F) are dispersed among collections of glycogen (× 8,000).

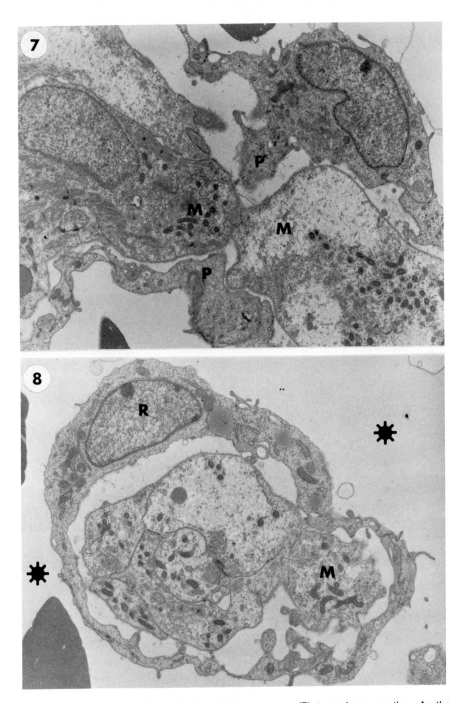

FIG. 7. Opposing endocardial cells direct their processes (P) toward one another. As the processes advance into the septum, the myocytes (M) of the septal core are separated. The atrial cavities are at the upper right and lower left (× 4,800).

FIG. 8. Subdivision of the septal tissue by the rounded endocardial cells (R) creates delicate cords of tissue which form the boundaries for the foramina secunda (*). Here a myocyte (M) is being separated from adjacent ones (× 6,000).

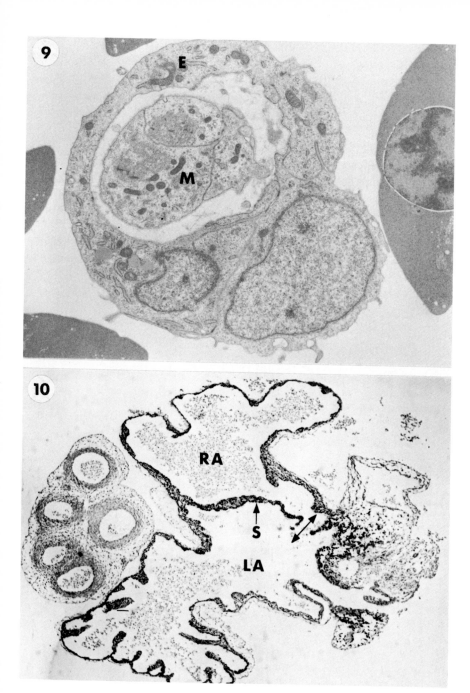

FIG. 9. The cords between foramina secunda may become quite small as illustrated in this field (compare cord with red blood cell at the right). These smaller cords are composed of one or two endocardial cells (E) surrounding one or more myocytes (M). A distinct subendocardial connective tissue space containing extracellular fibrils and interstitial bodies is present (× 6,000).

FIG. 10. Paraffin section of the right (RA) and left (LA) atria and their septum (S) (Best's carmine, Ehrlich's hematoxylin). There is intense staining of the cells of the septal core. Atrial walls are much less positive for glycogen. The aortic arches show no evidence of the stain. The dual-headed arrow traverses a foramen secundum (× 60).

to offer little resistance to the invading endocardial cell processes. The relationship of the cells of the septal core to the invading endocardium in the region of foramina secunda formation requires further morphological and biochemical analysis.

Free or phagocytized dead cells, and cells demonstrating clear-cut signs of irreversible degeneration, are uncommon in the area of the atrial septum that supports foramina formation. Their rarity indicates that they probably do not play a major role in foramina formation.

In summary, this study indicates that the rounded cells of the endocardium in the region of foramina secunda formation are the major cellular element involved in establishment of interatrial perforations. Programmed cell degeneration appears to play a minimal role in this process. Further studies concerning the mechanisms involved in stimulating the endocardial cell processes to invade the septal core are the emphasis of our ongoing studies.

REFERENCES

1. Chang, C. (1931): The formation of the interatrial septum in chick embryos. *Anat. Rec.,* 50: 9-22.
2. Hamilton, H. H. (1952): *Lillie's Development of the Chick,* 3rd. ed. Holt, Rinehart, and Winston, New York.
3. Hendrix, M. J. C., and Morse, D. E. (1977): Atrial septation. I. Scanning electron microscopy in the chick. *Dev. Biol.,* 57:345-363.
4. Karnovsky, M. J. (1965): A formaldehyde–glutaraldehyde fixative of high osmolality for use in electron microscopy. *J. Cell Biol.,* 27:137a-138a.
5. Los, J. A. (1971-72): The heart of the 5-day chick embryo during dilation and contraction. *Acta Morphol. Neerl. Scand.,* 9:309-335.
6. Morse, D. E. (1978): Scanning electron microscopy of the developing septa in the chick heart. *Birth Defects:* Original Article Series, XIV:91-107.
7. Odgers, P. N. B. (1935): The formation of the venous valves, the foramen secundum and the septum secundum in the human heart. *J. Anat.,* 69:412-422.
8. Patten, B. M. (1925): The interatrial septum of the chick heart. *Anat. Rec.,* 30:53-60.
9. Pexieder, T. (1975): Cell death in the morphogenesis and teratogenesis of the heart. *Adv. Anat. Embryol. Cell Biol.,* 51:11-100.
10. Preece, A. (1972): *A Manual for Histologic Technicians,* 3rd ed. Little, Brown and Company, Boston.
11. Quiring, D. P. (1933): The development of the sino-atrial region of the chick heart. *J. Morphol.,* 55:81-118.
12. Romanoff, A. L. (1960): *The Avian Embryo.* McMillan Company, London.
13. Wilson, J. G., Lyon, R. A., and Terry, R. (1953): Prenatal closure of the interatrial foramen. *Am. J. Dis. Child.,* 85:285-294.

DISCUSSION

Manasek: I would like to confirm that you can do very specific PAS staining on thick plastic sections. The finding that endocardial cells may be invasive is extraordinarily important; I have seen similar behavior in the embryonic ventricle. The myocardial cells have just been junction-separated, permitting ingrowth of the endocardium. There might be less complex reasons for the cell bulging, such as myocardial contraction.

Morse: Our choice of Best's carmine for glycogen staining was based on the same reservations concerning PAS specificity as were raised in the discussion of Dr. Bogenmann's paper. I am not quite sure that the rounding of cells is due to muscle contraction, because the mural endocardial cells of the atria are flattened.

De Vries: Are these small rounded cells endothelial cells?

Morse: We do not know the origin of those cells, but they most probably become rounded *in situ.*

Pexieder: The problem can be solved by a simple experiment. You can microdissect the atrial septum as we did with Dr. Rychter, impose an external stretching upon it, and see whether or not there will be a change in the number of rounded cells.

Dor: What do you find in the space between an endothelial cell and the enclosed myocyte?

Morse: We usually find cardiac jelly.

Fischman: Do you presume that these endothelial cells are subdividing muscle strands? What is the subsequent fate of the muscle strand if there is no phagocytosis?

Morse: That is a major question for us, because there is a decrease in the number of muscle cells in this area. Only 8 to 9 days after hatching do those thinned cords separating the foramina increase in size.

Los: Can we conclude that fusion and detachment of endothelial cells are reversible processes?

Morse: I do not think my evidence will support that.

Hurle: Did you find different amounts of microfilaments in the endocardial cells in the area of hole formation?

Morse: There seem to be more filaments in the rounded cells, particularly where they extend into the anchoring atrial septum.

Hurle: Can the rounded shape and the formation of foramina secunda be explained in terms of the blood flow in the atria?

Morse: We do not deny that there is an indirect hemodynamic effect here, as well as an effect caused by the dying cells. But it is not simply one phenomenon.

Clark: What happens to these cells when the foramina close after hatching?

Morse: They disappear long before that.

Fischman: Do you see any evidence that the muscle strands fixed at one end might be pulled by the contraction of the myocytes into the base of the strand?

Morse: No, we have not, but that would be a good mechanism for separation and creation of the foramina.

Markwald: The glycogen accumulation in the myocytes adjacent to the invaginating cells makes them look like nodal cells. Do you see anything that might turn cells into invasive types, such as a unique matrix property?

Morse: We do not find concentrations of glycogen in other atrial myocytes. The glycogen concentration body is always oriented against the endocardium. We have found only nicely formed collagen fibrils associated with these rounded cells. We have also frequently seen the interstitial bodies of Low in the subendocardial space in areas of foramina formation.

Perspectives in Cardiovascular Research, Vol. 5,
Mechanisms of Cardiac Morphogenesis and Teratogenesis,
edited by Tomas Pexieder. Raven Press, New York © 1981

Some Early Effects of Retinoic Acid on the Young Hamster Heart

I. M. Taylor

Department of Anatomy, University of Toronto, Toronto, M5S 1A8, Ontario, Canada

Pexieder (12) has pointed out that morphogenesis and teratogenesis of the heart are both multiparametric processes, of which the principal components are the proliferation of cells, the death of cells, cell population dynamics, and the secretion of glycosaminoglycans. All of these can be affected by vitamin A and related compounds, such as retinoic acid (18). In his monograph (12), Pexieder has summarized his earlier work (10,11) concerning the role of physiological cell death in the genesis of both normal and abnormal hearts. He has concluded that the most important and interesting foci of death are situated in the bulbar and atrioventricular cushions and in the aorticopulmonary septum. After experimental study of chick heart, he suggested that the prenecrotic cells found in the bulbar cushions represent a common target for the action of biophysical as well as chemical teratogens. Since then, Okamoto and Satow (7,8, 9,14,15) have described a focus of cell death in the conus ridge of normal embryonic rat heart and have demonstrated changes in the stage, size, and site of its appearance after whole-body neutron irradiation.

Retinoic acid has now been shown to have a profound effect on the developing hamster heart, since no less than 74% of fetuses surviving to term after exposure on day 8 of gestation have cardiac malformations (17,18). Of these 87% have a bulboventricular abnormality, such as double-outlet right ventricle (62%), classical transposition of the great vessels (14%), or an overriding aorta complex (11%).

Ultrastructural examination of treated hearts at intervals after exposure reveals the expected damage to cushion material in older specimens. However, it is remarkable that early death in day 8 treated embryos is observed predominantly in developing myocytes, rather than in the relatively undifferentiated mesenchymal cells which will form the cushions on day 9. This paper will therefore report the effects of retinoic acid on developing hamster heart prior to formation of the bulbar cushions.

MATERIALS AND METHODS

Golden Syrian hamsters of approximately 110 gm, obtained from Trenton Experimental Laboratory, were mated from 7 to 9 P.M. The following day was designated as day 0 of gestation. Mated animals were kept singly in wire cages at ambient temperature in a room with controlled light and dark periods of 12 hours each. Purina Lab Chow and tap water were provided *ad libitum.*

Twenty-seven mated animals were divided into three equal groups: untreated controls, corn-oil controls which received a single dose of a corn-oil vehicle, and retinoic acid-treated animals which received a single dose of retinoic acid suspended in corn oil. All applications were by gavage, and each animal received only a single treatment at the beginning of day 8. A dose of 80 mg of retinoic acid per kg maternal body weight was given.

The females were killed by prolonged chloroform anesthesia 5, 10, and 15 hours after treatment, and the uterine contents examined. Dead fetuses were excluded and the survivors fixed in formol saline. Following examination of the surface features of the heart, each embryo was photographed intact in ventral and right and left lateral views, in order to assess the size, relations, and shape of the heart.

The hearts from offspring of similar groups of animals were also examined by electron microscopy. They were obtained 2, 4, 6, 8, 12, 16, 18, or 24 hours after maternal treatment; only those hearts that were beating were processed. All specimens were fixed for 1 hour in cold 2% paraformaldehyde and 2% glutaraldehyde in 0.1 M phosphate buffer at pH 7.4. After postfixation in 1% osmium tetroxide, they were dehydrated in alcohol and embedded in Epon 812. Thin sections were stained with lead citrate and uranyl acetate and examined in a Philips 300 electron microscope.

RESULTS

The morphologic findings of Boyer (2) were confirmed for the period examined, and are summarized for day 8 of gestation.

Eight days after conception, the heart is a tube which normally bends towards the right (D-loop). The atrial and ventricular regions are clearly discernable while the endocardium and epimyocardium are widely separated. At 8.25 days, constrictions appear in the wall of the heart tube, which is thus delineated into sinus, atrial, ventricular, and bulbar regions. The heart is growing rapidly. By 8.5 days of gestation it bulges both ventrally and laterally so that it is about half again as wide as the trunk of the embryo. The bulboventricular sulcus forms at the site of the bend between the bulbus and the primitive ventricle, and trabeculae appear in parts of the walls of these two chambers. The truncus has not yet divided, but remains connected only to the bulbus.

The heart is still essentially a coiled tube by 9 days, and the atrial portion is its largest single part. However, the embryo has been growing more rapidly, so the heart no longer bulges laterally to any great extent, although its ventral prominence is still marked. The atrium is much thinner-walled than the ventricle, which by now possesses prominent trabeculae. It should be noted that the atrioventricular cushions are not large until day 9.5 and that the bulbar ridges make their appearance on day 10.

In the treated embryos, retarded growth of both the heart and embryo is constantly found 10 and 15 hours after administration of retinoic acid. Only a minority of treated hearts are clearly different in general shape from control specimens by 5 hours. More pronounced difference is always seen at 10 hours. In treated embryos, the heart tubes are nearly all D-looped, although a very few have anterior loops. Among the D-loops, a spectrum of types can be distinguished, determined by the position of the loop with respect to the coronal plane. It is noteworthy that no L-loop configurations have been seen in either controls, treated controls, or treated specimens. Both the untreated and treated control heart loops are nearly always found in the coronal plane, and very little variation is seen within those two groups.

To get some idea of the changes in the shape of the heart and the differences in length between various parts of treated and control hearts, the lengths of the atrium (AL), primitive ventricle (PV) and proximal bulbus (PB) were measured from the photographs. In addition, the outside width of the atrioventricular canal (AVC) was assessed, together with measurement of the angle made by a long axis bisecting the distal bulbus and truncus with the transverse plane. The angular measurement was made on ventral views of the embryo heart, but no correction was applied to compensate for any sloping of the bulbo-truncal axis with respect to the long axis of the embryo. All the photographic work was performed at a constant magnification, and the lengths recorded are in arbitrary units. No allowance was made for overall differences in embryo size between treated and control litters. Since no significant differences were found between the control and treated control series, they are classed together. A total of 30 hearts was measured for each of the 6 groups identified in Table 1. Very small or grossly atypical hearts were excluded from the study.

The calculated variances for retinoic acid-treated animals were always larger (in some cases as much as two-fold) than the controls. This indicates the increased variability found within the treated group of hearts, as compared to the control series. Earlier work (18) has shown that some of the hearts exposed to retinoic acid during the critical period of cardiac organogenesis will still be normal at term; this may be a reflection of the variability noted at this earlier stage of development.

An analysis of the differences between the means for each group of measurement was performed using small smaple size t-tests (Table 2). It can be seen that the overall size of the heart is decreased 10 hours after retinoic acid administration. More important, however, this treatment leads to a change in the relative proportional growth of the different parts of the heart. Hence, the overall shape of the organ, and particularly the bulboventricular loop, is markedly altered.

There are striking changes in the ultrastructural appearance of cells in the atrioventricular, ventricular, and bulbar myocardium. However, only minor effects, such as cell budding, have been observed in cells of the endocardium.

Two hours after administration of the drug to the mother, there may already be abnormal findings in both the myocardial and mesenchymal cells of fetuses. However, swelling of the plasma membrane associated with budding of cells,

TABLE 1. Range, mean, and variance of measurements[a] of various parts of the fetal hamster heart after administration of corn-oil vehicle (CO) or retinoic acid (RA) at the beginning of day 8 of gestation.

Day 8 + 5 hours

	CO			RA		
	Range	Mean	Variance	Range	Mean	Variance
AL	0.8	1.69	0.0598	0.7	1.71	0.0507
PV	0.9	2.07	0.0562	1.1	2.01	0.0785
PB	0.8	1.30	0.0387	0.8	1.33	0.0656
AVC	0.4	1.06	0.0101	0.5	1.09	0.0218
Angle[b]	19.0	29.06	27.0588	26.0	25.54	58.6230

Day 8 + 10 hours

	CO			RA		
	Range	Mean	Variance	Range	Mean	Variance
AL	0.8	1.92	0.0618	0.9	1.88	0.0556
PV	1.0	2.40	0.0775	0.8	2.17	0.0370
PB	1.1	1.65	0.1183	0.9	1.48	0.1200
AVC	0.6	1.36	0.0234	0.5	1.11	0.0153
Angle[b]	14.0	21.13	18.6850	29.0	24.20	49.7200

Day 8 + 14 hours

	CO			RA		
	Range	Mean	Variance	Range	Mean	Variance
AL	0.6	1.88	0.0389	0.6	2.09	0.0354
PV	0.8	2.37	0.0458	0.8	2.47	0.0837
PB	0.8	1.89	0.0678	1.1	1.71	0.1157
AVC	0.7	1.35	0.0226	0.5	1.22	0.0279
Angle[b]	15.0	25.38	17.9480	17.0	28.33	31.5150

Abbreviations for Tables 1 and 2: AL, atrial length; PV, length of primitive ventricle; PB, length of proximal bulbus; AVC, outer width of atrioventricular canal; Angle, angle between distal bulbus and truncus and the proximal bulbus and primitive ventricle.
[a] length in arbitrary units
[b] degrees

TABLE 2. *Mean differences between measurements on various parts of control and treated fetal hamster hearts at five-hour intervals after administration of compounds on day 8 of gestation.*

TIME	8 days, 5 hours	8 days, 10 hours	8 days, 15 hours
AL	0.2250	0.5398	3.0770*
PV	0.7160	3.4090*	1.2670
PB	0.0272	1.6680*	1.8500*
AVC	0.1276	5.8750*	3.4200*
Angle	1.6507*	1.7700*	1.7100*

* Significant difference if $t_{.05} > 1.645$

dilation of the rough endoplasmic reticulum, and accumulation of lipid droplets are the most obvious signs during the first 6 hours. Areas appear in which cytoplasmic organization is lost, accompanied by both intracellular and extracellular vesicles containing flocculent material (Figs. 1–3). There is also increasing separation of cells, and an apparent enlargement of the extracellular space.

After 12 to 24 hours, dying and dead myocardial cells are a prominent feature

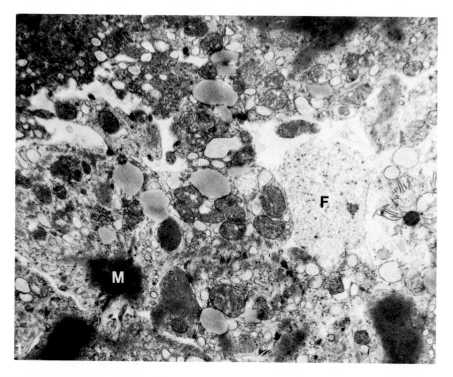

FIG. 1. Six hours after administration of retinoic acid on day 8, the myocytes in the atrioventricular canal region show obvious damage. Cell membranes are indistinct and there is flocculent material (F) in the intercellular space. The myofibrils (M) are becoming amorphous, and numerous vesicles and fat vacuoles are seen ($\times$ 9,000).

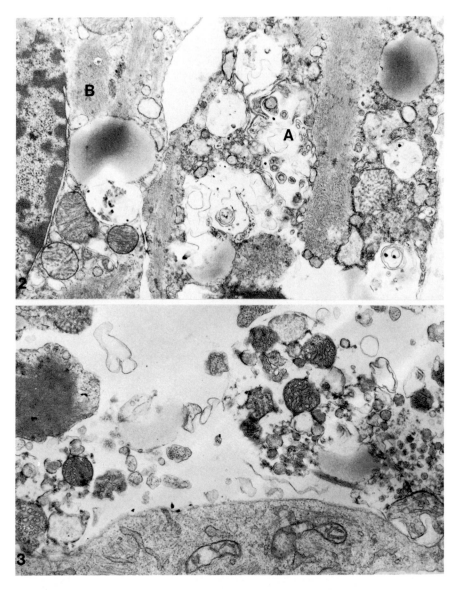

FIG. 2. Portions of 2 cells from the primitive ventricle 8 hours after treatment. The breakdown of organization in cell A is advanced. Nuclear chromatin is beginning to condense in cell B (× 16,188).

FIG. 3. Between 8 and 12 hours after giving retinoic acid, the intercellular spaces are full of cell debris, some of which is quite recognizable (× 16,188).

of the atrioventricular canal, the ventricular, and the bulboventricular region. Although such cells are also found under normal conditions, it should be emphasized that retinoic acid-treated hearts exhibited a much higher incidence of deaths than control specimens in any part of the heart that has been examined so far. Myocardial cells lose their polyribosomes, develop nuclear membrane irregularities, and fragment (Figs. 2–4). Their nuclei become abnormal. Most appear very pale; others become pyknotic and are then extruded. Such dead and dying cells can be found in groups throughout the myocardium, but they are especially noticeable in the atrioventricular canal and primitive ventricle. Similarly, some mesenchymal cells lose their ground cytoplasm, develop swollen or condensed mitochondria, and die.

In specimens 12 to 24 hours after maternal retinoic acid administration, it can be seen that portions of degenerating cells have been phagocytosed by healthy neighboring myocardial and mesenchymal cells. By 24 hours, many of the dead cells have been removed, and no traces remain in some areas except for the phagocytotic vacuoles (Fig. 5).

The retinoic acid-treated hearts seem to lag about 6 to 12 hours behind control hearts in terms of both their general appearance and their myofibrillar development. However, 24 hours after treatment, the vast majority of cells display profuse glycogen deposits, as well as the abundant rough endoplasmic reticulum that is typically found in the fetal heart.

DISCUSSION

It has previously been shown (17,18) that retinoic acid is a potent cardiac teratogen in hamsters. Although only 74.4% of the total live fetuses that are treated on day 8 can be shown on day 14 to have abnormal hearts, this incidence is higher than the frequencies observed following the use of many other chemical teratogens. Furthermore, 87% of those live animals in which abnormalities can be demonstrated possess some sort of bulboventricular malformation. These malformations include double-outlet right ventricle and transposition, which are found in 62% and 14% respectively, the remaining 11% consisting of the overriding aorta complex.

At present, there is a lack of agreement concerning the pathogenesis of bulboventricular malformations, although they are no longer considered to represent simple arrests of development at different stages. Rather, they are believed by many to be caused by maldevelopment of the conus, reflecting different combinations of excessive, normal, or reduced conal rotation and absorption, and of septal migration (1,5,6). Others, such as Van Mierop and Wiglesworth (19), hold that abnormal fusion of malformed conotruncal ridges is also involved in certain malformations of this type. However, the fact that a single agent can produce many different bulboventricular malformations by a single treatment at different points within the 48-hour period between day 7 and 9 seems to

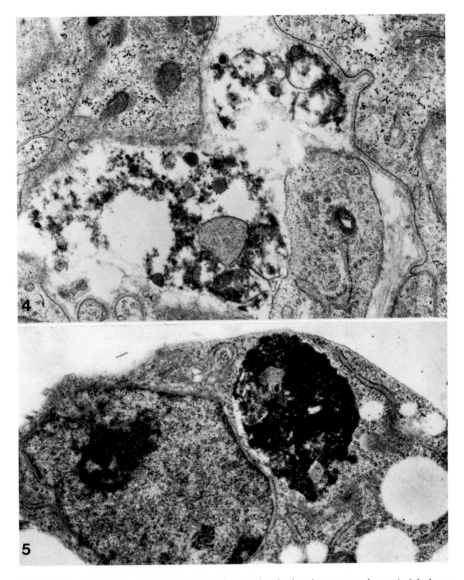

FIG. 4. Later, this debris loses its organization, and only the dense granular material shown here remains in the intercellular space (× 16,188).

FIG. 5. Both organized and disorganized material is phagocytosed by myocardial and mesenchymal cells, such as the one shown here (× 16,188).

indicate the presence of a fundamental link common to all the malformations observed.

Pexieder (12) recognizes that cell death is only one of several processes occurring in the developing heart, but he believes that the point of least resistance lies in the bulbar and atrioventricular cushions. In particular, he suggests that the foci of death of undifferentiated mesenchyme observed in these areas at certain stages of cardiogenesis have a morphogenetic role, and that their intensity and topography normally depend on hemodynamic factors. Moreover, he suggests that those cells in the bulbar cushions that are prenecrotic may represent a common target for the action of biophysical and chemical teratogens. Such agents may increase or decrease the amount of cell death normally observable in any particular part of the heart.

In a previous study, Taylor et al. (17) reported greatly increased numbers of dying and dead mesenchymal cells in the atrioventricular and bulbar cushions, and especially in the proximal portions of the latter structures. In the present study, the ultrastructure of hearts prior to formation of the cushion is under consideration; here, too, damage and death are noticeable, but in this case involving myocytes found in both the atrioventricular canal and the primitive ventricle. It would therefore seem reasonable to direct attention to both the muscular and cushion components of the developing atrioventricular and bulboventricular areas when considering possible mechanisms of teratogenesis.

Shenefelt (16) has suggested that the teratogenic effect of retinoic acid does not persist for very long, since considerable differences in the types and rates of malformation are produced by treatments only 6 hours apart. Furthermore, Desmukh et al (3) have shown that maternal blood and liver retinoic acid levels remain elevated and roughly constant for between 1 and 4 hours after administration, and then drop off rapidly. Roberts and DeLuca (13) also found maximal levels 3 to 4 hours after intake, and then a rapid decline as the acid was metabolized.

It may be, therefore, that the considerable effect on mesenchymal cells in the atrioventricular and bulbar cushions noted in 8-day treated embryos at much later stages of examination (18) is not due to the direct effect of retinoic acid (or possibly its metabolites). Instead, it may be indirect, a hemodynamically produced result of the earlier myocardial damage. Furthermore, even when the myocardium has apparently recovered from the primary insult, myofibrillar development is slowed by approximately 12 hours after treatment with retinoic acid. This delay, when combined with the widespread death of myocardial cells, is quite likely to affect the functional capacity of the heart, and may also contribute to any defects produced. In addition, administration of retinoic acid and related compounds is associated with development of abnormal vasculature in the limbs of the offspring (4). If this is also true of the pharyngeal arches, this, too, may lead to the secondary development of cardiac abnormalities.

ACKNOWLEDGMENTS

I wish to acknowledge the excellent technical assistance of C. G. T. Watterson and to thank Miss Pam Gale for her secretarial services. This work was supported by the Medical Research Council of Canada.

REFERENCES

1. Anderson, R. H., Wilkinson, J. L., Arnold, R., and Lubkiewicz, K. (1974): Morphogenesis of bulboventricular malformations. 1. Consideration of embryogenesis in the normal heart. *Br. Heart J.,* 36:242-255.
2. Boyer, C. C. (1953): Chronology of development for the golden hamster. *J. Morphol.,* 92:1-37.
3. Desmukh, D., Malathi, P., Rao, K., and Ganguly, J. (1964): Absorption of retinoic acid (vitamin A acid) in rats. *Ind. J. Biochem.,* 1:164-166.
4. Fraser, B. A. (1977): The relationship of aberrant vasculogenesis to retinoic acid induced dysmelia in the hamster fetus. Presented at the *5th International Conference on Birth Defects,* August 21-27, Montreal.
5. Goor, D. A., Dische, R., and Lillehei, C. W. (1972): The conotruncus. I. Its normal inversion and conus absorption. *Circulation,* 46:375-384.
6. Lev, M., Bharati, S., Meng, C. C., Liberthson, R. R., Paul, M. H., and Idriss, F. (1972): A concept of double outlet right ventricle. *J. Thorac. Cardiovasc. Surg.,* 64:271-281.
7. Okamoto, N. (1977): Programmed cell death in bulbar cushion of developing heart. In: *Gene–Environment Interaction in Common Disease,* edited by E. Inoue and H. Nishimura, pp. 89-94. University of Tokyo Press, Tokyo.
8. Okamoto, N. (1977): Embryological basis of the transposition complexes. *Teratology.,* 16:100.
9. Okamoto, N., and Satow, Y. (1975): Cell death in bulbar cushion of normal and abnormal developing heart. In: *Developmental and Physiological Correlates of Cardiac Muscle,* edited by M. Lieberman and T. Sano, pp. 51-65. Raven Press, New York.
10. Pexieder, T. (1972): The tissue dynamics of heart morphogenesis. 1. The phenomena of cell death. A. Identification and Morphology. *Z. Anat. Entwickl. Gesch.,* 137:270-284.
11. Pexieder, T. (1972): The tissue dynamics of heart morphogenesis. 1. The phenomena of cell death. B. Topography. *Z. Anat. Entwickl. Gesch.,* 138:241-253.
12. Pexieder, T. (1975): Cell death in the morphogenesis and teratogenesis of the heart. *Adv. Anat. Embryol. Cell Biol.,* 51:1-100.
13. Roberts, A. and DeLuca, H. (1967): Pathways of retinol and retinoic acid metabolism in the rat. *Biochem. J.,* 102:600-605.
14. Satow, Y., Okamoto, N., Hidaka, N., and Akimoto, N. (1977): Electron microscopic observation on the fate of conus swelling of rat embryonic heart. *Teratology,* 16:120.
15. Satow, Y., Okamoto, N., Hidaka, N., Akimoto, N., and Miyabara, S. (1978): Intracellular mechanism of teratogenesis of embryonic heart. In: *Morphogenesis and Malformation of the Cardiovascular System,* edited by G. C. Rosenquist and D. Bergsma, pp. 251-271. Alan R. Liss, Inc., New York.
16. Shenefelt, R. E. (1972): Morphogenesis of malformations in hamsters caused by retinoic acid: Relation to dose and stage of treatment. *Teratology,* 5:103-118.
17. Taylor, I. M., Agur, A., and Wiley, M. J. (1978): Retinoic acid-induced malformations of the heart. Presented at the July Meeting of the *Anatomical Society of Great Britain and Ireland,* Glasgow.
18. Taylor, I. M. (1979): The effect of retinoic acid on the developing hamster heart—an ultrastructural and morphological study. In: *Advances in the study of Birth Defects,* Vol. III, edited by T. V. N. Persaud, pp. 119-134. MTP Press, Lancaster.
19. Van Mierop, L. H. S., and Wiglesworth, F. W. (1963): Pathogenesis of transposition complexes. II. Anomalies due to faulty transfer of the posterior great artery. III. True transposition of the great vessels. *Am. J. Cardiol.,* 12:226-239.

DISCUSSION

De Vries: It is necessary to exclude retinoic acid toxicity as the cause of death of mesenchymal cells. I would think that the metabolism of the myocardial cells would be significantly different from that of the mesenchymal cells.

Taylor: There is no structural evidence of damage in the mesenchymal cells we have looked at.

De Vries: My suggestion is that you might very well see the effect significantly later in a cell of different metabolic type.

Fischman: Retinoic acid in low concentration increased the formation of tight junctions between epithelial cells. It might be very interesting to explore retinoic acid effects on the junctions between these myocardial cells.

Taylor: It is not simply a tight junction which is affected. An increase in the number of gap junctions and desmosomes was also reported in heart fibroblasts in culture. The increased adherence of cells will limit their motility.

De Haan: Do you know what 80 mg/kg of retinoic acid does to the mother?

Taylor: If the treatment is done properly (no lung injection), all the fetuses survive. Those who did not were obviously severely damaged and were excluded from this study.

Extracellular Matrix

Perspectives in Cardiovascular Research, Vol. 5,
Mechanisms of Cardiac Morphogenesis and Teratogenesis,
edited by Tomas Pexieder. Raven Press, New York © 1981

Extracellular Matrix: Introduction

Francis J. Manasek

Department of Anatomy, The University of Chicago, Chicago, Illinois 60637

Although, to my knowledge, no quantitative data exist to support the concept that extracellular matrix is the largest compartment of the very early developing heart, those of us who have spent many hours working with these early stages generally agree that this concept is correct. In this section, we will explore current studies of this major part of the developing heart.

What are the functions of this compartment? What are its properties and composition? In general terms, we know some answers to these questions. Functions at the biomechanical level have been explored and related to early pumping efficiency; the composition has been inferred, at least in part, from studies of isotope incorporation and histochemistry; physical properties are being listed as attempts to discern them directly are improved.

Although it is not my function to review exhaustively the history of studies of cardiac jelly, it is my prerogative to play prophet and attempt to identify the areas of future investigation that may provide the greatest insight into the relationship between extracellular matrix and cardiac morphogenesis.

Unique problems are associated with the cardiac jelly of early hearts. It is clear that most of the constituent macromolecules, e.g., collagen, glycosaminoglycans, and glycoproteins, are asymmetrical molecules. How do these asymmetrical structures become ordered in an environment that imposes upon them significant stress resulting both from myocardial contraction and from bending? How does such an interaction regulate further developmental events? Clearly, cushion development and endocardial remodeling involve intimate interaction between cells and matrix.

Endocardial cushion cells migrate into the extracellular matrix. Is the matrix instructive or is it neutral? By instructive, I mean, does it contain not only directional information but does it also select the cells that will migrate and act to regulate further their development, as well as to direct their translocation?

What I am implying by these remarks is that we are asking holistic questions; in order to answer them, however, we must first understand molecular and subcellular levels. Only then can we begin to understand the vastly more complex interactions between matrix components and the reactions between matrix and cells.

Finally, in our holistic scheme, we sense the remarkable fragility of cardiovascular morphogenesis. Many experimental manipulations alter the normal developmental sequence. How many of these are analogues of spontaneously occurring events that result in "normal" congenital malformations? Perhaps one of the most challenging problems to be examined experimentally is demonstration that the etiology of a spontaneous malformation can be related, mechanistically, to a similar malformation induced experimentally.

With the recent exciting expansion of work in the area of cardiovascular development, many new approaches to the matrix have been initiated. Let us see what is new in the field of cardiac jelly.

Perspectives in Cardiovascular Research, Vol. 5,
Mechanisms of Cardiac Morphogenesis and Teratogenesis,
edited by Tomas Pexieder. Raven Press, New York © 1981

The Importance of Extracellular Matrix Components in Development of the Embryonic Chick Heart

Carlos Argüello López and Marta Servín Martínez

Venezuelan Institute of Cardiology, Department of Cell Biology, Caracas, 104 Venezuela

Only recently has the extracellular compartment (8) in the embryonic heart been taken into consideration as an important component in development of this organ (15). The origin of the macromolecules that constitute the extracellular matrix (ECM) in early chick heart seems to derive mainly from myoblasts and myocytes (16). Later, the endocardium and the endocardial cushion cells of the cono-truncal and atrioventricular canal (AV canal) appear to synthesize some of the matrical components of these regions (20,21,22). The macromolecules already identified in the ECM, during the early development of the embryonic heart, are glycosaminoglycans (GAGs) (7,19,20,24), glycoproteins (18), and type *I*-like collagen (12). Among the GAGs that have been shown to be synthesized by the myocytes are hyaluronic acid (HA), chondroitin (Ch), chondroitin sulfate (ChS), and undersulfated chondroitin (17). These findings contribute to a new concept of the developing cardiac muscle cell; thus "in addition to being muscle, it is a secretory cell, much in the same way as a fibroblast" (16). In fact, a study of the development of the truncus in chick embryo (1) has shown that myocardial cells are actually able to differentiate into fibroblasts. A similar process has also been observed in the myocardium of the AV canal (2). However, the myocardium of the AV canal is believed to lose its continuity with the atrial and ventricular muscle by an invasion of connective tissue cells (endocardial and subepicardial) located at both sides of the myocardium (26). Because it is important to clarify this problem, we will present in the first part of this work a sequential study of the changes that take place in the myocardium of this region.

Intimately related to the differentiation of the myocardium are the other developmental processes occurring in the AV canal, including formation and migration of the endocardial cushion cells derived from the endocardium (21,23) and elaboration of the extracellular matrix. The evidence presented by Markwald (22) indicates that the endocardium and the endocardial cushion cells are responsible for synthesis of HA and ChS, and that the myocardium does not play an important role in these processes (20). Since we have previously observed that the myocardial layer of the truncus is able to synthesize some ECM (1), we wanted to determine if the same process takes place in the AV canal. In order to visualize which cells contribute to elaboration of the ECM, different cationic substances were utilized for light and electron microscopy.

Attempts have been made to evaluate the importance of the ECM in development of the heart by the use of substances such as salicylates, which inhibit the incorporation of $^{35}SO_4$ groups to GAGs (6) and produce cardiac malformations (5). However, it remains unknown how the malformations are produced. In the final part of our work, we present the results of several experiments designed to determine how salicylates affect development of the AV canal region in embryonic chick heart.

MATERIALS AND METHODS

Preparation of Embryonic Hearts for Light and Electron Microscopy Study

Three to 14-day (9) embryonic chick hearts, whose degree of development was determined according to de la Cruz et al. (4), were removed from the embryos and washed with salt solution (30). For histochemical study of the ECM components of the AV canal region, the hearts were dissected to facilitate the penetration of the various cationic substances used to retain and visualize the GAGs. Reaction with 0.1% toluidine blue O (TBO) (28), 1 mg/ml ruthenium red (RR) (14), or 1% cetylpyridinium chloride (22) was performed at the same time as fixation with 2.5% glutaraldehyde in 0.1 M cacodylate buffer, pH 7.2, for 1 to 2 hrs. In the case of cationized ferritin (3) or alcian blue (AB) (29), the reaction was done after fixation with the glutaraldehyde. The specimens were washed twice with saline solution and then treated with 1.5 mg/ml of cationized ferritin in PBS (phosphate buffer saline), pH 7.0, for 30 min at 0°C. Staining with an aqueous solution of 1% AB adjusted either to pH 1.0 or 2.5 with 1N HCl was done for 2 hrs at room temperature. Tissues were postfixed in 1% osmium tetroxide, and then dehydrated in increasing concentrations of ethanol and embedded in Epon 812. Thin sections of 1 μm were stained with 1% TBO in 1% borax. The ultra-thin unstained sections were examined with a Hitachi 300 electron microscope.

Treatment with N-acetylsalicylic acid (NASA): Two- and 3-day-old chick embryos were injected through the air sac with 0.1 ml of a sterile solution of NASA (1×10^{-5} mol). Since NASA was dissolved in 96% ethanol and isotonic NaCl (1:5), the controls consisted of eggs injected with 0.1 ml of this solution. After 48 or 72 hrs of further incubation at 37.5°C, the eggs were opened in a saline solution; the hearts were removed and carefully examined under a stereoscopic microscope. The treated and control hearts were fixed in 2.5% glutaraldehyde containing 0.1% of TBO or processed with AB as described above.

RESULTS

Development of the Atrioventricular Canal

In the 3-day chick embryo heart the AV canal possesses a thick layer of myocardium, which is continuous with the atrium and ventricle and divided into two layers. One layer is two cells thick and external, and the other is three to four cells thick and internal, facing the cardiac jelly (Fig. 1a). The layers are connected by myocardial cells which lie in between them. It is of interest, and probably related to the slow conduction velocity exhibited by the AV canal (33), that the inner and external cells of this region acquire radial and circular arrangements, respectively. At this time, the endocardial cushion cells are forming from the endocardium (23) and the cardiac jelly constitutes the main compartment (Fig. 1a). In the 4th day, the epicardium forms and covers the myocardium. The endocardial cushion cells proliferate and migrate far from the endocardium (Fig. 1b). At about the 5th day, the dorsal and ventral endocardial cushions reach their maximum size and the mesenchymal cells cover almost the entire area of the cushions, except for a small region close to the myocardium (Fig. 1c). The endocardial cells draw together and begin to fuse as described by Hay and Low (10). Until this stage of development, we have found no difference between the myocardial cells from the dorsal, ventral, or lateral portions of the AV canal, as observed in the mouse by Virágh and Challice (34). From day 5.5 to 6, the endocardial cushions have already fused, and the cushion cells fill the space previously close to the myocardium. Interestingly enough, at this stage the inner cells of the myocardium, particularly those near a trabeculated portion of the ventricle, begin to separate from each other and migrate toward the cushions (Fig. 1d). These cells, when observed under the electron microscope, can be recognized inside the cushions by their content of myofibrils (2). Even though the subepicardial and cushion cells are close to the myocardium, we did not observe the invasion described by Patten (26). Also evident at this stage (Fig. 1d), and clearly observable at 6.5 days, is that the myocardium bends toward the fused cushions (Fig. 1e). This leads to a reduction of the distance that separates the atrial and ventricular muscle. The myocardial cells continue separating and migrate far from each other, until a clear interruption forms between the myocardium of the AV canal and the ventricular muscle (Fig. 1e). The subepicardial cells proliferate and move toward the space left by the myocardium (Fig. 1e) to form the connective tissue between the auricle and ventricle (Fig. 1f).

Histochemical Study of the Extracellular Matrix of the AV Canal

Light microscopy: (A) Alcian blue (AB) used at pH 2.5 stained ECM more strongly than at pH 1.0, and this was particularly true for the early stages

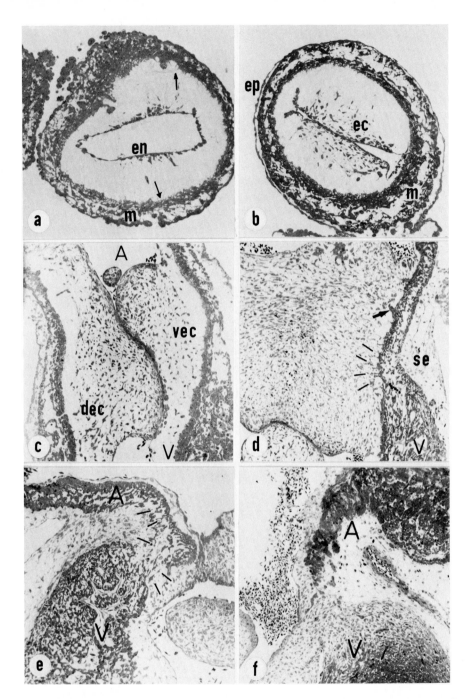

FIG. 1. Development of the AV canal in the embryonic chick heart. Transverse section of the AV canal. **a:** 3 days *(Arrow).* Material stained with alcian blue pH 2.5 (× 150). **b:** 4 days (× 120). Longitudinal section of the AV canal. **c:** 5 days (× 80). **d:** 5.5 to 6 days *(Arrow).* Myocardial cells migrating into the cushion tissue (× 80). **e:** 6.5 days (× 100). **f:** 14 days (× 90). Lines indicate areas of myocardial cell separation.

Abbreviations: A, atrium; bl, basal lamina; dec, dorsal endocardial cushion; ec, endocardial cushion cells; em, extracellular matrix; en, endocardium; ep, epicardium; m, myocardium; sc, subepicardial cells; V, ventricle; vec, ventral endocardial cushion.

described in our study. At the beginning of the period of endocardial cushion formation (3 days), the material stained was filamentous and lay close to the myocardium. However, the 1 μm sections do not permit clear differentiation of the staining in the endocardium (Fig. 1a). In the 4th day, the intensity of staining increases, both close to the myocardium and to the newly formed endo-

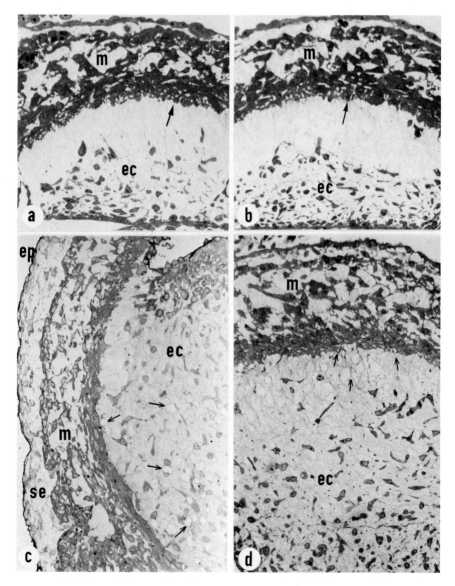

FIG. 2. Alcian blue and toluidine blue O stain of AV canal cushions. **a:** Alcian blue pH 1.0. 4-day heart (× 300). **b:** Alcian blue pH 2.5. 4-day heart (× 270). **c:** Toluidine blue O, 5 days (× 240). **d:** Alcian blue pH 2.5. 5 days (× 400). Arrows indicate stained extracellular matrix.

cardial cushion cells (Fig. 2a and 2b). At day 5 at both pHs, we observed the most intense staining of the endocardial cushion matrix. This formed a very complex net of filamentous and granular material around the myocardium and mesenchymal cells (Fig. 2d). (B) Toluidine blue O (TBO): Staining with TBO confirmed the findings with AB, but the material close to the myocardium appears granular rather than filamentous. Different structures within the matrix frequently observed with this procedure are large, rounded vesicles, sometimes associated with mesenchymal cells (Fig. 2c).

Electron microscopy: Since in the 3 to 3.5 day embryonic heart there are few cells in the endocardial cushion, we believed this was a more suitable stage to study, if in fact the myocardial cells were producing some matrical components and if they are different from those of the endocardial cushion cells. (A) Alcian blue: When AB at pH 2.5 was used, an electron-dense reaction in the form of bundles constituted of very fine fibrils was observed on the myocardial cell membrane (Fig. 3c). Some bundles were connected to each other and remained attached to the membrane by long, thin fibrils (Fig. 3c). As seen with the light microscope, large complexes of this material extend far from the myocardium. In contrast, the endocardial cushion cells and the endocardium showed scanty reaction either on the cell surface or close to the cells (Fig. 4c). At pH 1.0, instead of the bundles of fibrillar material, particles of about 25 nm and a few fibrils of 6 nm were observed. Again, the reaction was more intense close to the myocardium. (B) Toluidine blue O: The inner layer of the myocardium gave a strong reaction on the surface membrane constituting the basal lamina. Close to this layer, an amorphous granular material was evident (Fig. 3d). In addition, TBO penetrated well and stained the intercellular space in the myocardium (Fig. 3d). The endocardial cushion cells also gave a reaction, but this was less intense and took the form of large particles of about 100 to 200 nm. Some of these particles were in contact with the membrane; others were free in the ECM, and were comprised of short and thick fibrils held together by an amorphous material (Fig. 4d). (C) Ruthenium red: This has been the most widely used cation in the ultrastructural characterization of the cell surface and extracellular matrix components. In our case, RR gave very satisfactory results when used together with the fixative. The myocardial basal lamina was very well shown; a central fibrillar structure was recognized, as well as some granular and filamentous materials associated with it. The matrix close to the myocardium contains fibrils of about 10 nm in diameter, to which 10 to 20 nm particles are attached. Thin fibrils of 3 to 4 nm form connections between the thick fibrils (Fig. 3a). The endocardial cushion cells present irregularly distributed 10 to 20 nm particles on the cell membrane, and the matrix contains small aggregates of these (Fig. 4a). (D) Cationized ferritin: Another cation used in the study of molecules with negative charges dissociated at neutral pH is cationized ferritin (3). In our study, we tested whether this procedure would give new information about the structure and organization of the ECM. The inner myocardial cells showed discontinuous labeling on the cell surfaces. Close

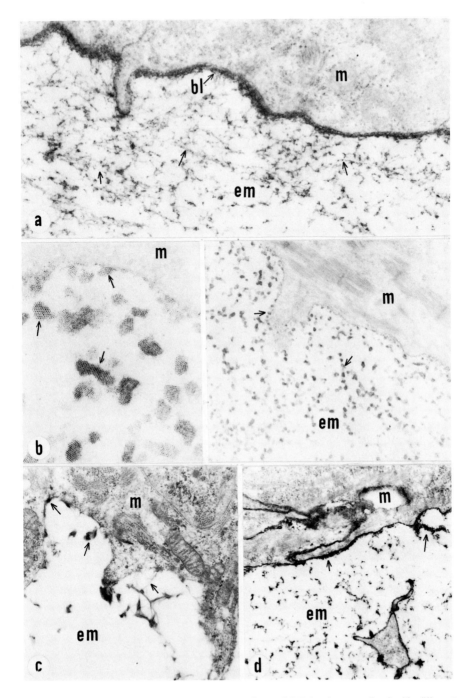

FIG. 3. Extracellular matrix close to the myocardium of 3.5-day heart stained with different cations. **a:** Ruthenium red (× 17,500). **b:** Cationized ferritin (× 50,000). **c:** Alcian blue pH 2.5 (× 13,600). **d:** Toluidine blue O (× 7,000). Arrows indicate extracellular matrix components.

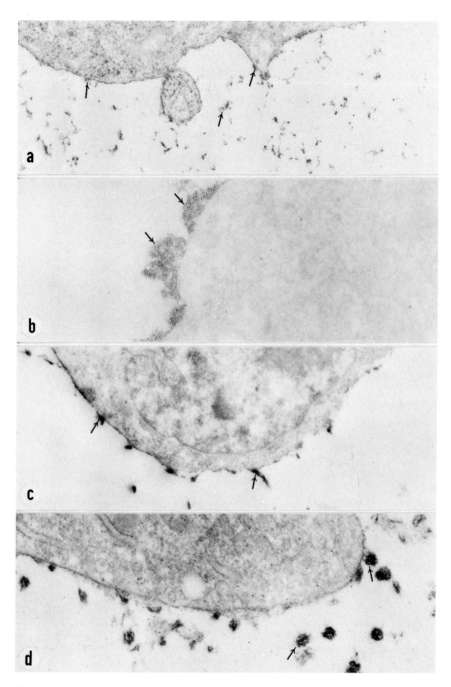

FIG. 4. Extracellular matrix close to the endocardial cushion cells of 3.5-day heart. **a:** Ruthenium red (× 10,500). **b:** Cationized ferritin (× 42,500). **c:** Alcian blue pH 2.5 (× 11,000). **d:** Toluidine blue O (× 21,600). Arrows indicate ECM components.

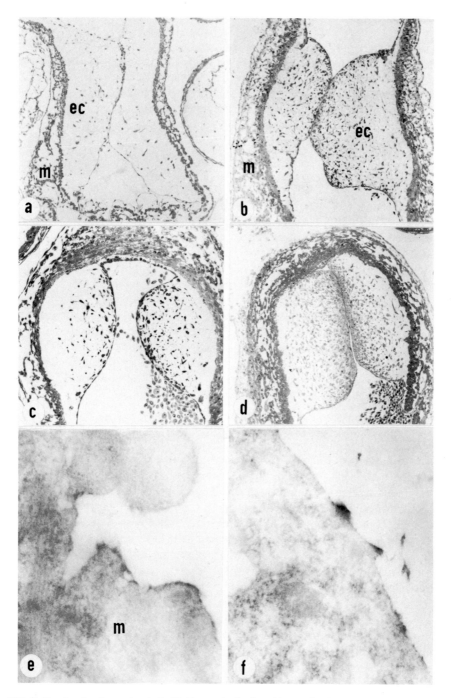

FIG. 5. Hearts of embryos treated with N-acetylsalicylic acid. **a:** 4-day heart of a treated embryo (× 90). **b:** 4-day heart control (× 64). **c:** 5-day heart of a treated embryo (× 120). **d:** 5-day heart control (× 86). **e:** Ultrastructure of muscle. **f:** Endocardial cushion cells of a 4-day embryo treated with N-acetylsalicylic acid and stained at pH 2.5 (× 25,700).

to these cells, abundant particles of 120 to 130 nm were distributed without any particular arrangement in the matrix (Fig. 3b). Under high magnification, these particles were seen to be formed of regularly arranged granules of 5.6 nm, having an intergranular space of 4.2 nm. It is of interest that the particles present on the cell surface also have this arrangement (Fig. 3b, left). The endocardial cushion cell surface, although heavily labeled with cationized ferritin, did not present any particular arrangement (Fig. 4b).

N-acetylsalicylic Acid Experiments

The percentage of survival of 2-day embryos treated with 180 μg/0.1 ml of NASA was around 50% after 2 days. We could distinguish defects related to the growth of the cono-truncal portion of the heart, as well as an enlargement of the AV canal region. When sections of 1 μm were made (Fig. 5a), the endocardial cushion of the AV canal extended from the ventricles into the atrium, and the number of cells in the cushion decreased dramatically as compared with the controls (Fig. 5b). In addition, the myocardium and the epicardium were poorly developed. When 3-day embryos were treated, the survival rate rose to 60%, although the endocardial cushions of the AV canal and cono-truncal regions were similarly affected. The endocardial cushions showed a reduced size and few cushion cells (Fig. 5c), as compared with the control (Fig. 5d). Under the electron microscope, we observed a reduction in the ECM close to the myocardium (Fig. 5e) and the cushion cells (Fig. 5f).

DISCUSSION

In the early stages (10 to 13) of embryonic chick heart, the most important morphogenetic events are formation of the bulboventricular loop and elaboration of the cardiac jelly. During this period, the heart is composed of endocardium and myocardium. Later, at about stage 17, two new components are formed: the epicardium and the cells of the endocardial cushions of the cono-truncus and the AV canal. The endocardial cushion cells have been shown to develop from the endocardium (21,23), but what causes these cells to proliferate only in such regions is unknown. Manasek (16) speculated that regional compositional differences in the ECM of the heart may provide the stimulus for such proliferation. A very critical period in the morphogenesis of chick heart is around 5 to 6 days, at which time fusion of the cono-truncal and AV canal cushions occurs. Equally important is the differentiation of the wall of the truncus (1) and the AV canal (2), in which the muscle is changed into connective tissue.

In an attempt to understand the importance of the ECM in development of the AV canal, embryos from 3 to 14 days were studied. Our observations of development of the AV canal region, and particularly of the myocardial layer, showed that the discontinuity between the atrium and the ventricle is produced by separation and migration of the myocardial cells into the cushion tissue

(Fig. 1), rather than by invasion of fibroblasts, as was proposed by Patten (26). These changes in the myocardial layer were previously suggested to be related to the influence of the ECM. In the case of the AV canal, before we arrive at any conclusion we must further analyze our results.

Histochemical study of the AV canal region with the various cations used showed that the strongest reaction of the ECM was observed close to the myocardium, rather than in the cushion cells (Fig. 2,3,4). If these findings reflect differences in capacity for synthesis among the cells, we can assert that the contribution of the myocardium is important to the formation of the endocardial cushion matrix, and consequently that it has secretory activity. In addition to the quantitative differences in the matrix previously described, there were qualitative ultrastructural differences which probably indicate that the myocardium and the cushion cells are synthesizing different kinds of extracellular molecules (Fig. 3,4). The evidence presented by Orkin and Toole (25) has shown that the main GAG synthesized by the embryonic chick heart during days 3 to 5 is hyaluronic acid; this was the period in which we observed higher labeling with the cations. In the case of the rat, Markwald (22) has demonstrated the existence of HA in the premigratory matrix of the bulbus cordis. From these observations, it seems likely that the matrix close to the myocardium is rich in HA. On the other hand, the cushion cells seem to have a matrix formed of chondroitin sulfate, since they presented a positive reaction in the form of particles 10 to 20 nm diameter with Alcian blue at pH 1.0 and with ruthenium red in other systems. These particles have been associated with the presence of ChS (11,32). The evidence so far available in various systems (13,31) indicates that high molecular weight hyaluronic acid stimulates cell proliferation and plays an important role in cell migration (27,31). Whether or not the matrix close to the myocardium stimulates separation and migration of the cells remains to be experimentally determined. Similarly, it becomes very interesting to establish whether that matrix stimulates the endocardial cells to proliferate and migrate toward the myocardial layer, since the matrix provides a concentration gradient in that direction.

In the initial work of Gessner (5) on the effect of salicylates on development of the heart, only embryos of about 17 days were examined. We believed it important to determine the effects produced by these drugs in the earlier stages. Our results demonstrate that NASA has a dramatic effect in the embryo. It causes a high rate of mortality, such as was reported by Gessner (5) for sodium salicylate. However, some of the embryos that survived the treatment were shown to have defects in the formation of the cushion cells (Fig. 5), as well as in the matrix (Fig. 5). Interpretation of these findings requires further investigation to clarify whether or not NASA inhibits the synthesis of other GAGs, such as hyaluronic acid, which appears to be more important during the stages we studied. Considering the types of modifications observed in the heart, we could expect to see important malformations related to development of the AV canal. The malformations described by Gessner (5) were more related to defects of the outflow tract. This probably means that the most severe malformations were not detected because the embryos died.

In summary, we can say that the AV canal is a good system for study of several of the basic developmental processes *in vivo*. These processes include cell differentiation, proliferation, migration, and interaction. It seems probable that ECM is produced by the myocardial layer and the endocardial cushion cells. ECM is an important compartment that probably influences differentiation of the myocardial layer of the AV canal. It may also stimulate cell proliferation and migration, since inhibition of acid mucopolysaccharide synthesis prevents cushion-cell proliferation.

ACKNOWLEDGMENTS

We are greatly indebted to Dr. A. Anselmi for his support and encouragement of this research program. The authors also wish to thank Prof. Carlos Herrera and Carlos Ayesta for excellent photographic assistance and the facilities of the Department of Photography, Faculty of Science, U.C.V. We wish to express our thanks to the staff and friends of our laboratory, Héctor Arrechedera, María Antonia Suárez, Silvia Moros, and E. Arciniegas. We gratefully acknowledge the critical review of the manuscript by Dr. K. Dawidowicz.

REFERENCES

1. Arguello, C., de la Cruz, M. V., and Sánchez, C. (1978): Ultrastructural and experimental evidence of myocardial cell differentiation into connective tissue cells in embryonic chick heart. *J. Mol. Cell. Cardiol.,* 10:307-315.
2. Arguello, C., and Servín, M. (1978): Ultrastructural and experimental evidence of myocardial cell differentiation into connective tissue cells in the atrioventricular canal of embryonic chick heart. *III International Conference on Differentiation. Differentiation and Neoplasia.* University of Minnesota, Minneapolis.
3. Danon, D., Goldstein, Y., and Skutelsky, E. (1972): Use of cationized ferritin as a label of negative charges on cell surfaces. *J. Ultrastruct. Res.,* 38:500-510.
4. de la Cruz, M. V., Muñoz-Armas, S., and Muñoz Castellanos, L. (1972): *Development of the chick heart.* Johns Hopkins University Press, Baltimore and London.
5. Gessner, I. H. (1970): Some biochemical and anatomic effects of sodium salicylate on the chick embryo heart. In: *Pathophysiology of Congenital Heart Disease,* edited by F. H. Adams, H. J. C. Swan, and V. E. Hall, pp. 17-26. University of California Press, Berkeley, Los Angeles, and London.
6. Gessner, I. H., and Bostrom, H. (1965): "In vitro" studies on S-sulfate incorporation into the acid mucopolysaccharides of chick embryo cardiac jelly. *J. Exp. Zool.,* 160:283-290.
7. Gessner, I. H., Lorincz, A. E., and Bostrom, H. (1965): Acid mucopolysaccharide content of the cardiac jelly of the chick embryo. *J. Exp. Zool.,* 160:291-298.
8. Grobstein, C. (1975): Developmental role of intercellular matrix: Retrospective and prospective. In: *Extracellular Matrix Influences on Gene Expression,* edited by H. C. Slavkin and R. C. Greulich, pp. 9-16. Academic Press, New York.
9. Hamburger, B., and Hamilton, H. L. (1951): A series of normal stages of the chick embryo. *J. Morphol.,* 88:49-92.
10. Hay, D. A., and Low, F. N. (1972): The fusion of dorsal and ventral endocardial cushions in the embryonic chick heart: A study in fine structure. *Am. J. Anat.,* 133:1-24.
11. Hay, E. D. (1977): Interactions between the cell surface and extracellular matrix in corneal development. In: *Cell and Tissue Interactions,* edited by J. W. Lash and M. M. Burger, pp. 115-137. Raven Press, New York.

12. Johnson, R. C., Manasek, F. J., Vinson, W. C., and Seyer, J. M. (1974): The biochemical and ultrastructural demonstration of collagen during early heart development. *Dev. Biol.,* 36:252-271.
13. Lippman, S. M. (1968): Glycosaminoglycans and cell division. In: *Epithelial Mesenchymal Interactions,* edited by R. Fleischmajer and R. E. Billingham, pp. 208-229. Williams and Wilkins Co., Baltimore.
14. Luft, J. H. (1966): Fine structure of capillary and endocapillary layer as revealed by ruthenium red. *Federation Proc.,* 25:1773-1783.
15. Manasek, F. J. (1975): The extracellular matrix: A dynamic component of the developing embryo. In: *Current Topics in Developmental Biology,* edited by A. A. Moscona and A. Monroy, pp. 35-102. Academic Press, New York.
16. Manasek, F. J. (1976a): The extracellular matrix of the early embryonic heart. In: *Developmental and Physiological Correlates of Cardiac Muscle,* edited by M. Lieberman and T. Sano, pp. 1-20. Raven Press, New York.
17. Manasek, F. J. (1976b): Macromolecules of the extracellular compartment of embryonic and mature hearts. *Circ. Res.,* 38:331-337.
18. Manasek, F. J. (1976c): Glycoprotein synthesis and tissue interactions during establishment of the functional embryonic chick heart. *J. Mol. Cell. Cardiol.,* 8:389-402.
19. Manasek, F. J., Reid, M., Vinson, W., Seyer, J., and Johnson, R. (1973): Glycosaminoglycan synthesis by the early embryonic chick heart. *Dev. Biol.,* 35:332-348.
20. Markwald, R. R., and Adams Smith, W. N. (1972): Distribution of mucosubstances in the developing rat heart. *J. Histochem. Cytochem.,* 20:896-907.
21. Markwald, R. R., Fitzharris, T. P., and Adam Smith, W. N. (1975): Structural analysis of endocardial cytodifferentiation. *Dev. Biol.,* 42:160-180.
22. Markwald, R. R., Fitzharris, T. P., Bank, H., and Bernanke, D. H. (1978): Structural analysis on the matrical organization of glycosaminoglycans in developing endocardial cushions. *Dev. Biol.,* 62:292-316.
23. Markwald, R. R., Fitzharris, T. P., and Manasek, F. J. (1977): Structural analysis of endocardial cushion tissue development. *Am. J. Anat.,* 148:85-120.
24. Ortíz, C. E. (1958): Estudio histoquímico de la gelatina cardíaca en el embrión de pollo. *Arch. Inst. Cardiol. Méx.,* 28:244-262.
25. Orkin, R. W., and Toole, B. P. (1978): Hyaluronidase activity and hyaluronate content of the developing chick embryo heart. *Dev. Biol.,* 66:308-320.
26. Patten, B. M. (1956): The development of the sinoventricular conduction system. *Michigan M. Bulletin.,* 22:1-21.
27. Pratt, R. M., Larsen, M. A., and Johnston, M. C. (1975): Migration of cranial neural crest cells in a cell-free hyaluronate-rich matrix. *Dev. Biol.,* 44:298-305.
28. Shepard, N., and Mitchell, N. (1976): Simultaneous localization of proteoglycan by light and electron microscopy using toluidine blue O: A study of epiphyseal cartilage. *J. Histochem. Cytochem.,* 24:621-629.
29. Spicer, S. S., and Henson, J. G. (1967): Methods for localizing mucosubstances in epithelial and connective tissues. In: *Meth. Achievm. Exp. Pathol.,* edited by E. Bajusz and G. Jasmin, pp. 78-112. S. Karger, Basel and New York.
30. Spratt, N. T. (1947): Development "in vitro" of the early chick blastoderm explanted on yolk albumen extract saline–agar substrata. *J. Exp. Zool.,* 106:345-365.
31. Toole, B. P., Okayama, M., Orkin, R. W., Yoshimura, M., Muto, M., and Kaji, A. (1977): Developmental roles of hyaluronate and chondroitin sulfate proteoglycans. In: *Cell and Tissue Interactions,* edited by J. W. Lash and M. M. Burger, pp. 139-154. Raven Press, New York.
32. Trelstad, R. L., Hayashi, K., and Toole, B. P. (1974): Epithelial collagens and glycosaminoglycans in the embryonic cornea. *J. Cell. Biol.,* 62:815-830.
33. Van Mierop, L. H. S. (1967): Location of the pacemaker in chick embryo heart at the time of initiation of heart beat. *Am. J. Physiol.,* 212:407-415.
34. Virágh, Sz., and Challice, C. E. (1977): The development of the conduction system in the mouse embryo heart. I. The first embryonic AV conduction pathway. *Dev. Biol.,* 56;382-396.

DISCUSSION

Fitzharris: I would suspect that 99% of the cases of your myocardial migration are small finger-like projections of myocardium that reach into the matrix. What you have presented does not demonstrate, at least to me, migration of myocardial cells into the extracellular matrix area.

Arguello: It is very difficult to follow all of the sequences of the migration of the myocardial cells. Can you suggest any other method of demonstrating their migration or its absence? How can you explain the interruption of the AV region?

Fitzharris: Serial sections at a light microscopic level will demonstrate to you that much of the material is really projections from the myocardium in terms of ingrowth of the myocardial wall, rather than outgrowth and delamination of individual cells as we see in the seeding of the cushion tissue cells.

De Vries: There is no question about the continuity of the strands of the myocardium in the atrioventricular canal. But I thought that the matrix is formed by the trabecular muscle growing in.

Markwald: I did find great fun in choosing inhibitors. Dr. Pexieder has already indicated problems with inhibitors, especially for the matrix. From my experience with salicylates, I have to conclude that their effects are not sufficiently specific to state that we are lacking a particular glycosaminoglycan. Giving salicylate as a teratogen to affect the matrix may hit cell migration and proliferation as well. The final effect is a decreased number of AV cushion cells present. The results I will present suggest that removal of glycosaminoglycans causes piling up of the cushion cells underneath the endocardium. For this reason, I have almost convinced myself that the endocardium is a source of cushion tissue cells through the first 90 hours of avian development. I have no evidence that myocardium can contribute cells to the cushion tissue. It needs to be demonstrated in a very convincing fashion. It would require initial demonstration that myocytes moving into this tissue dedifferentiate—a process that is very difficult to accept.

Perspectives in Cardiovascular Research, Vol. 5,
Mechanisms of Cardiac Morphogenesis and Teratogenesis,
edited by Tomas Pexieder. Raven Press, New York © 1981

Synthesis and Distribution of Glycopeptides and Glycosaminoglycans in Cultures of Embryonic Heart Cells

Francis J. Manasek, Joan Lacktis, James Aiton*, and Melvyn Lieberman*

Department of Anatomy, The University of Chicago, Chicago, Illinois 60637;
*Department of Physiology, Duke University Medical Center,
Durham, North Carolina 27706

Early cardiac morphogenesis depends upon regulated interaction between cells and their environment, as well as among the cells themselves. The immediate environment for heart cells during the formative stages of heart morphogenesis is a relatively abundant extracellular matrix. The materials in this matrix are largely products of the developing myocardium during early development (9,10). Initially acellular, the extracellular space, called the cardiac jelly, becomes populated by cushion cells derived from the endocardium (12,14). Recent studies (13) have suggested that these mesenchymatous cushion cells modify the composition of the cardiac jelly as they migrate through it.

Central to the general problem of interactions of cells with both their environment and with other cells is the synthesis and elaboration of extracellular and cell surface macromolecules. Most cells contain, as a functional part of the outer plasmalemmal surface, a layer of carbohydrate-rich material called, variously, the cell coat or glycocalyx. This material is present on the surfaces of embryonic heart cells (5,6,9) and is altered by known teratogens (15). Cell-surface materials are dynamic and turn over. Furthermore, there is evidence that they are shed into the cells's surroundings (8). In addition, many embryonic cells, regardless of their phenotype (including developing heart cells), elaborate collagens, glycosaminoglycans, and non-collagenous glycoproteins.

As part of our systematic studies of the control of cardiac morphogenesis, we have investigated the relationship between the cell-surface material and the extracellular environment. In this paper, we report on a quantitative study of the distribution of radioisotopically labeled anionic saccharides synthesized by embryonic heart cells in a controlled culture environment.

We specifically tested the hypothesis that embryonic heart cells are able to respond to alterations in their environment. We demonstrate that surface components, identifiable as anionic glycopeptides and glycosaminoglycan polysaccharides, are shed into the medium, but that such release is not uniform and depends upon the composition of the medium. Thus, exchange between surface and medium is not a simple "shedding" process but rather is a regulated phenomenon.

MATERIALS AND METHODS

Cell cultures: Cells were harvested from 11-day-old chick embryos according to the method of Horres et al. (7). Cultures were grown in Falcon No. 3008 plates; each well was inoculated with 1 ml suspension containing 2.5×10^5 cells/ml.

Glucosamine (GlcN) labeling: ^{3}H-GlcN (NEN, 30 Ci/mM) was dried and redissolved in appropriate medium (either fresh or "conditioned") to a final activity of 600 μCi/ml.

Labeling was carried out under the following conditions:

Continuous labeling: Medium was removed from confluent cultures, which were rinsed once with balanced salt solution (BSS). Fresh medium containing ^{3}H-GlcN was added, and incubation continued for periods ranging up to 32 hours.

Chase: Confluent cultures were labeled as above for 24 hours. Medium was then decanted, cultures washed with BSS, and fresh, unlabeled medium added. Cultures were reincubated and harvested after 1 and 9 hours.

Labeling with conditioned medium: Medium was harvested from confluent cultures. ^{3}H-GlcN was dissolved in this medium and used to label cultures. In this way, cultures were exposed to ^{3}H-GlcN in conditioned rather than fresh medium.

Analysis of labeled molecules: Analyses were performed as described earlier (11,15).

RESULTS

Time Course of Synthesis and Distribution of Labeled Molecules

Separate identical cultures were labeled with ^{3}H-GlcN. Label was introduced by preparing fresh medium and adding ^{3}H-GlcN to a final concentration of 600 μCi/ml. Cultures were rinsed once and then received fresh medium containing ^{3}H-GlcN. Incubations were stopped at 3,6,9,24, and 32 hours and, for each time, medium and surface molecules were analyzed on diethyl aminoethyl cellulose (DE-52). A typical chromatograph of surface material is seen in Fig. 1. An initial radioactive peak represents neutral or positively charged moieties, as well as unincorporated glucosamine.

The first major set of peaks representing anionic materials (Peaks A) is distinctly separate from the second (Peaks B). A series of peaks elute at higher LiCl concentrations (above 0.15 M) and represent glycosaminoglycan polysaccharides, with hyaluronate eluting first and then chondroitin sulfates. Prolonged incubation with label does not result in qualitatively different labeled molecules, as judged by this criterion.

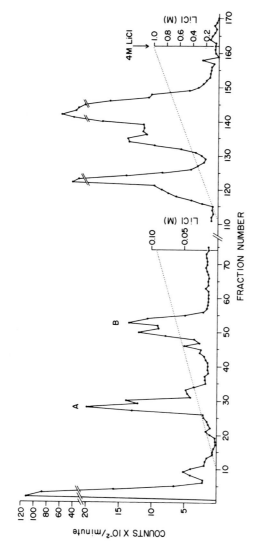

FIG. 1. Tryptic digestion of labeled cell surface molecules separated on DE-52. Cultures had been labeled for 6 hours. After an initial elution of radioactive material, two characteristic complex peaks elute, identified as A and B. The second LiCl gradient results in recovery of hyaluronate (HA) (ca. fraction 120) and chondroitin sulfate (ChS) eluting between fraction 132 and 150. This is a typical elution pattern which does not change qualitatively with incubation time.

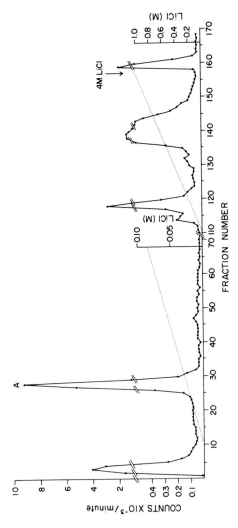

FIG. 2: DE-52 elution of medium after 6 hours incubation. Peak A is prominent, but no Peak B material is detected. The medium contains HA, ChS, and a significant peak eluting with 4 M LiCl. This peak represents H.

Similar analysis of the medium resulted in the profile shown in Fig. 2. Peak B, present on the surface (Fig. 1), is absent from the medium and was not recovered even after 32 hours of incubation. Again, there are no qualitative changes detected over a 32-hour labeling period.

The accumulation of label, administered at time 0, in various surface and medium moieties, is shown in Fig. 3 and 4.

To test for culture viablity for the period of the experiment, parallel, unlabeled cultures were maintained under identical conditions and labeled 24 hours after the experiment was begun. These cultures were harvested 8 hours later. The levels of recorded labeled moieties strongly suggest that leveling off of incorporation does not result from a time-dependent loss of synthetic activity by the cultures.

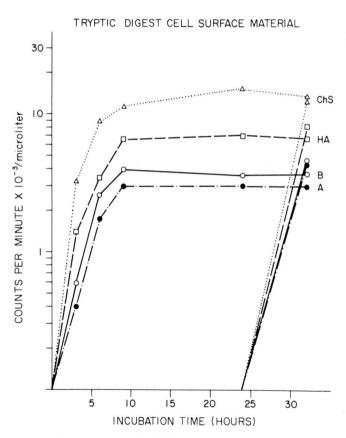

FIG. 3: Time course incorporation of ³H-GlcN into cell-surface materials. Identical, parallel cultures were labeled at the same time. Each point represents a pair of cultures withdrawn for analysis. Twenty-four hours after the start of the experiment, label was added to a previously unlabeled culture. The resulting incorporation shows that the plateau is not the result of time-dependent cessation of synthesis.

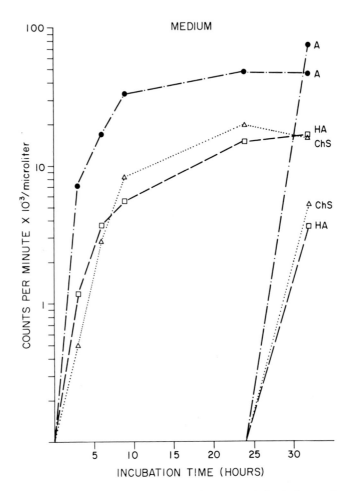

FIG. 4: Similar to Fig. 3, except representing accumulation in the medium.

Release of Surface Molecules into Fresh Medium

Cultures were incubated with ^{3}H-GlcN for 24 hours, washed briefly to remove free GlcN and incubated with fresh medium without additional ^{3}H-GlcN. Incubations were terminated at both 1 and 9 hours after introduction of label, and both labeled cell-surface and medium molecules were examined. In this experimental design, we can examine the fate of molecules present at the time the cells were first subjected to fresh medium, since these molecules have already been labeled.

Cell-associated molecules are not qualitatively different after 1 or 9 hours (Fig. 5) of labeling. The medium contains freshly liberated glycosaminoglycans (Fig. 6) even after 1 hour. Medium Peak A is prominent, and we detect for the first time the unequivocal presence of Peak B glycopeptides in the medium.

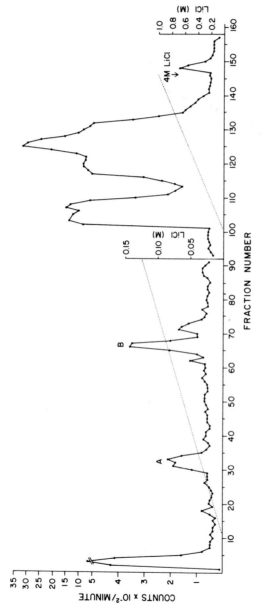

FIG. 5: Cultures were labeled for 24 hours; the medium was then replaced with fresh, unlabeled medium. Cultures were harvested after 1-hour and 9-hour exposure to fresh medium. This elution pattern (1-hour exposure) is representative of surface material recovered in this experiment.

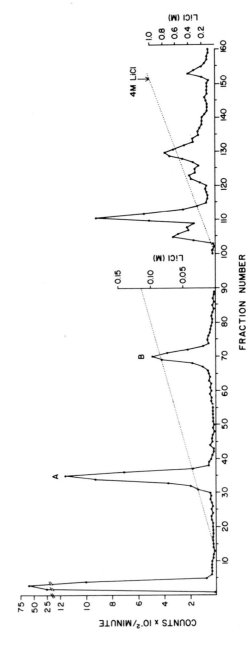

FIG. 6: Medium recovered from same experiment as Fig. 5. Note presence of Peak B.

A substantial Peak B is seen in the medium after 1 hour exposure to fresh, unlabeled culture medium. This peak is relatively smaller and almost absent in medium exposed for 9 hours (Fig. 7). Continued elaboration of glycosaminoglycans has occurred (compare Fig. 7 and 6).

Labeling in the Presence of "Conditioned" Medium

Medium was removed from cultures and replaced with medium obtained from parallel cultures. We added ^{3}H-GlcN (600 μCi/ml) to this "conditioned" medium. Cultures labeled with "conditioned" medium were incubated for 10 hours. Synthesis of surface-associated material is qualitatively similar (Fig. 8) to that synthesized in the presence of fresh medium (Fig. 1). However, the conditioned medium contains relatively little labeled glycosaminoglycan, despite its abundant presence on the surface (Fig. 9). Medium Peak B is absent from the medium, but Peak A is present (Fig. 9).

DISCUSSION

In this study, our analysis depends upon the presence of radioactive tracers in the molecules we wish to examine. Hence, we detect only those synthesized in the presence of label, and we cannot measure those molecules synthesized before label is added or after it is removed. We can, however, make inferences based upon our experimental results. For example, the first group of experiments clearly shows that cultured heart cells synthesize glycosaminoglycans and elaborate them into the medium. We can therefore surmise that the "conditioned" medium employed in the last set of experiments contained similar molecules, although we did not detect them (since they were unlabeled). Similarly, this medium would have contained unlabeled Peak A.

We can thus, in the case of the first and second set of experiments, trace the passage of labeled molecules from the cell into new medium devoid of any such molecules, and, in the last set of experiments, determine the effect, if any, of the pre-existence of these molecules on synthesis and release.

Cultured heart cells from 11-day embryos synthesize glycosaminoglycans and elaborate them into the medium. In this respect, they are similar to very early myocardial cells *in situ* (9). In the present study, we discern evidence that there are two separate and discrete compartments for glycosaminoglycans. Clearly, some are secreted into the medium. However, the amount of glycosaminoglycan in the medium does not increase indefinitely, but reaches a plateau level after about 10 hours. Our experiments with "conditioned" medium (which presumably contains plateau levels of glycosaminoglycans) show that very little newly synthesized glycosaminoglycan is added. However, glycosaminoglycan synthesis is not shut off. Rather, glycosaminoglycan production continues, but the newly synthesized molecules are restricted largely to the cell-surface compartment. Relatively small numbers of new molecules are found in the medium.

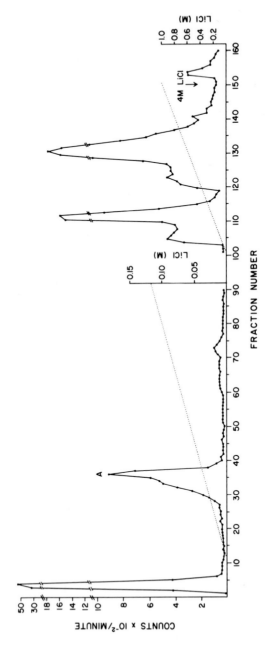

FIG. 7: Medium from 24-hour labeled culture that had been exposed to fresh medium for 9 hours. There has been continued "shedding" of glycosaminoglycans into medium, but Peak B glycopeptides are virtually absent. This suggests that B moieties are cleared, since they are initially released into fresh medium (Fig. 6).

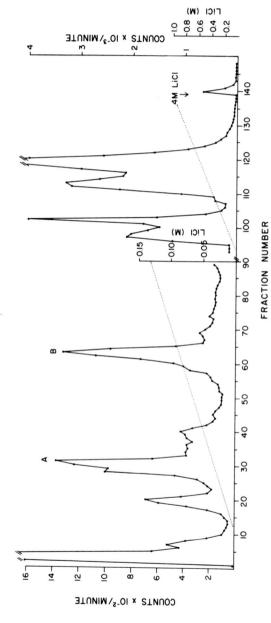

FIG. 8: Tryptic digest from surface of cells incubated with label contained in conditioned medium. Elution profile qualitatively similar to that of Fig. 5.

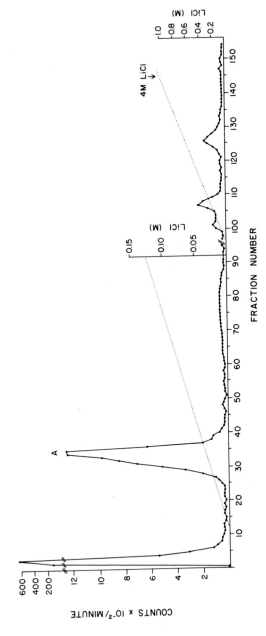

FIG. 9: Medium from same experiment as Fig. 8. Note absence of Peak B glycopeptides and low level of medium glycosaminoglycans.

The fact that there is, in the presence of conditioned medium, rapid new synthesis of surface-associated molecules indicates that the observed plateau is not the result of exhaustion of some essential nutrient from the medium.

Collectively, these data show that heart cells respond to their environment by altering the elaboration of newly synthesized molecules, but that their surface glycosaminoglycans remain qualitatively unaffected. After 24 hours of labeling, our experiments show that cells do not add significant glycosaminoglycans to the medium. However, if we replace this medium with fresh medium, there is a rapid (1 hour or less) release of glycosaminoglycan, indicating a rapid mobilization of the surface compartment. Thus, heart cells are capable of rapid response to environmental change.

Since synthesis continues even though there is little secretion into the medium, and there is no appreciable further accumulation of glycosaminoglycan, there must be turnover. We tested this directly by introducing label into "conditioned" medium at time intervals that corresponded to times along the plateau region in Figure 3. In each case, there was new synthesis of surface glycosaminoglycan. Since there is turnover, there is probable reutilization of breakdown products. This reutilization makes it difficult to determine true synthesis rates. We speculate that in heart cells, as in other cells (4), reutilization of surface-coat materials involves endocytosis, and that such endocytotic activity is constantly occurring. Earlier studies (9), in which heart cell-surface coats were stained *in situ* with ruthenium red, failed to demonstrate evidence of significant endocytotic activity in young (up to stage 16) hearts. However, phagocytosis has been demonstrated in cultured heart cells (3), and, in our laboratories, the authors have preliminary evidence for extensive endocytosis *in vitro*. We do not yet know whether endocytosis is age-dependent or is induced by culture conditions.

The glucosamine-labeled glycopeptides that elute at low ionic strengths appear similar to those that were detected earlier by means of fucose-^{3}H labeling (15) and to those synthesized by a variety of embryonic cell types (1). We do not detect all the surface-associated glycopeptides in the medium, and under most conditions employed in this study only Peak A glycopeptides appeared in the medium in significant amounts. This could mean that the other glycopeptides either are not elaborated into the medium or that they are present only in very small quantitites. We detected a significant Peak B in the medium when pre-labeled cells were exposed to fresh medium for 1 hour. Under these conditions, cells with labeled surface molecules were challenged by fresh medium that did not contain any shed cell surface moieties. The fact that labeled surface glycopeptides were detected after a brief period (1 hour) indicates that they can be rapidly released. However, B-glycopeptides disappear from the medium rather rapidly, since after 9 hours the total radioactivity in the medium Peak B groups is less than it was at 1 hour. We do not detect appreciable Peak B glycopeptides when label is introduced along with fresh medium, since the pre-existing Peak B molecules (which would be rapidly shed into the medium) are unlabeled and hence not detected. We do not know whether the transitory nature of Peak B in the medium is the result of degradation, incorporation into other molecules, or removal by the cells themselves. However, it is intriguing to note that its presence in medium is short-lived and that it is not a normal component of conditioned medium.

The use of extended gradients in the present study has enabled us to detect these differences which were not detected by Kapeller et al. (8) in a similar study. These workers, also using ion exchange chromatography, concluded that surface- and medium-recovered moieties were similar.

Shedding of B-glycopeptides is clearly a response to changes in the medium, but such medium challenges do not seem to elicit synthesis of remarkably different molecules. The presence of Peak A in the experiments using labeled conditioned medium suggests that these glycopeptides are also turning over. There is no net accumulation, yet labeled moieties appear, indicating continued synthesis.

The shedding of surface molecules into fresh medium may be considered a form of damage to the cell surface coat. Damage was studied earlier by Buck and Warren (2), who induced changes in the cell surface coat by means of enzymatic digestion. Their studies showed that damaged surface molecules are not "repaired" but rather are replaced. Damage, for example, caused by desialyation by means of neuraminadase, did not increase the rate of synthesis of new, replacement molecules. Seemingly, synthesis continued at a constant rate. Buck and Warren analyzed tryptic fragments on the basis of size, by means of Sephadex G-50 chromatography. Our present study separates moieties on the basis of charge, and we are consequently able to distinguish between glycosaminoglycan polysaccharide and surface glycopeptides. The rate of shedding did not appear to vary strikingly among these components, as measured by the accumulation of newly synthesized molecules in non-conditioned medium.

We conclude with a note of caution. Although this study has elucidated some aspects of the responses of embryonic heart cells to changes in environment and has clarified some of the relationships between cell surface coat and matrix, we cannot yet relate this to heart development at a tissue or organ level. It is tempting to speculate, but we need more data.

ACKNOWLEDGMENTS

This work was supported by USPHS grants HL 13831 and HL 12157 and by the North Carolina Heart Association.

REFERENCES

1. Brown, J. C. (1972): Cell surface glycoprotein I: Accumulation of a glycoprotein on the outer surface of mouse LS cells during mitosis. *J. Supramol. Struct.,* 1:1-7.
2. Buck, C. A., and Warren, L. (1976): The repair of the surface structure of animal cells. *J. Cell Physiol.,* 89:187-200.
3. Garfield, R. E., Chacko, S., and Blose, S. (1975): Phagocytosis by muscle cells. *Lab. Invest.,* 33:418-427.

4. Grinnell, F., Tobleman, M. Q., and Hakhenbrock, C. R. (1975): The distribution and mobility of anionic sites on the surfaces of baby hamster kidney cells. *J. Cell Biol.,* 66:470-479.
5. Gros, D., and Challice, C. E. (1975): The coating of mouse myocardial cells. A cytochemical electron microscopical study. *J. Histochem. Cytochem.,* 23:727-744.
6. Gros, D., Mocquard, J.-P., Challice, C. E., and Schiével, J. (1975): Evolution de la surface des cellules myocardiques de la souris au cours de l'ontogenèse. *J. de Microscopie,* 23:249-270.
7. Horres, C. R., Lieberman, M., and Purdy, J. E. (1977): Growth orientation of heart cells on nylon monofilaments. *J. Memb. Biol.,* 34:313-329.
8. Kapeller, M., Gal-Oz, R., Grover, N. B., and Doljanski, F. (1973): Natural shedding of carbohydrate-containing macromolecules from cell surface. *Exp. Cell Res.,* 79:152-158.
9. Manasek, F. J. (1975): The extracellular matrix of the early embryonic heart. In: *Developmental and Physiological Correlates of Cardiac Muscle,* edited by M. Lieberman and T. Sano, pp. 1-20. Raven Press, New York.
10. Manasek, F. J. (1976): Macromolecules of the extracellular compartment of embryonic and mature heart. *Circ. Res.,* 38:331-337.
11. Manasek, F. J., and Cohen, A. (1977): Anionic glycopeptides and glycosaminoglycans synthesized by embryonic neural tube and neural crest. *Proc. Natl. Acad. Sci. USA,* 74:1057-1061.
12. Markwald, R. R., and Fitzharris, T. P. (1977): Structural analysis of endocardial cushion tissue development. *Am. J. Anat.,* 148:85-120.
13. Markwald, R. R., Fitzharris, T. P., Bolender, D. L., and Bernanke, D. H. (1979): Structural analysis of cell:matrix association during the morphogenesis of atrioventricular cushion tissue. *Dev. Biol.,* 69:634-654.
14. Patten, B. M., Kramer, T. C., and Barry, A. (1948): Valvular action in the embryonic chick heart by localized apposition of endocardial masses. *Anat. Rec.,* 102:299-311.
15. Satow, Y., and Manasek, F. J. (1977): Direct effects of trypan blue on cardiac extracellular macromolecule synthesis. *Lab. Invest.,* 36:100-105.

DISCUSSION

De Haan: Is Peak B of smaller molecular weight than Peak A?

Manasek: It elutes on the basis of its charge; it is slightly more negatively charged. It is very difficult to size.

De Haan: When you challenge your washed cells with conditioned medium, they do not release Peak B?

Manasek: That is correct.

De Haan: When you challenge them with non-conditioned medium they release Peak B and clear it. Why do they not respond to the cleared medium as if it were non-conditioned medium?

Manasek: Peak B may not be the stimulus. Peak B may be a response to another stimulus, which might be mucopolysaccharide content. We do not know what the stimulus is.

Markwald: Could not a factor in the serum, which is used up in the conditioned medium, represent an alternative to matrix feedback? An antigen glycoprotein over which we have no control?

Manasek: Yes, that is very true, but the point is that the cells respond to a change in environment by altering what they do with their matrix molecules.

Fischman: Do you consider these proteins integral membrane proteins, or are they part of some glycocalyx outside the cell?

Manasek: They are probably part of the glycocalyx; the trypsin treatment removes them. What we have seen is probably turnover of the glycocalyx. There was a difference between surface material and medium material. It is not simply a shedding.

De Vries: Did you detect any hyaluronate in the matrix? Have you done any work on the sol–gel relationship of different glycoproteins in the fusion of various cushions?

Manasek: No, I have not. We did some experiments with Dr. Nakamura with native cardiac jelly. It retains the shape of the heart even in the absence of cells.

Perspectives in Cardiovascular Research, Vol. 5,
Mechanisms of Cardiac Morphogenesis and Teratogenesis,
edited by Tomas Pexieder. Raven Press, New York © 1981

Localization of Fucose-Containing Substances in Developing Atrioventricular Cushion Tissue

*Don A. Hay and **Roger R. Markwald

*Department of Anatomy, The University of New Mexico School of Medicine, Albuquerque, New Mexico 87131 and **Department of Anatomy, Texas Tech University School of Medicine, Lubbock, Texas 79049*

Between 3 and 6 days of incubation (Hamburger–Hamilton stages 19 to 28) (6), the atrioventricular (AV) canal of the embryonic chick heart is the site of progressive development of gelatinous swellings termed endocardial cushions. At three days of incubation (stage 19), the presumptive AV region of the simple tubular heart is comprised of a luminal layer of cells (endocardium), an intermediate, acellular zone of extracellular matrix (cardiac jelly), and an outer peripheral layer of muscle (myocardium). Eventually, the cardiac jelly becomes populated with mesenchymal-like cells termed cushion tissue (CT) cells, which originate by delamination from the endocardium (21,22,28). The CT cells subsequently migrate through the cardiac jelly to the periphery of cushion, where they contact the myocardium and thus contribute to the formation of dorsal and ventral cushion pads. The cushions progressively enlarge, approach one another, and finally fuse during stages 27 to 28 (7,8,12). One significance of the cushion tissues is that they contribute to the septum intermedium, an integral portion of the membranous interventricular (IV) septum. Maldevelopment of cushion tissue can thus contribute to an IV septal defect or an AV valvular defect (32).

The factors responsible for regulating CT morphogenetic events have not been determined. However, most CT activities occur in close association with extracellular macromolecules identified as glycosaminoglycans (GAG), protein-polysaccharides, and collagen (22,23,24). Modifications in the composition and structural ordering of these macromolecules accompany changing CT cell migratory or secretory activities and are thus suggestive of potential causal interrelationships. This supposition is consistent with recent studies reporting that extracellular macromolecules may mediate genetic expression in morphogenesis (31).

---

* *Present address:* Department of Anatomy, The University of Florida College of Medicine, Gainesville, Florida 32610.

GAG and collagen have such limited molecular heterogeneity and are so ubiquitously distributed that it is likely that these substances provide only general regulative information, e.g., a motility or mitotic stimulus, and do not provide a tissue-specific stimulant that might selectively direct the formation of cushion tissue (14). Manasek (15,17,18) has recently identified extracellular glycoprotein (GP) in the cardiac jelly of early embryonic hearts, stages 12 to 14. Because of its greater molecular heterogeneity, GP would be a better candidate for such a tissue-specific stimulant. It remains to be determined whether or not GP is also present in cardiac jelly during CT formation and, if so, what its sources are and how it is assembled into the matrix. Using structural methods including ^{3}H-fucose radioautography, we present data that indicate GP is secreted into cardiac jelly during CT cell migration from three potential sources, and that it is structurally associated with both GAG and collagen-like microfibrils.

MATERIALS AND METHODS

Transmission Electron Microscopy

Excised hearts from 3.5- to 5.5-day chick embryos (stages 21 to 27) were immersed in 2% glutaraldehyde in 0.065 M cacodylate buffer, pH 7.2 to 7.4, containing 1% tannic acid for 2 hours at room temperature. Tissues were subsequently rinsed and osmicated in buffered 2% OsO_4 containing tannic acid. A V canals were isolated by microdissection, dehydrated, and embedded in Epon 812 by a routine procedure (21). Thin and thick (0.5 to 1.0 μ) sections were obtained using a Porter-Blum ultramicrotome, stained with uranyl acetate (UA) and lead citrate (LC), and examined in a Zeiss 10 electron microscope operated at 60 KV or in a JEOL 1000 high-voltage electron microscope (High Voltage EM Laboratory, Boulder, Colorado).

To remove GP and any associated matrix, excised AV canals fixed in glutaraldehyde/tannic acid were treated with a 100 μg trypsin/ml in 0.1 M phosphate buffer or 50 μg/ml testicular hyaluronidase (Sigma Type I) in 0.1 M sodium potassium, phosphate buffer, pH 5.5 for 10 minutes to 1 hour at 37°C in a gassed shaker water bath. Controls were incubated in buffer alone. Protease activity of the hyaluronidase was previously tested and found to have less than 0.5% of the proteolytic activity of trypsin (23). After incubation, specimens were rinsed, osmicated, and prepared for Epon embedment, as described above.

Scanning Electron Microscopy

Specimens for scanning electron microscopy (SEM) were fixed as described above in glutaraldehyde/tannic acid, postfixed in osmium, dehydrated in graded ethanols, transferred in absolute ethanol to a critical point dryer, and dried in liquid CO_2. Dried hearts were microdissected, using glass needles, to expose the interior of cushion pads, mounted on aluminum studs, coated with gold–

palladium in a Geico (Hitachi) sputter-coater, and examined in a Hitachi S500 SEM operated at 25 KV.

Radioautography

Three groups of embryos (3 per group) were incubated at 3.5, 4.5, and 5.5 days, respectively. Each embryo was given a single dose of 400 μCi of L-(^{3}H) fucose (12.06 Ci/mM; New England Nuclear) by dripping the isotope solution directly on the embryo and continuing incubation for 3 hours. The embryos were removed, placed in petri dishes containing 37°C Tyrode's buffer (pH 7.3), washed thoroughly, and staged (stages 21, 24, 25, and 27). Several milliliters of fresh Tyrode's buffer were microperfused through the common cardinal vein prior to perfusion with Tyrode's solution containing 2.5% glutaraldehyde (pH 7.3). Hearts were excised and placed in fresh fixer at room temperature for 2.5 hours. After buffer rinsing and post-fixation in cacodylate buffered 2% OsO_4 (1.5 hours), the hearts were immersed in 1% tannic acid for 30 minutes (30). After rinsing in 1% sodium sulfate, each heart was stained *en bloc* with saturated UA, dehydrated in graded ethanols, and embedded in Epon 812. Hearts taken from embryos not exposed to ^{3}H-fucose were prepared as described above and were used as method controls.

For light microscopic radioautography, 1.0 μm thick sections were cut and coated with full-strength Kodak NTB2 emulsion. For electron microscopic radioautography, gold sections were placed on both formvar-coated and uncoated grids and covered with Ilford L-4 emulsion diluted 1:2 with deionized water, using Caro's (2) loop technique. After suitable exposure (2 weeks for thick sections, 5 weeks for thin sections), the emulsions were developed using D19. The thick sections were stained in methylene blue–Azure II, while grids were stained with UA and LC. The radioautographs were examined in a Phillips 200 electron microscope operated at 60KV.

RESULTS

Normal Morphologic Observations

A representative light microscopic cross-section of the AV canal region is shown in Fig. 1a. At all stages examined, each cushion tissue pad displayed migrating cushion tissue cells at variable distances from the progenitive endocardium.

After fixation in glutaraldehyde/tannic acid, a major non-microfibrillar component of the cardiac jelly was an amorphous deposit of variable extent and density. In both colonized (postmigratory) and non-colonized (premigratory) matrix, this electron-dense component was most frequently localized into small foci, forming a centroid from which radiated 5 to 10 nm filaments and low-density, wispy material (Fig. 1b,c). This association of low- and high-density materials occurred free in the matrix space or superimposed upon microfibrils (Fig. 1b). Isolated electron-dense amorphous foci were also deposited irregularly

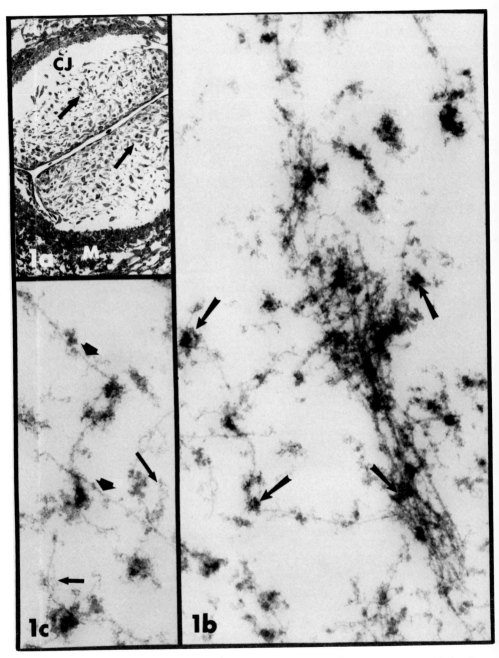

FIG. 1. a: Cross-section through the AV canal showing both cushion pads at stage 23. In all stages studied, cushion cells *(arrows)* were present in the cardiac jelly (CJ); (M) myocardium. **b:** Cardiac jelly fixed in glutaraldehyde/tannic acid. Note the electron-dense foci *(arrows)* from which extend low-density, wispy material and 5–10 nm filaments. **c:** Higher magnification of dense material with associated low-density material *(thin arrows)* and 5–10 nm filaments *(short arrows)*. (a) × 150; (b) × 30,000; (c) × 45,000.

upon individual microfibrils or along the course of microfibrillar bundles (Fig. 1 and 2). In addition, large, more attenuated ribbon-like deposits of highly electron-dense material were observed, particularly in premigratory matrix. In high voltage EM, a fibrillar substructure was evident in some portions of this material. Highly structured, banded, and unbanded microfibrils coated with low-density, granular substances contacted or permeated this material (Fig. 3). The motility processes of migrating cushion cells were usually in direct association with some form of the electron-dense amorphous material (Fig. 4).

Treatment with testicular hyaluronidase did not degrade any of the electron-dense components but removed the 5 to 10 nm filaments and the low-density material associated with the central foci of electron-dense matrix (Fig. 5).

Short-term (10 to 30 minutes) trypsin digestion also removed the same material as degraded by testicular hyaluronidase (Fig. 6). Longer trypsin digestion (30 minutes to 1 hour) removed all matrix components except banded microfibrils (Fig. 7).

Radioautographic Observations

Fucose label was found distributed throughout the cushion pad of all stages examined, both in the extracellular matrix and within all cell types (Fig. 8 through 13). When the various cell types were visually compared for differences in label incorporation, the myocardium from each period appeared most active (Fig. 10,12,13). Although silver grains were not evenly dispersed within the matrix, there appeared to be no particular regional concentration. Indeed, even the extracellular matrix between myocardial cells exhibited little additional accumulation of label and was frequently devoid of label (Fig. 10,12,13).

In the AV cushion matrix, fucose uptake occurred primarily in trypsin-sensitive, amorphous, electron-dense components at all stages examined (Fig. 14 through 16). However, some grains occurred over the low-density filamentous components associated with the dense matrical material, over unbanded or irregularly banded microfibrils, or over areas devoid of any visible structure (Figures 14 through 16).

DISCUSSION

In recent years, considerable emphasis has been placed upon cardiac extracellular matrix and upon the identification of matrical components. This is the result of increasing evidence that the extracellular macromolecules may act as "biological stimulants" mediating genetic expression in tissue interactions (9,11,14,29). Type I collagen (10) and GAG, such as hyaluronate (19,20,26), chondroitin sulfate (4,5,19,20,27), and heparin/heparan sulfate (4,5,19) have been identified in cardiac jelly. In cushion tissue morphogenesis, roles have been proposed for some of these macromolecules in contact guidance, motility activation, and cytodifferentiation (22). Recently, Manasek (15,17) reported the presence of

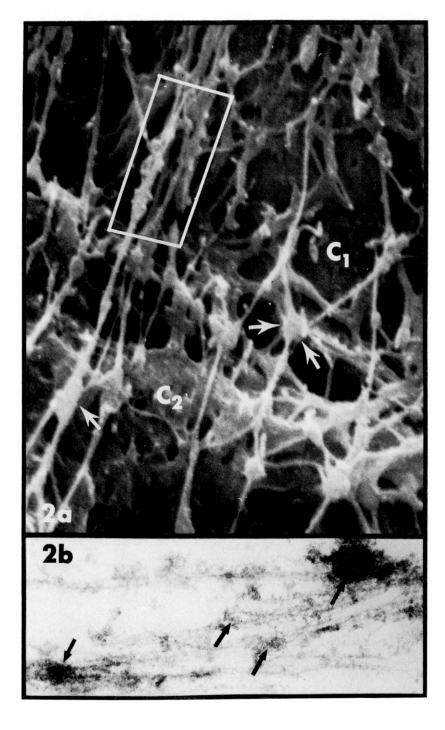

GP in early embryonic cardiac matrix. The potential of GP for greater molecular heterogeneity than that offered by either collagen or GAG raises the possibility that GP may function as a tissue-specific extracellular stimulant. Thus, one significance of our demonstration of extracellular fucose-containing material in direct structural association with CT cells is that it identifies an extracellular component that could initiate the morphogenetic events leading to CT formation in specific regions (AV canal and bulbus cordis) of the heart (21).

Without chemical analysis, the uptake of ^{3}H-fucose into cushion constituents, as demonstrated by our morphologic techniques, does not obligatorily prove GP composition, although for other tissues, previous workers have indicated such proof (1,3). Manasek's biochemical studies (15,18) of fucose macromolecules separated by pronase digestion and elution on Sephadex G-50 columns from embryonic chick hearts during an age range encompassing our study (3 to 18 days) strongly suggest that the cardiac jelly material labeled with fucose contains GP.

The principal matrical constituent labeled with ^{3}H-fucose in this study was trypsin-sensitive, amorphous, electron-dense material which closely resembled interstitial bodies described by Low (13). Identification of this component as GP is particularly relevant to the unidentified mechanisms by which individual cardiac matrix molecules (collagen, GAG, etc.) are integrated into specific structural associations (23). These complex macromolecular orderings endow cardiac jelly with the capacity to retain its shape even after removal of its epithelial coverings, and to reversibly expand and contract in response to changes in ionic strength (24,25). Extracellular glycoproteins are the logical choice for promoting macromolecular ordering in cardiac jelly, since they both covalently and non-covalently interact with GAG to form large macromolecular aggregates (18). Our morphological data support Manasek's biochemical observations (18) by demonstrating that ^{3}H-fucose is incorporated into material structurally interfaced to testicular hyaluronidase-sensitive substances visualized by the mordant action of tannic acid (30). Presumably, one or more of these components, either the 5 to 10 nm filaments or associated low-density material, is GAG. Since brief trypsin treatment also removed hyaluronidase-sensitive material, it is likely that these components are covalently linked to glycoprotein, which probably retards their dissolution. In a related study (23) of cardiac jelly using cetylpyridinium chloride to minimize GAG dissolution in aqueous fixatives, electron-dense amorphous material similar to that observed in this study was linked to 3 nm filaments identified as hyaluronate, and granules (not readily seen after glutaraldehyde/tannic acid fixation) identified as chondroitin sulfate-protein.

FIG. 2. (a): SEM of matrix corresponding to Fig. 1b. Microfibrils are irregularly studded with an amorphous substance *(small arrows)* correlating with electron-dense material, as seen in HVEM. Motility processes from two cushion cells (C_1, C_2) are enmeshed with matrix similar to that seen in Fig. 1c. **b:** HVEM of matrix equivalent to that enclosed within the box of Fig. 2a. Arrows denote the frequent association of electron-dense material with 20–40 nm collagen-like microfibrils. (a) × 51,200; (b) × 36,000.

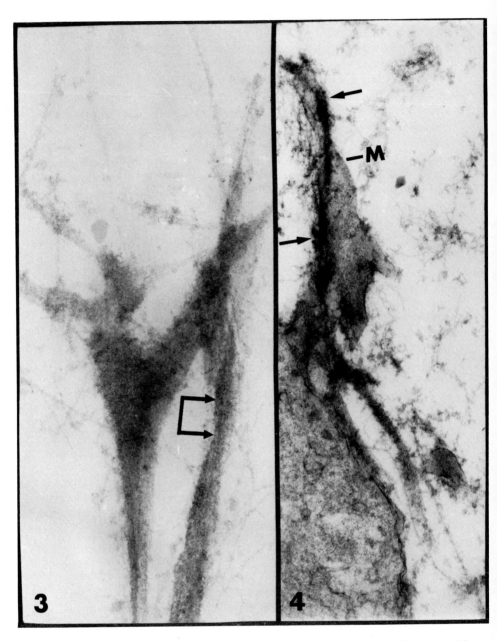

FIG. 3. HVEM. This electron-dense component has a fibrillar substructure *(arrows)* and is organized into elongated strands. Note that 20–40 nm microfibrils contact or permeate the dense strands (× 36,000).

FIG. 4. HVEM. A motility appendage (M) from a migrating cushion cell is in direct structural contact *(arrows)* with the variable forms of the electron-dense component (× 22,800).

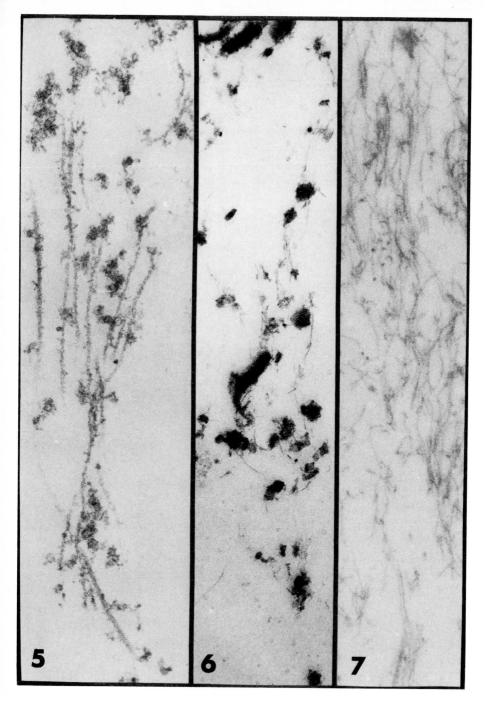

FIG. 5. TEM of testicular hyaluronidase-treated matrix. Note the low-density material and 5–10 nm filaments are removed. The electron-dense material and punctate deposits on the microfibrils persist (× 90,000).

FIG. 6. Brief (10–30 min) trypsin treatment. As in Fig. 5, components (especially the low density material) associated with the dense foci are removed (× 116,000).

FIG. 7. Trypsin treatment for 30–60 min. Note that most electron-dense material and all associated components are removed, leaving only 20–40 nm collagen-like microfibrils usually collapsed upon cell surfaces (× 48,000).

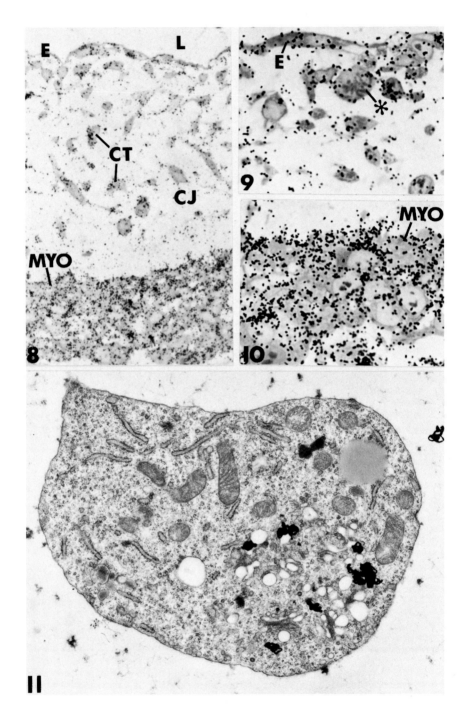

Fucose-labeled electron-dense components were also observed, morphologically associated with collagen-like microfibrils. This association suggests that a fucosylated GP with collagen-binding properties is secreted into cardiac jelly. The migration of AV cushion cells is accompanied by progressive alignment of randomized microfibrils into polarized matrical bundles or tracks, utilized as a migratory template (24). If the source of this collagen binding-associated glycoprotein is the migrating CT cells themselves, this could explain the alteration in spatial orientation of premigratory microfibrils accompanying CT cell migration. Alternatively, the collagen-associated GP may facilitate cell attachment to the microfibrils. Work is currently in progress to determine if fibronectin, a fucosylated collagen-binding glycoprotein (33), is present in cardiac jelly.

Three potential sources of fucosylated GP were identified: endocardium, myocardium, and migrating cushion cells. However, it is not possible using radioautographic data, even if pulse studies had been done, to establish conclusively which cells actually released the labeled material into cardiac jelly. Potentially, some or all of the labeled material localized in Golgi apparati and secretory vesicles could be destined for incorporation into the cell surface, rather than actually being released into the matrix. This appeared to be the case with the myocardium. Prior to cushion tissue formation (stages 12 to 14), the myocardium was the principal source of cardiac jelly GP (16,17), but after CT formation (stage 21), most myocardially incorporated label was localized at cell surfaces. Cardiac jelly contiguous with the myocardium exhibited no gradient of labeled material and, even after a 3-hour labeling period, was often devoid of label. This suggests a shift in myocardial production of GP from one of extracellular release to one of intracellular (cell surface) utilization. Finally, while the myocardium visually appeared to be the most heavily labeled cell type, quantitative comparisons (e.g., by grain counting) would be meaningless, since the endogenous pool sizes for fucose are unknown (14). Lectin tracers may clarify cellular origins of extracellular glycoprotein if the latter are found to be heterogenous in composition.

FIG. 8–10. Light microscopic radioautographs of ^{3}H-fucose incorporation in the AV cushions at stage 21 (3.5 days). Silver grains *(black dots)* are distributed within each cell type (endocardium, E; cushion tissue cells, CT; myocardium, MYO), as well as within the cardiac jelly (CJ). In Fig. 9, a labeled CT cell is undergoing mitosis *(asterisk)*. Note the dense population of grains over the myocardial cells, but no noticeable accumulation of silver grains in the matrix adjacent to the myocardium. Heart lumen (L), Fig. 8, × 500; Fig. 9, × 1,100; Fig. 10, × 1,200.

FIG. 11.* Cushion cell, stage 21. ^{3}H-fucose incorporation is commonly observed in Golgi complexes and related vesicles (× 14,500).

* Fig. 11 and 14 originally appeared in Hay, D. A.: Development and fusion of the endocardial cushions. In: *"Morphogenesis and Malformation of the Cardiovascular System."* edited by G. C. Rosenquist and D. Bergsma New York: Alan R. Liss for The National Foundation—March of Dimes, BD:OAS XIV(7), 1978.

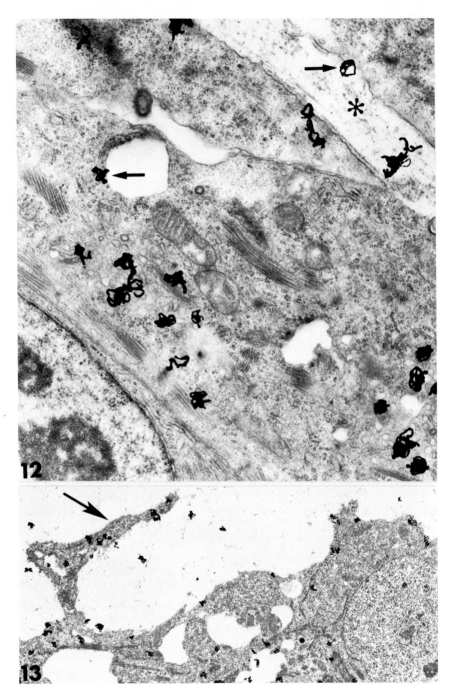

FIG. 12. Myocardial cells, stage 21. Heavy labeling is noted throughout the myocardium at this stage, particularly in Golgi complexes (microvesicles) and at the cell periphery *(arrows)*. A smaller amount of label is found in the surrounding extracellular matrix *(asterisk)* ($\times$ 20,500).

FIG. 13. Myocardium at junction of cushion matrix, stage 25. ^{3}H-fucose labeling is frequently concentrated in cellular processes *(arrow)*. The label is heavy over plasmalemmae, but relatively sparse over the myocardial basal lamina and adjacent cardiac jelly ($\times$ 4,800).

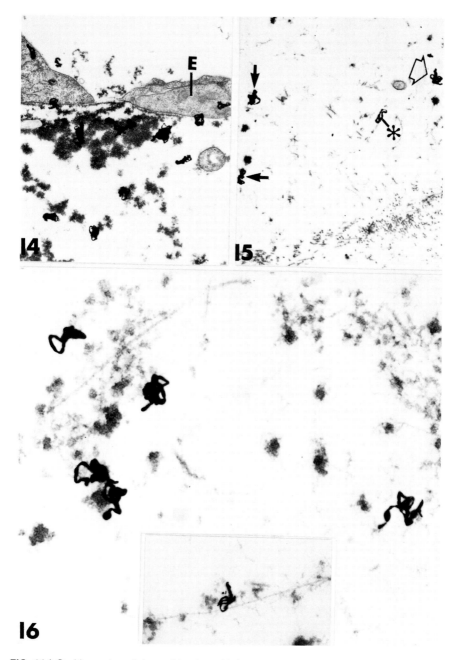

FIG. 14.* Cushion extracellular matrix, stage 21. Large aggregates of electron-dense material just beneath the endocardium (E) are heavily labeled (× 12,000).

FIG. 15 and 16. Extracellular matrix, stage 21. The distribution and density of labeling within cushion cardiac jelly varies from one region to another with no noticeable pattern. In Fig. 15, electron-dense clusters *(arrows),* the 5–10 nm filamentous material *(clear arrow)* and an electron lucent area *(asterisk)* are labeled. In Fig. 16, most of the labeling is confined to electron-dense aggregates. Inset: a collagenous-like microfibril is in direct contact with labeled electron-dense material. Fig. 15, × 13,500; Fig. 16, × 29,500. Inset, × 37,000.

To summarize, the secretion of fucosylated glycoproteins into cardiac jelly could serve either to act as a catalyst for matrix maturation, i.e., to modify or coordinate post-translational self-assembly or integrative qualities (14), or to provide "tissue-specific" cues for CT formation.

ACKNOWLEDGMENTS

The authors are grateful to Dr. Frank Manasek for helpful discussions, to Patricia Cooper, Ann Munger, and Jayne Krook for their valuable technical assistance, and to Cecile Bishop for typing the manuscript. Support was provided, in part, by grants-in-aid from the Wisconsin Heart Association, the University of Wisconsin–Stevens Point Foundation, NIH Grant #HL-19136, and a NIH travel grant to the High-Voltage Electron Microscopy Laboratory, Boulder, Colorado.

REFERENCES

1. Bekesi, J. G., and Winzler, R. J. (1967): The metabolism of plasma glycoproteins. Studies on the incorporation of L-fucose-1-14-C into tissue and serum in the normal rat. *J. Biol. Chem.*, 242:3873-3879.
2. Caro, L. G. (1969): A common source of difficulty in high-resolution radioautography. *J. Cell Biol.*, 41:918-919.
3. Coffey, J. W., Miller, O. N., and Sellinger, O. Z. (1964): The metabolism of L-fucose in the rat. *J. Biol. Chem.*, 239:4011-4017.
4. Gessner, I. H., Lorincz, A. E., and Bostrom, H. (1965): Acid mucopolysaccharide content of the cardiac jelly of the chick embryo. *J. Exp. Zool.*, 160:291-298.
5. Gessner, I. H., and Bostrom, H. (1965): In vitro studies on ^{35}S-sulfate incorporation into the acid mucopolysaccharides of chick embryo cardiac jelly. *J. Exp. Zool.*, 160:283-290.
6. Hamburger, V., and Hamilton, H. L. (1951): A series of normal stages in the development of the chick embryo. *J. Morph.*, 88:49-92.
7. Hay, D. A., and Low, F. N. (1972): The fusion of dorsal and ventral endocardial cushions in the embryonic chick heart: A study in fine structure. *Am. J. Anat.*, 133:1-24.
8. Hay, D. A. (1978): Development and fusion of the endocardial cushions. In: *Birth Defects: Original Article Series*, Vol. XIV, No. 7, edited by G. C. Rosenquist and D. Bergsma, pp. 69-90. Alan R. Liss, Inc., New York.
9. Hay, E. D. (1977): Cell-matrix interaction in embryonic induction. In: *International Cell Biology 1976–1977*, edited by B. R. Brinkley and K. R. Porter. Rockefeller University Press, New York.
10. Johnson, R. C., Manasek, F. J., Vinson, W. C., and Seyer, J. M. (1974): The biochemical and ultrastructural demonstration of collagen during early heart development. *Dev. Biol.*, 36:252-271.
11. Lash, J. W., and Vasan, M. S. (1977): Tissue interactions and extracellular matrix components. In: *Cell and Tissue Interactions*, edited by J. W. Lash and M. M. Burger, pp. 101-114. Raven Press, New York.
12. Los, J. A., and van Eijndthoven, E. (1973): The fusion of the endocardial cushions in the heart of the chick embryo. *Z. Anat. Entwickl.-Gesch.*, 141:55-75.
13. Low, F. N. (1970): Interstitial bodies in the early chick embryo. *Am. J. Anat.*, 128:45-56.
14. Manasek, F. J. (1975): The extracellular matrix: A dynamic component of the developing embryo. In: *Current Topics in Developmental Biology*, Vol. 10, edited by A. A. Moscona and A. Monroy, pp. 35-102. Academic Press, New York.
15. Manasek, F. J. (1976): Glycoprotein synthesis and tissue interactions during establishment of the functional embryonic chick heart. *J. Mol. Cell Cardiol.*, 8:389-402.
16. Manasek, F. J. (1976): Heart development: Interactions involved in cardiac morphogenesis.

In: *The Cell Surface in Animal Embryogenesis and Development,* edited by G. Poste and G. L. Nicholson, pp. 545-598. Elsevier-North Holland, Amsterdam.

17. Manasek, F. J. (1976): The extracellular matrix of the early embryonic heart. In: *Developmental and Physiological Correlates of Cardiac Muscle,* edited by M. Lieberman and T. Sano, pp. 1-20. Raven Press, New York.

18. Manasek, F. J. (1977): Structural glycoproteins of the embryonic cardiac extracellular matrix. *J. Mol. Cell Cardiol.,* 9:425-439.

19. Manasek, F. J., Reid, M., Vinson, W., and Johnson, R. (1973): Glycosaminoglycan synthesis by the early embryonic chick heart. *Dev. Biol.,* 35:332-348.

20. Markwald, R. R., and Adams Smith, W. M. (1972): Distribution of mucosubstances in the developing rat heart. *J. Histochem. Cytochem.,* 20:896-907.

21. Markwald, R. R., Fitzharris, T. P., and Adams Smith, W. N. (1975): Structural analysis of endocardial cytodifferentiation. *Dev. Biol.,* 42:160-180.

22. Markwald, R. R., Fitzharris, T. P., and Manasek, F. J. (1977): Structural development of endocardial cushions. *Am. J. Anat.,* 148:85-120.

23. Markwald, R. R., Fitzharris, T. P., Bank, H., and Bernanke, D. H. (1978): Structural analyses on the matrical organization of glycosaminoglycans in developing endocardial cushions. *Dev. Biol.,* 62:292-316.

24. Markwald, R. R., Fitzharris, T. P., Bolender, D. L., and Bernanke, D. H. (1979): Structural analysis of cell: Matrix association during the morphogenesis of atrioventricular cushion tissue. *Dev. Biol.,* 69:634-654.

25. Nakamura, A., and Manasek, F. J. (1978): Experimental studies of the shape and structure of isolated cardiac jelly. *J. Embryol. Exp. Morph.,* 43:167-183.

26. Orkin, R. W., and Toole, B. P. (1978): Hyaluronidase activity and hyaluronate content of the developing chick embryo heart. *Dev. Biol.,* 66:308-320.

27. Ortiz, E. C. (1958): Estudio histoquimico de la gelatina cardiaca en el embryion de pollo. *Arch. Inst. Cardiol. Mex.,* 28:244-262.

28. Patten, B. M., Kramer, T. C., and Barry, A. (1948): Valvular action in the embryonic chick heart by localized apposition of endocardial masses. *Anat. Rec.,* 102:299-312.

29. Reddi, A. H. (1976): Collagen and cell differentiation. In: *Biochemistry of Collagen,* edited by G. N. Ramachandran and A. H. Reddi, pp. 449-478. Plenum Publishing Corp., New York.

30. Simionescu, N., and Simionescu, M. (1976): Galloylglucoses of low molecular weight as mordant in electron microscopy. I. Procedure and evidence for mordanting effect. *J. Cell Biol.,* 70:608-621.

31. Slavkin, H. C., and Greulich, R. C. (1975): *Extracellular Matrix Influence on Gene Expression.* Academic Press, New York.

32. Van Mierop, L. H. S., Alley, R. D., Kausel, H. W., and Stranahan, A. (1962): The anatomy and embryology of endocardial cushion defects. *J. Thorac. Cardiovasc. Surg.,* 43:71-96.

33. Yamada, K. M., Hahn, L. E., Olden, K. (1979): Structure and function of the fibronectins. *J. Supramol. Structure,* Suppl. 3:413.

DISCUSSION

Fischman: Did you try to do any pulse-chase experiments?

Hay: Yes, in pilot studies. This particular one was ³H-labeling, as we were primarily interested in which cells incorporate fucose and where it can be found in the matrix.

Fischman: In view of Dr. Manasek's findings on the turnover of glycopeptides, I feel concerned with the problem of fucose reutilization.

Hay: I did an experiment in which the tissue was incubated with fucose for 30, 60, and 90 minutes. There was a basically similar distribution over the Golgi zone, cell surface, and in the matrix. Only the amount of silver grains increased.

Perspectives in Cardiovascular Research, Vol. 5,
Mechanisms of Cardiac Morphogenesis and Teratogenesis,
edited by Tomas Pexieder. Raven Press, New York © 1981

Localization of Collagen Types in the Embryonic Heart and Aorta Using Immunohistochemistry

Mary J. C. Hendrix

Department of Anatomy, Harvard Medical School, Boston, Massachusetts 02115

It is well known that deviations occurring during cardiac morphogenesis critically affect the connective tissue component of the extracellular matrix. To facilitate a better understanding of birth defects in this area, it is essential that the constituents of this functionally important compartment be identified morphologically and biochemically, and that these approaches be correlated by immunohistochemistry and other cytochemical methods.

Collagen, the most common protein of many different connective tissues, occurs in vertebrates in the form of at least five, and probably more, genetically distinct molecules (7,24,30). Type I collagen, initially found in bone and skin, occurs as a major or minor constituent of most embryonic and adult connective tissues. Type II collagen has been isolated from cartilage by Miller and Matukas (25), from notochord by Linsenmayer et al. (14), from vitreous by Swann et al. (35), Newsome et al. (29), and Smith et al. (33), and from the primary embryonic chick corneal stroma by Linsenmayer et al. (15). Type III collagen has been detected in skin, blood vessels, and other tissues containing reticular fibers (24), and type IV collagen occurs in basement membranes (7,12). A new collagen, designated AB_2, has recently been isolated and characterized from basement membranes by Chung et al. (4), and from various embryonic muscles by von der Mark and von der Mark (41).

During development of the embryonic heart, several events occur involving the formation and remodeling of the extracellular matrix. A compartment of extracellular matrix, known as cardiac jelly, separates the outer developing myocardium from the inner endocardium. This specialized compartment has been shown to contain glycosaminoglycans, hyaluronate, chondroitin sulfate, type I-like collagen, and other glycoproteins (18–21). Development of the collagenous framework in the avian heart has been analyzed using hydroxyproline assays by Woessner et al. (42), who suggested that the increasing proportion of collagen in the growing heart was related to the increasing mechanical strength of the heart.

Many studies have dealt with collagen and its significance in aging myocardium with respect to cardiac disease. Many discrepancies exist in the literature concerning this topic. Lenkiewicz and associates (13) suggest that collagen does increase with age, but only in the subendocardial and subepicardial zones. Mohan and Radha (27) reported an accumulation of insoluble collagen and a decrease in salt-extractable collagen in aging cardiac muscle. By hydroxyproline assay, it has been estimated that the concentration of collagen is higher in the right ventricle than in the left ventricle in the normal heart (3,5). Ventricular hypertrophy is accompanied by an increase in the total mass of collagen, but age has no effect on ventricular concentration of collagen.

More recently, several pathological disorders involving collagen biosynthesis and/or malformation have received considerable attention. Iwatsuki et al. (9) showed that collagen synthesis and deposition are increased in arteries, where blood pressure is elevated, but not in veins, where pressure is only slightly elevated. Some of the disorders characterizing Hurler's syndrome are cardiovascular lesions, including cardiac valvular deformities. It has been postulated that elevated levels of dermatan sulfate in Hurler's syndrome lead to an abnormally high synthesis of collagen and to its polymerization in intracellular loci (31). As a final example of collagen involvement in cardiac pathology, there have been experiments that showed an increase in myocardial hydroxyproline during myocardial infarction (11).

Within the past five years, investigators have begun to isolate more than one collagen type in the heart using carboxymethyl-cellulose chromatography, cyanogen bromide cleavage with fractional salt separation, and SDS-gel electrophoresis. Bovine cardiac muscle collagen has been characterized as consisting of both types I and III (23,28). Mannschott and associates (22) reported the presence of types I and III collagen in pig heart valves. Using immunohistochemistry, Bashey et al. (2) also identified types I and III collagen in bovine heart valve.

Recent investigations by von der Mark et al. (38-40) have utilized rhodamine- and fluoresceine-conjugated antibodies and immunofluorescence for the localization of collagens in tissues, and have confirmed and extended biochemical studies of the distribution of collagens, especially in embryonic avian tissues. It is of considerable interest to compare avian cardiac development with morphogenesis of the other embryonic tissues that have already been studied biochemically and by immunofluorescence. We will also compare avian tissues with human and other mammalian tissues because of the possible existence of species differences in collagen distribution. Using rhodamine- and ferritin-conjugated collagen antibodies, we hope to gain some understanding of the distribution and developmental significance of the many different genetically determined collagen types in cardiac development.

MATERIALS AND METHODS

For immunohistochemical localization of collagen types, tissues were treated with antibodies using a double-layered sandwich technique as described by Sternberger (34). Hearts dissected from 12-day chick embryos of the White Leghorn strain and 16-week-old human fetuses were immersed in 1% formaldehyde fixative buffered with 0.2 N cacodylate for 30 minutes at room temperature. The tissues were rinsed extensively in phosphate-buffered saline (PBS) and free aldehyde groups were quenched overnight in 0.15 M Tris HCl, pH 7.4. For immunofluorescent studies, the tissue was quick-frozen to liquid N_2 temperature and 8 μm sections of the entire heart were cut on a cryostat, placed on albumin-coated slides, and treated with testicular hyaluronidase in PBS (4,000 U/ml) for 30 minutes at 37°C.

Subsequently, the sections were treated with one of the primary collagen antibodies, either concentrated or diluted with PBS, for 1 hour at room temperature, followed by several washes of PBS. The secondary antibody, consisting of rhodamine-conjugated IgG fraction of goat anti-rabbit IgG, rabbit anti-guinea pig IgG, or rabbit anti-goat IgG (Cappel Laboratories; diluted 4:1,500 with PBS), was reacted with the sections in the dark for 1 hour. The sections were rinsed thoroughly as before, and were then coated with glycerol:PBS (90:10) before attaching coverslips. Slides were viewed in a Zeiss photomicroscope III, using the rhodamine filter set.

For electron microscopic studies, chick hearts fixed in an identical manner were sliced into minute pieces with a razor or vibratome, treated with hyaluronidase, and then incubated 4 hours in the primary antibody at room temperature. After extensive washing at 4°C, ferritin-conjugated goat anti-rabbit IgG or rabbit anti-goat IgG (Miles Corp.; 1:50 dilution) was reacted with the tissues for another 4 hours at room temperature, followed by a 2 to 4 hour wash at 4°C. Tissues were then prepared for transmission electron microscopy by embedding in Spurr resin and thin sections were viewed in a JEOL 100B or 100S.

Primary collagen antibodies were obtained from Drs. Klaus von der Mark, Helga von der Mark, Waltraud Dessau, and Rupert Timpl (see below). Secondary antibodies were purchased from Miles Corp. and Cappel Labs. With the help of Dr. Thomas F. Linsenmayer, Developmental Biology Laboratory, Massachusetts General Hospital, the commercial preparations were further purified by ion-exchange chromatography, as described by Rikihisa et al. (32).

Controls, which are essential in evaluating the specificity of results from antigen–antibody reactions, included: (1) omitting the primary collagen antibody and treating only with the secondary ferritin conjugate to test for non-specific ferritin binding, and (2) substituting preimmune rabbit, guinea pig, or goat IgG for the primary collagen antibody, followed by treatment with the appropriate ferritin conjugate.

The preparation of the various chick collagens, the production of subsequent antibodies, and the specificity of the immunizing agents and antisera have been previously established, as indicated below.

1. Rabbit anti-Chick I	Antibodies prepared by Dr.
2. Rabbit anti-Chick II	Klaus von der Mark [Max-
3. Guinea Pig anti-Chick I	Planck-Institut für Biochemie,

4. Guinea Pig anti-Chick II   München, Germany (38)].
5. Goat anti-Chick III   Antibody prepared by Dr. Wal-
                              traud Dessau (Max-Planck-In-
                              stitut für Biochemie, München,
                              Germany).
6. Rabbit anti-Chick AB_2 Antibody prepared by Drs.
                              Helga and Klaus von der Mark
                              [Max-Planck-Institut für Bio-
                              chemie, München, Germany
                              (41)].
7. Rabbit anti-Calf I   Antibodies prepared by Dr.
8. Rabbit anti-Calf III   Rupert Timpl (Max-Planck-In-
                              stitut für Biochemie, München,
                              Germany).

RESULTS AND DISCUSSION

Immunofluorescent studies reveal that types I and III collagen occur together in the connective tissue compartments of the heart tissues and adjacent aorta from 12-day chick embryo and 16-week-old human fetus. The human fetal heart (Fig. 1e,f, 2a-c) showed a pattern of distribution of calf collagens I and III similar to that obtained with the chick collagens used for staining embryonic chick heart (Fig. 1a-d, 2d). It is of interest to note that human heart tissues did not cross-react with antibodies specific for chick collagens. Type AB_2 collagen is distributed along the surfaces of the avian cardiac muscle cells and also occurs in the extracellular spaces (Fig. 2e,f). Type II collagen is not found in chick heart tissues (Fig. 3a,b) and probably not in human. (Rabbit anti-calf collagen II is not available at this time.) All controls were negative for non-specific rhodamine staining (Fig. 3c).

At the electron microscopic level, ferritin-labeled antibodies reveal the presence of types I and III collagen primarily in striated fibrils (20 to 50 nm in diameter), as shown in Fig. 3d and 3e; however, some non-striated fibrils also labeled with anti-collagens I and III. In the aorta, type III collagen occurs not only in striated and non-striated fibrils, but also in close association with elastic laminae (Fig. 3f). The presence of AB_2 collagen is confirmed in amorphous-

---

FIG. 1. Light micrographs of sections of aorta and heart atrium (AT) and ventricle (V) from 12-day-old chick embryos and 16-week-old human fetuses, stained by the indirect immuno-fluorescence method using antibodies against chick and calf collagens followed by rhodamine-conjugated γ-globulin (diluted 4:1500). **(a)** Goat anti-chick type I collagen (0.15 mg/ml); chick aorta in close association with a portion of atrial roof (× 100). **(b)** Goat anti-chick type III collagen (0.17 mg/ml); chick aorta (× 110). **(c)** Goat anti-chick I collagen (0.15 mg/ml); chick heart. Note the staining of the connective tissue components between the atrium and ventricle (× 100). **(d)** Goat anti-chick III collagen (0.17 mg/ml); BV, blood vessels located within the chick ventricle (× 100). **(e)** Rabbit anti-calf I collagen (0.14 mg/ml); human fetal heart (× 60). **(f)** Rabbit anti-calf III collagen (0.15 mg/ml); human fetal ventricle; S, cardiac skeleton (× 60).

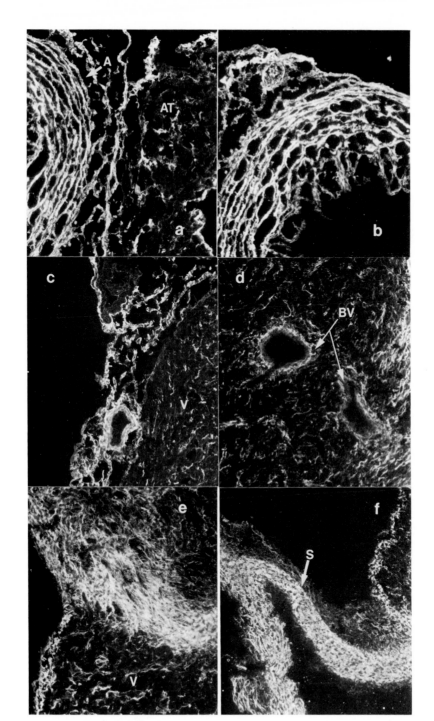

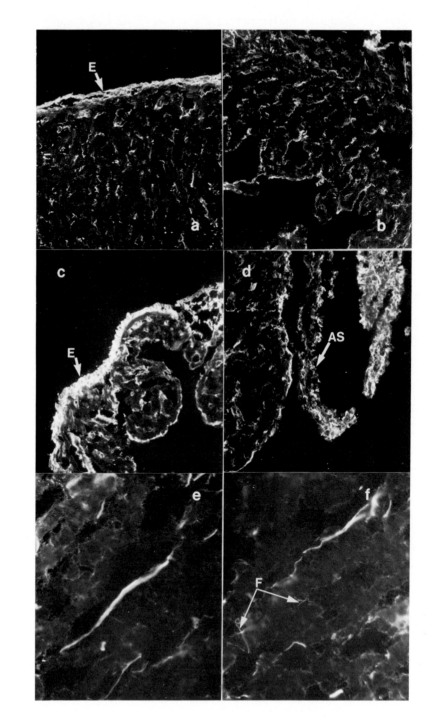

appearing matrix materials on the cell surface and in fibrils, as shown in Fig. 4. The controls were negative for non-specific ferritin labeling. At the electron microscopic level, it is clear that cardiac and vascular collagens are not confined to striated fibrils, but occur extensively throughout the matrix.

Several questions raised by this study will be the topic of subsequent experiments. One concerns the distribution of the different collagens in the early heart. Our immunohistochemical results confirm the presence of types I and III collagen in the heart, as shown biochemically by McClain (23), Mannschott et al. (22), and Bashey et al. (2), and in the aorta by Miller et al. (26) and Epstein (6). However, it is interesting to note that the biochemical findings of Johnson et al. (10) reported only type I in the very early chick embryonic heart. We will subsequently explore the possibility that type I is the first of the collagen types to appear in the developing heart. The present study concentrated only on 12-day chick embryos and 16-week-old human fetuses, in which both collagen types were clearly evident.

The coexistence of types I and III collagen in the same regions of the cardiac matrix during development is reminiscent of the distribution of two different collagen types (I and II) in the developing corneal stroma (7,8,40), and raises the possibility that one collagen fibril may contain both types of collagen. On the other hand, types I and III collagens may occur in separate fibrils that have different functions in the heart. Type I may provide tensile strength to the skeleton of the heart, whereas type III could be associated with the proteoglycan of the cardiac matrix and provide resiliency to the connective tissue compartment. It should be possible in the future to judge the relation of collagen types to each other by double-labeling experiments.

Another point of interest revolves around the synthesis of these collagen types. Most of the cardiac jelly macromolecules are synthesized by the developing myocardium (16-21). When type III appears, is it synthesized by fibroblasts? Manasek (16-21) has suggested that some of the collagen is produced by the myocardium and has shown secretory organelles within this compartment of the developing heart. Arguello et al. (1) have shown myocardial cells of the developing heart to acquire a fibroblastic phenotype. Production of extracellular macromolecules continues throughout the differentiation of the myocardium into cardiac muscle, but gradually decreases as the heart reaches maturity (21). At which stage is the production of collagen types I and III decreased? Is

---

FIG. 2. Light micrographs of sections of chick and human fetal heart, stained by the indirect immunofluorescence method using antibodies against chick and calf collagens and rhodamine-conjugated γ-globulin (diluted 4:1500). **(a)** Rabbit anti-calf I collagen (0.14 mg/ml); E, ventricular epicardium ($\times$ 60). **(b)** Rabbit anti-calf III collagen (0.15 mg/ml). Note connective tissue components of human fetal trabeculae ($\times$ 60). **(c)** Rabbit anti-calf I collagen (0.14 mg/ml); E, atrial epicardium ($\times$ 60). **(d)** Rabbit anti-chick I collagen (0.13 mg/ml); AS, atrial septum in proximity to chick ventricle ($\times$ 100). **(e)** Rabbit anti-chick AB_2 collagen (0.12 mg/ml); chick. Note stain on surfaces of cardiac muscle cells ($\times$240). **(f)** Rabbit anti-chick AB_2 collagen (0.12 mg/ml); chick; F, fibrils in the extracellular space ($\times$ 240).

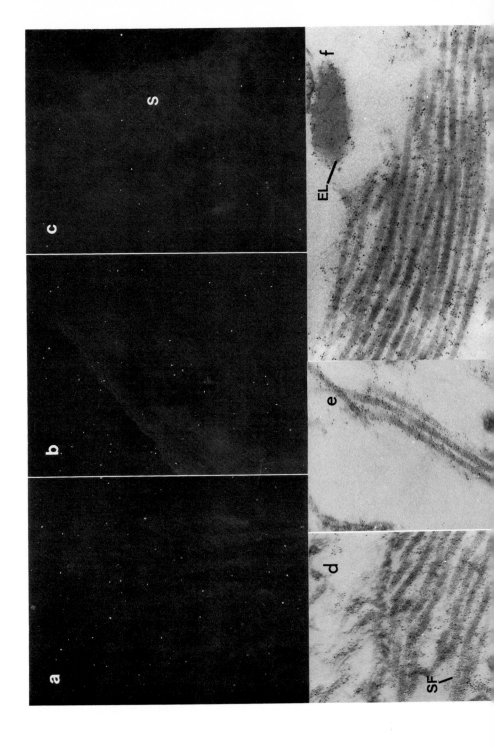

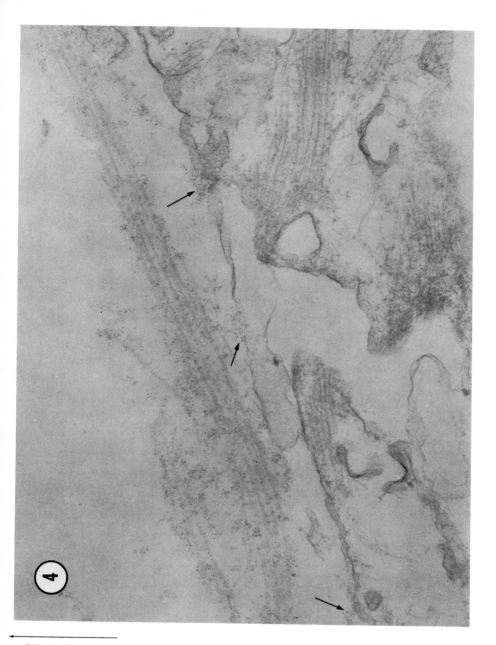

FIG. 3. Light **(a,b,c)** and electron **(d, e, f)** micrographs showing indirect immunofluorescence staining and ferritin labeling of heart tissues from chick and human fetus, using antibodies against chick and calf collagens followed by rhodamine- or ferritin-labeled IgG (rhodamine IgG diluted 4:1500; ferritin IgG diluted 1:50). Rabbit anti-chick type II collagen (0.16 mg/ml) does not stain **(a)** chick aorta (× 270) or **(b)** chick ventricle (× 270). **(c)** PBS control and rhodamine-conjugated goat anti-rabbit IgG is negative for non-specific rhodamine staining over human cardiac skeleton(s) (× 225). **(d)** Chick ventricle connective tissue stained with rabbit anti-chick I collagen (0.13 mg/ml) and ferritin-conjugated goat anti-rabbit IgG; SF, striated fibrils (× 45,000). **(e)** Goat anti-chick III collagen (0.17 mg/ml) and ferritin-conjugated rabbit anti-goat IgG-labeled collagen fibrils in the extracellular matrix of chick cardiac muscle (× 45,000) and **(f)** in the chick aorta (× 56,250); EL, elastic lamina.

there an equal distribution of these collagens in the mature heart or is one collagen type turned off and another type continually produced?

With the recent development of antibodies to specific collagen types (36-41) the new knowledge gained regarding the origin and distribution of the different collagen types secreted into the extracellular matrix will contribute to our understanding of tissue interactions in the embryo. Understanding the normal role of collagen in embryonic matrices will also promote our understanding of abnormal differentiation in cardiac anomalies and various pathological states.

ACKNOWLEDGMENTS

This research was supported by a United States Public Health Service Fellowship, HL-05682, to M. J. C. H. and a research grant, HD-00143, to Dr. Elizabeth D. Hay, in whose laboratory the work was conducted. The author is most grateful to Dr. Elizabeth D. Hay for her helpful suggestions and critical reading of this manuscript.

REFERENCES

1. Arguello, M., de la Cruz, V., and Sanchez, C. (1978): Ultrastructural and experimental evidence of myocardial cell differentiation into connective tissue cells in embryonic chick heart. *J. Mol. Cell Cardiol.,* 10:307-315.
2. Bashey, R. E., Bashey, H. M., and Jimenez, S. A. (1978): Characterization of pepsin-solubilized bovine heart-valve collagen. *Biochem. J.,* 173:885-894.
3. Caspari, P. G., Newcomb, M., Gibson, K., and Harris, P. (1977): Collagen in the normal and hypertrophied human ventricle. *Cardiovas. Res.,* 11:554-558.
4. Chung, E., Rhodes, K., and Miller, E. J. (1976): Isolation of three collagenous components of probable basement membrane origin from several tissues. *Biochem. Biophys. Res. Commun.,* 71:1167-1174.
5. Chvapil, M., Rakušan, K., Wachtlova, M., and Poupa, O. (1966): Collagen in the heart of wild and domesticated animals. *Gerontol.,* 12:144-154.
6. Epstein, E. H., Jr. (1974): $\alpha1(III)_3$ Human skin collagen. *J. Biol. Chem.,* 249:3225-3231.
7. Hay, E. D., Linsenmayer, T. F., Trelstad, R. L., and von der Mark, K. (1979): Origin and distribution of collagens in the developing avian cornea. *Curr. Top. Eye Res.,* 1:1-35.
8. Hendrix, M. J. C., Hay, E. D., von der Mark, H., and von der Mark, K. (1978): Electron microscopic localization of collagen types in the embryonic chick cornea and tibia utilizing ferritin-conjugated antibodies. *J. Cell Biol.,* 79:150.
9. Iwatsuki, K., Cardinale, G. J., Spector, S., and Udenfriend, S. (1977): Hypertension: Increase of collagen biosynthesis in arteries but not in veins. *Science,* 198:403-504.
10. Johnson, R. C., Manasek, F. J., Vinson, V., and Seyer, J. (1974): The biochemical and ultrastructural demonstration of collagen during early heart development. *Dev. Biol.,* 36:252-271.

FIG. 4. Electron micrograph of a section of chick cardiac muscle stained with rabbit anti-chick AB_2 collagen (0.12 mg/ml) and ferritin-conjugated goat anti-rabbit IgG (diluted 1:50). Collagen fibrils and amorphous matrix materials *(arrows)* associated with muscle cell surfaces are labeled (× 60,000).

11. Judd, J. T., and Wexler, B. C. (1975): Prolyl hydroxylase and collagen metabolism after experimental myocardial infarction. *Am. J. Physiol.,* 228:212-216.

12. Kefalides, N. A. (1975): Basement membranes: Structural and biosynthetic considerations. *J. Invest. Dermatol.,* 65:85-92.

13. Lenkiewicz, J. E., Davies, M. J., and Rosen, D. (1972): Collagen in human myocardium as a function of age. *Cardiovas. Res.,* 6:549-555.

14. Linsenmayer, T. F., Trelstad, R. L., and Gross, J. (1973): The collagen of chick embryo notochord. *Biochem. Biophys. Res. Comm.,* 53:39-45.

15. Linsenmayer, T. F., Smith, G. N., and Hay, E. D. (1977): In vitro synthesis of two collagen types by embryonic chick corneal epithelium. *Proc. Natl. Acad. Sci. USA,* 74:39-43.

16. Manasek, F. J. (1968): Embryonic development of the heart. I. A light and electron microscopic study of myocardial development in the early chick embryo. *J. Morphol.,* 125:329-366.

17. Manasek, F. J. (1970): Histogenesis of the embryonic myocardium. *Am. J. Cardiol.,* 25:149-168.

18. Manasek, F. J., Reid, M., Vinson, W., Weyer, J., and Johnson, R. (1973a): Glycosaminoglycan synthesis by the early embryonic chick heart. *Dev. Biol.,* 35:332-348.

19. Manasek, F. J. (1973b): Some comparative aspects of cardiac and skeletal myogenesis. In: *Developmental Regulation,* edited by S. Coward, pp. 193-218. Academic Press, New York.

20. Manasek, F. J. (1975): The extracellular matrix of the early embryonic heart. In: *Developmental and Physiological Correlates of Cardiac Muscle,* edited by M. Lieberman and T. Sano, pp. 1-20. Raven Press, New York.

21. Manasek, F. J. (1976): Heart development: Interactions involved in cardiac morphogenesis. In: *The Cell Surface in Animal Embryogenesis and Development,* edited by G. Poste and G. L. Nicolson, pp. 545-598. North-Holland Pub., New York.

22. Mannschott, P., Herbage, D., Weiss, M., and Buffevant, C. (1976): Collagen heterogeneity in pig heart valves. *Biochim. Biophys. Acta,* 434:177-183.

23. McClain, P. E. (1974): Characterization of cardiac muscle collagen. *J. Biol. Chem.,* 249:2303-2311.

24. Miller, E. J. (1976): Biochemical characteristics and biological significance of the genetically-distinct collagens. *Mol. Cell Biochem.,* 13:165-192.

25. Miller, E. J., and Matukas, V. J. (1969): Chick cartilage collagen: A new type of α1 chain not present in bone or skin of the species. *Proc. Natl. Acad. Sci. USA,* 64:1264-1268.

26. Miller, E. J., Epstein, E. H., Jr., and Piez, K. (1971): Identification of three genetically distinct collagens by cyanogen bromide cleavage of insoluble human skin and cartilage collagen. *Biochem. Biophys. Res. Commun.,* 42:1024-1029.

27. Mohan, S., and Radha, E. (1975): Collagen in aging muscles. *Experientia,* 31:1181-1183.

28. Morris, S. C., and McClain, P. E. (1972): Heterogeneity in the cyanogen bromide peptides from striated muscle and heart valve collagen. *Biochem. Biophys. Res. Commun.,* 47:27-34.

29. Newsome, D. A., Linsenmayer, T. F., and Trelstad, R. L. (1976): Vitreous body collagen. *J. Cell Biol.,* 71:59-67.

30. Piez, K. (1976): Primary structure. In: *Biochemistry of Collagen,* edited by G. N. Ramachandran and A. H. Reddi, pp. 1-44. Plenum Press, New York.

31. Renteria, V. G., and Ferrans, V. J. (1976): Intracellular collagen fibrils in cardiac valves of patients with Hurler's syndrome. *Lab. Invest.,* 34:263-272.

32. Rikihisa, Y., Ohkuma, S., and Mizuno, D. (1976): Elimination of nonspecific binding to plasma membranes in indirect immunoferritin technique. *Cell Struc. Funct.,* 1:251-258.

33. Smith, G. N., Jr., Linsenmayer, T. F., and Newsome, D. A. (1976): Synthesis of type II collagen in vitro by embryonic chick neural retina tissue. *Proc. Natl. Acad. Sci. USA,* 73:4420-4423.

34. Sternberger, L. A. (1979): *Immunoferritin and Immunocolloid Methods: Immunocytochemistry.* Wiley and Sons, New York.

35. Swann, D. A., Constable, S. J., and Harper, E. (1972): Vitreous structure. III. Composition of bovine vitreous collagen. *Invest. Ophthalmol.,* 11:735-738.

36. Timpl, R. (1976): Immunological studies on collagen. In: *Biochemistry of Collagen,* edited by G. N. Ramachandran and A. H. Reddi, pp. 319-375. Plenum Press, New York.

37. Timpl, R., Wick, G., and Gay, S. (1977): Antibodies to distinct types of collagens and procollagens and their application in immunohistology. *J. Immunol. Meth.,* 18:165-182.

38. von der Mark, H., von der Mark, K., and Gay, S. (1976a): Study of differential collagen

synthesis during development of the chick embryo by immunofluorescence. I. Preparation of collagen type I and type II specific antibodies and their application to early stages of the chick embryo. *Dev. Biol.,* 48:237-249.

39. von der Mark, K., von der Mark, H., and Gay, S. (1976b): Study of differential collagen synthesis during development of the chick embryo by immunofluorescence. II. Localization of type I and type II collagen during long bone development. *Dev. Biol.,* 53:153-170.
40. von der Mark, K., von der Mark, H., Timpl, R., and Trelstad, R. L. (1977): Immunofluorescent localization of collagen types I, II and III in the embryonic chick eye. *Dev. Biol.,* 59:75-85.
41. von der Mark, H., and von der Mark, K. (1979): Isolation and characterization of collagen A and B chains from chick embryos. *FEBS* Lett., 99:101-105.
42. Woessner, J. F., Jr., Bashey, R. I., and Boucek, R. J. (1967): Collagen development in heart and skin of the chick embryo. *Biochim. Biophys. Acta,* 140:329-338.

DISCUSSION

Manasek: Can you prove to us that your antibodies are reacting with collagen in the embryo and that they are doing so specifically?

Hendrix: We have tried to correlate the immunofluorescent studies at the light microscope with the electron microscopic studies and ferritin labeling of the same piece of tissue. As far as the specificity is concerned, these studies are all based on biochemistry done by Dr. Klaus von der Mark.

Manasek: When you do immunodiffusion, how many precipitin lines can be seen when you react one of those antibodies with the crude extract of the embryonic heart?

Hendrix: We have not done biochemical studies for the heart. I was only theorizing on preliminary results based on previous investigations.

Kulikowski: Have you observed any staining after absorbing the antibodies to II and III type collagen with an antigen to type I collagen?

Hendrix: So far, we have done blocking experiments, in which we take, for example, type I collagen antigen and react it with the collagen type I antibody to precipitate it and then present it to the tissue.

Kulikowski: What about staining with the heterologous antigen or antibody?

Hendrix: The data on specificity of all these antibodies have been published by Dr. Klaus von der Mark in *Developmental Biology.*

Manasek: In none of those papers was the purity of the antigen shown, even at immunodiffusion. The question of what the antibody is specific to is very important.

Hendrix: We have performed double-staining, which is a good indication when you have two different antibodies to two different collagen types. In tibia, where we have type I collagen in the perichondrium and type II in the cartilage, we have seen double-staining of these two areas.

Manasek: Why did you not simply do Ouchterlony?

Fischman: Ouchterlony would not be a very good method for this particular antigen. The polymer form of collagen in a diffusion system might preclude interpretation of the result. Do you believe that testicular hyaluronidase is a good method to expose all antigenic sites? I would assume the antigenic sites to be rather masked, inaccessible to the entry of an eventual antibody. Negative results may then represent a problem.

Hendrix: Initially, we did not treat the tissue with hyaluronidase and we did not get any fluorescence. It is really necessary to add hyaluronidase for better penetration.

Fischman: You are assuming that after the hyaluronidase pretreatment the antigen was equally exposed, but that might not be the case.

Hendrix: If there is no collagen type II, despite the presence of type I and III and hyaluronidase pretreatment, there will be no staining.

Clark: Can you speculate on the relationship of the suspected presence of different collagen types and the problem of atrial septum formation as mentioned by Dr. Morse?

Hendrix: The first thing we want to speculate on is which cells are producing this collagen, and at what time. In the atrial septum, formation of holes is accompanied by disappearance of collagen type I and III.

Perspectives in Cardiovascular Research, Vol. 5,
Mechanisms of Cardiac Morphogenesis and Teratogenesis,
edited by Tomas Pexieder. Raven Press, New York © 1981

Endocardial Shape Change in the Truncus During Cushion Tissue Formation

Timothy P. Fitzharris

Department of Anatomy, Medical University of South Carolina,
Charleston, South Carolina 29403

The endocardium has been considered the primary source of cushion tissue (CT) in the developing heart (6,9), although this concept has never been experimentally established. Assuming that the early endocardium does provide cellular progeny for CT morphogenesis, there remains the basic question of how the cells for this new mesenchymal population arise without disrupting the epithelial integrity of the parent endocardium. In order to approach this problem in a reproducible and quantitative fashion, we have devised a method that enables us to arbitrarily, but systematically, divide the truncus into five sections (Fig. 1). The region adjacent to the aortic arch has been designated Station 1 (St. 1), and the juncture of the truncus with the ventricle has been designated Station 5 (St. 5). Lines drawn through these two stations converge to form an angle. Bisection of this angle, followed by bisection of the two remaining angles, yields St. 3, 2, and 4, respectively. This arbitrary but reproducible method can be applied to the truncus at any stage of development to yield cross-sections which can be compared with respect to each other, or with similar stations from younger or older embryos. Using this method, recent investigations have demonstrated

SECTIONING STATIONS

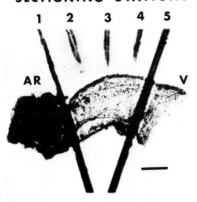

FIG. 1. A flat embedded conotruncus from a stage 15 chick embryo, which has been scribed for sectioning by the station technique (AR = aortic arch region; V = ventricle; Bar = 100 μm). (Reprinted with permission from Wistar Press).

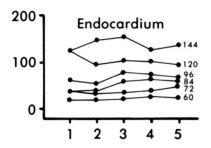

FIG. 2. Total number of nuclei present in the endocardium at each station from 60 hr of development through 144 hr. (Ordinate = number of nuclei; Abscissa = station number). (Reprinted with permission from Wistar Press).

differential mitotic indices for the endocardium and myocardium during CT formation (14). Although the number of cells comprising the endocardium at each stage of development remains fairly uniform along the length of the truncus (Fig. 2), the tissue displaying the greatest mitotic activity is the endocardium (Fig. 3B). This period of activity coincides with the initial appearance of CT in the truncus. It is reasonable to assume that most of the daughter cells are released subjacent to the endocardium, thus becoming CT by virtue of their new position (Fig. 3A). A smaller percentage of the daughter cells would remain in their original location, in order to prevent depletion of the endocardium through growth. Other potential sources for CT have been suggested, such as myocardium and splanchnic mesoderm (1,2). However, those suggestions do not negate the role of the endocardium in contributing to CT formation as described. Rather, they point out the potential heterogeneity of origin of CT,

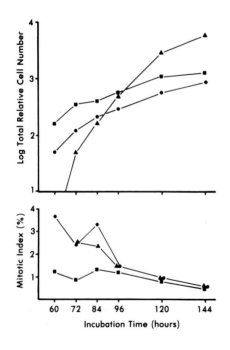

FIG. 3. Growth of major tissue types in the entire truncus. Ordinate: **(Top)** Logarithm of the relative total number of each cell type present, estimated by multiplying the sum of the nuclei in all station averages by the lengths in millimeters of each truncus. **(Bottom)** Mitotic indices of the major cell types (*triangle,* mesenchyme; *circle,* endocardium; *square,* myocardium). Abscissa: hours of incubation. (Reprinted with permission from Wistar Press).

a circumstance that may play a major role in the differentiation of adult structures (15).

In addition to the rise in mitotic activity, the endocardium undergoes very characteristic shape changes during CT formation (Fig. 4). From its initial tubular formation at stage 7 and 8 through stage 12 of development, the endocardium in cross-section is basically round or slightly elliptical in contour. From stage 13 through the formation of CT (approximately stage 24 to 25), the endocardium acquires an unusual configuration, with projections termed "flutes" arching into the cardiac jelly and approaching the myocardium (Fig. 5). With CT formation basically completed, the endocardium resumes a more oval contour with very few, if any, flutes remaining (Fig. 4, lower row). Formation of flutes seems to presage the appearance of CT, since most of the initial cells, or "pioneer cells," according to Markwald et al. (8), appear subjacent to and in association with a flute.

Why would this shape change be involved in the seeding of CT cells into the cardiac jelly space? If cushion cells arose by mitotic seeding and delamination of existing endocardial cells, the epithelial integrity of the endocardium would be disrupted, allowing uncontrolled flow of ions and other soluble components into and out of the cardiac jelly matrix. Since matrical organization and composition are very important in normal development (5,7,10,11), such an alteration

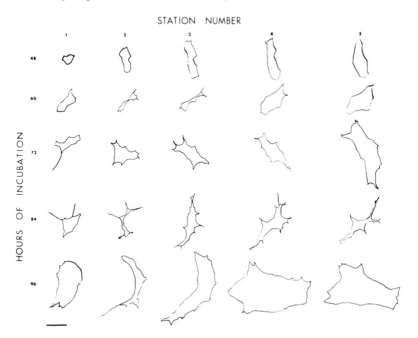

FIG. 4. Line drawings of the endocardial luminal surface in cross-section of chick embryos incubated from 48 to 96 hr of development, according to the sectioning technique illustrated in Fig. 2. The most prominent shape changes occur at 72 and 84 hr, when cushion tissue formation is well in progress. Bar = 100 μm.

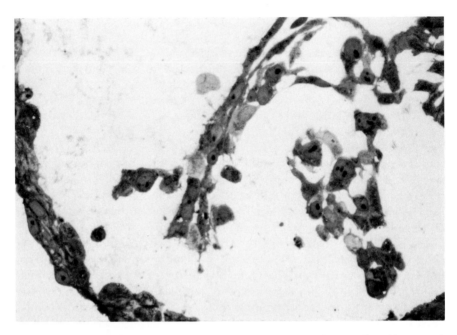

FIG. 5. A light micrograph of a flute from st. 4 of a 72-hr truncus (stage 18) arching towards the myocardium (M). Note the initial appearance of cushion tissue (CT) subjacent to the endocardium, and a possible former flute (right-hand side) which has already delaminated, leaving only a small infolding from the lumen (L). (CJ = cardiac jelly space) (× 245).

could lead to maldevelopment. Flutes form to accommodate the loss of cells from the endocardium while maintaining an intact epithelium, presumably allowing the following sequence of events to occur: the endocardium comes into contact with itself over a large area of its luminal surface, giving many cells the opportunity to form membranous complexes along the length of a flute; the cells deepest in the matrix can then lose their epithelial associations and delaminate, without disrupting the overlying epithelium; cell division in other regions of the endocardium provides a source of cells which "flow" towards a flute in a continuous process of replacement/displacement (Fig. 6). In this manner, cells can leave the endocardium without disrupting the morphological and, presumably, the physiological integrity of the endocardium.

How do flutes form and maintain their unique shape? It has been demonstrated that isolated cardiac jelly (9) is a viscoelastic solid which, when deformed, will resume its normal shape. To form a flute, then, one of two conditions must be met: either the extracellular matrix must be removed to allow the endocardium to arch towards the myocardium, or the matrix must be compressed by a process which would involve a continuous expenditure of energy in order to resist the viscoelastic forces (Fig. 7). If the matrix were compressed, a plausible means of achieving this condition would be an active interaction between endocardial cells and components of the matrix known as fiber tracts (10). Such

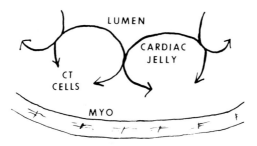

FIG. 6. The proposed dynamic role of endocardial shape change, flute formation, and morphogenesis of cushion tissue cells (CT).

fiber tracts, running from the underside of the endocardium all the way to the myocardium, can be easily visualized in the scanning electron microscope (Fig. 8). These fiber tracts could be utilized by endocardial cells in the following manner: filopodia would probe deep into the matrix and attach to the tracts; following attachment, filopodial contraction, as a result of an interplay of microfilaments and other cytoskeletal elements, would cause the endocardium to arch towards the myocardium; repeating the process of attachment followed by contraction, a flute would be formed by compression of the underlying matrix. Since most of these fiber tracts are composed of collagen, their tensile strength would be affected by β-aminopropionitrile (BAPN), an agent that suppresses extracellular cross-linking of collagen (13). When embryos are incubated with 500 μg of BAPN, total embryonic development proceeds normally and flute formation is unaffected in the heart, indicating that the fiber tracts are probably

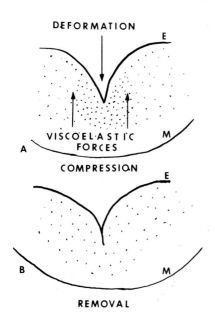

FIG. 7. A schematic presentation of two possible mechanisms involved in flute formation. **(A)** An active generation of force by the endocardium, compressing the underlying cardiac jelly *(heavily stippled area)* by actively probing the matrix with filopodia which would interact with the matrical components. **(B)** Formation of a flute by active enzymatic removal of the matrix, which would not involve compression of the underlying matrix but could still involve the active participation of filopodia.

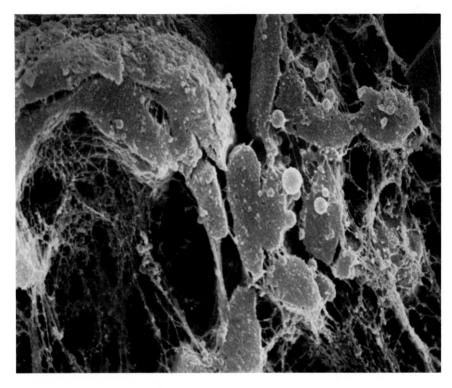

FIG. 8. A scanning electron micrograph of station 4 of an 84-hr chick embryo truncus illustrating a flute, initial CT tissue formation subjacent to the flute, and the matrical fiber tracts which run from the endocardium towards the myocardium ($\times$ 8,960).

not involved in anchoring the endocardium to the myocardium to resist viscoelastic forces (3). Additional biochemical studies have demonstrated that BAPN effects collagen cross-linking by shifting the ratio of soluble to insoluble collagen, by forming more of the soluble fraction.

In contrast, the endocardium has been shown to possess a high level of hydrolytic activity, as evidenced by a positive acid phosphatase reaction (Fig. 9). Much, but not all, of the acid phosphatase activity is found in the endocardial cells which comprise the flute. Although this histochemical test demonstrates only general hydrolytic activity, it has been demonstrated biochemically (12) that one of the major hydrolytic enzymes present in the chick heart at this time is hyaluronidase. Since much of the matrix is comprised of hyaluronate and chondroitin sulfate at this time (4), it is reasonable to assume that flutes form by selectively removing the matrix which is interposed between the endocardium and myocardium.

Even though CT forms selectively in the truncus and atrioventricular (AV) canal in association with a defined shape change in the endocardium, there is another defined shape change in the ventricle that is not associated with formation of a separate population of mesenchyme. Trabeculation is a coordinated process

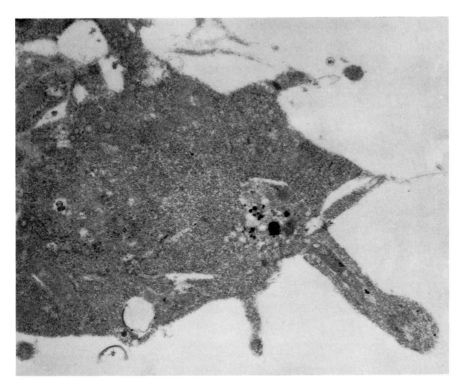

FIG. 9. A transmission electron micrograph of the matrical side of the endocardium from a 72 hr, station 4 truncus, showing a positive reaction for acid phosphatase, indicating general hydrolytic activity in the presence of lysosomes ($\times$ 16,000).

which involves similar, but smaller and more numerous, infoldings of the endocardium. These eventually come to lie in apposition to a muscular core of myocardial tissue with very little, if any, interposing matrix (6). This biphasic pattern of cytodifferentiation, i.e., prospective CT endocardium in the truncus and AV canal vs. mural endocardium in the atria and ventricles, has not been experimentally explored to determine whether the capacity to form a mesenchymal cell population is acquired (induced) by the adjacent myocardium or matrix, or whether it is a capacity that is lost as a result of similar but negative inductive factors. Elucidation of these basic tissue interactions will require mapping of the potential regional matrical or cellular characteristics that precede these events in normal cardiogenesis. With this information, we may be able to understand the events that lead to endocardial cushion defects.

ACKNOWLEDGMENTS

The author would like to thank Robert L. Ashcraft for his dedication and expert technical assistance. This work was supported in part by a grant-in-aid, American Heart Association (79-1039) and a travel grant from the Health Sciences Foundation, Medical University of South Carolina.

REFERENCES

1. Adams Smith, W. N. (1963): The site of action of trypan blue in cardiac teratogenesis. *Anat. Rec.,* 147:507-524.
2. Chang, C. (1932): On the reaction of the endocardium to the bloodstream in the embryonic heart, with special reference to the endocardial thickenings in the atrioventricular canal and the bulbus cordis. *Anat. Rec.,* 51:253-265.
3. Fitzharris, T. P., Markwald, R. R., and Dunn, B. E. (1979): Effects of BAPN on early heart development. *J. Mol. Cell Cardiol. (in press).*
4. Markwald, R. R., and Adams Smith, W. N. (1972): Distribution of muco-substances in the developing rat heart. *J. Histochem. Cytochem.,* 20:896-907.
5. Markwald, R. R., and Fitzharris, T. P. (1974): Early endocardial development in the rat. *Anat. Rec.,* 178:411-412.
6. Markwald, R. R., Fitzharris, T. P., and Adams Smith, W. N. (1975): Structural analysis of endocardial cytodifferentiation. *Dev. Biol.,* 42:160-180.
7. Markwald, R. R., Fitzharris, T. P., Bank, H., and Bernanke, D. H. (1978): Structural analyses on the matrical organization of glycosaminoglycans in developing endocardial cushions. *Dev. Biol.,* 62:292-316.
8. Markwald, R. R., Fitzharris, T. P., Bolender, D. L., and Bernanke, D. H. (1979): Structural analysis of cell:matrix association during the morphogenesis of atrioventricular cushion tissue. *Dev. Biol.,* 69:634-654.
9. Markwald, R. R., Fitzharris, T. P., and Manasek, F. J. (1977): Structural development of endocardial cushions. *Am. J. Anat.,* 148:85-120.
10. Nakamura, A., and Manasek, F. J. (1978): Cardiac jelly fibrils: Their distribution and organization. In: *Birth Defects,* original article series, Vol. XIV, Number 7, edited by G. C. Rosenquist and D. Bergsma, pp. 229-250. Alan R. Liss, Inc., New York.
11. Nakamura, A., and Manasek, F. J. (1978): Experimental studies of the shape and structure of isolated cardiac jelly. *J. Embryol. Exp. Morph.,* 43:167-183.
12. Orkin, R. W., and Toole, B. P. (1978): Hyaluronidase activity and hyaluronate content of the developing chick embryo heart. *Dev. Biol.,* 66:308-320.
13. Pinnell, S. R., and Martin, G. R. (1968): The cross-linking of collagen and elastin: Enzymatic conversion of lysine in peptide linkage to α-aminoadipic-S-semialdehyde (allysine) by an extract from bone. *Proc. Nat. Acad. Sci.,* 61:708-716.
14. Thompson, R. P., and Fitzharris, T. P. (1979): Morphogenesis of the truncus arteriosus of the chick embryo heart: The formation and migration of mesenchymal tissue. *Am. J. Anat.,* 154:545-556.
15. Thompson, R. P., and Fitzharris, T. P. (1979): Morphogenesis of the truncus arteriosus of the chick embryo heart: Tissue reorganization during septation. *Am. J. Anat.,* 156:251-264.

DISCUSSION

De Vries: I would suggest another interpretation for the reorientation of endothelial cells. It may be the result of elastic forces active in the endothelium versus the compression from contraction of the myocardium.

Fitzharris: Even a myocardial contraction that starts that way along a tube will give, within a given radius and direction, the same compressional force.

De Vries: You are describing the matrix as not symmetrical. This, together with an asymmetrical distribution of cells, will change the whole elastic module right there.

Manasek: The analysis of forces in tissues as complex as this one, in which there are very large deformations and many anisotropic structures superimposed, is extremely difficult and risky.

Clark: Did you control for the effect of contraction on the folding of the noncompressible cardiac jelly? Did you fix in diastole or in systole?

Fitzharris: The specimens were all fixed in maximal contraction.

Clark: That makes interpretation of the folding more difficult, since the non-compressible jelly has to go some place.

Fitzharris: Yes, except that one would not expect to find prealigned fibrils in the matrix. With each heart folding its own way, you would expect every heart to be different, but we found fairly reproducible shaping. Even in the mutant axolotl heart of Dr. Lemanski, which barely beat, you still got the shape changes occurring in the matrix.

Rychter: Did you take into account the change in heart function between the 2nd and 3rd e.d. when interpreting the sudden change in cell shape? On the 2nd e.d., the heart works on the principle of a peristaltic wave, whereas on the 3rd e.d. the bulbus functions as a separate cavity. Did you observe any difference between the proximal and distal parts of the bulbus, since in the distal part there is material entering the heart from the body of the embryo?

Fitzharris: From the comparison of station 1 to station 5, I would infer that there are greater shape changes closer to the ventricle than up by the arches. I will make the supposition that in the distal part there would be a mixed population of cells derived from both the aortic arches and the endocardium. Closer to the ventricle, most of the mesenchyme would be endocardially derived.

Hurle: Can you explain the difference between the radial orientation of cardiac jelly in pictures by Dr. Manasek and its amorphous appearance in your photographs?

Fitzharris: This is due to differences in fixation and staining procedures used. I would like to stress that all of the micrographs actually available do not show how the matrix looks. Under *in vivo* conditions the cardiac jelly is totally saturated with water and ions, whereas here it is totally dehydrated.

Fischman: In a number of embryonic systems, cell migration seems to be correlated with regional differences in hyaluronate concentration and associated hydration of the matrix. Is there any evidence in cardiac jelly, first of all, for regional differences in hyaluronic acid concentration, and second, is it associated with the region of endothelium migration? Assuming that we have in the myocardial layer a secretory epithelium which is releasing the cardiac jelly materials, is there any evidence for a difference in the myocardial cell ultrastructure that suggests differential secretory activity?

Manasek: There have been too few attempts at actual compositional analysis to allow for the idea that there is a hyaluronate gradient that somewhat directs cells.

Markwald: Our experiments with lysozyme polygenic serotonin have shown that the cells remove the hyaluronate as they move into the matrix. In tri-dimensional cultures, where we have stripped the endocardium away, seeding will take place as long as serum, which contains a lot of hyaluronate, is present. In the absence of serum, very little seeding takes place. If you add hyaluronate, seeding does occur. Treatment with hyaluronate of cells that have already moved into the matrix increases the cells' perimeters and the depth of their penetration. But it may also have an indirect effect, by localizing ions.

Fitzharris: By the aortic arches, most of the so-called fiber tracts are longitudinally oriented along the heart tube axis. At the midpoint they become radially oriented. There is a differential directional activity of the fiber tracts. With the glycoprotein technique presented by Dr. Hay, I have observed a differential deposition of glycoprotein material towards the area in which the ventricular trabeculation is occurring, and few, if any, mesenchymal tissues are invading.

Perspectives in Cardiovascular Research, Vol. 5,
Mechanisms of Cardiac Morphogenesis and Teratogenesis,
edited by Tomas Pexieder. Raven Press, New York © 1981

Structural Analyses of 6-Diazo-5-Oxo-L-Norleucine Effects upon Early Cushion Tissue Morphogenesis

Roger R. Markwald and David H. Bernanke

Department of Anatomy, Texas Tech University School of Medicine, Lubbock, Texas 79430

The primary or simple tubular heart consists of two epithelia separated by a broad acellular zone known as cardiac jelly. The latter is produced by the myocardium (19) and represents one of the larger accumulations of extracellular macromolecules in the early embryo. The composition of the jelly includes glycosaminoglycans (GAG), collagen, and glycoprotein (8,10,11,17,19,20). Although various hemodynamic functions have been attributed to cardiac jelly, in this study we are investigating whether the components of cardiac jelly are causally or casually related to the formation of atrioventricular (AV) endocardial cushions, the primordia of valvular and membranous septal tissues (1).

Three major events comprise early cushion tissue development; (a) selective activation of AV endocardium (as opposed to ventricular mural endocardium), which involves hypertrophy and reorientation of the endocardium, acquisition of secretory potential, and the formation of motility characteristics; (b) an epithelial–mesenchymal transformation of the activated endocardium into mesenchymal progeny, termed cushion tissue (CT) cells; and (c) the motility and directed cell movement of the seeded CT cells towards the myocardium to form cushion pads (3,21,22).

Our specific hypothesis is that one or more of the early events of CT formation is mediated by extracellular macromolecules produced by the myocardium. To test the hypothesis, embryonic hearts were treated *in vivo* with 6-diazo-5-oxo-L-norleucine (DON). This substance is known to block the formation of glucosamine via inhibition of a specific transaminase which catalyzes the transfer of the amino group from L-glutamine to fructose-6 phosphate (4,6,7). Creating a glucosamine deficiency has been reported to decrease the synthesis of GAG (5,16,26,29) and to alter the development of mesenchymal tissues (8,12). In the present study, we have observed that when DON was administered 24 hours prior to endocardial activation, the initial step of CT formation, the AV endocardium failed to acquire locomotive appendages, an event accompanied by reduced CT cell formation and abnormal population of the cardiac jelly.

MATERIALS AND METHODS

DON Injections

Fertilized White Leghorn eggs obtained from the Texas A & M Poultry Science Department were incubated at 37.5°C at 60% humidity. At 48 hours, 10 μg (78 embryos), 20 μg (36 embryos), and 50 μg (30 embryos) DON/0.1cc sterile water was administered by dripping onto the vitelline circulation through a small window in the shell. Controls (110 embryos) received either sterile water or DON plus glucosamine (GSA) (5 times the amount of DON). Incubation was continued until 72 to 76 or 90 to 96 hours, after which embryos were removed, placed in warm Tyrode's solution, and staged (9). Additional embryos were collected and staged at the time of injection.

Light Microscopy

Excised hearts were fixed for 2 hours in 2% glutaraldehyde, with or without 1% cetylpyridinium chloride (CPCL) buffered with 0.065 M sodium cacodylate, pH 7.2 to 7.4, rinsed, dehydrated, embedded in glycol methacrylate in a consistent manner with the apex directed downward, serially sectioned at 2 μ through the AV canal, and viewed with Nomarski or brightfield optics. Ten embryos from each group were additionally processed as follows: three sections spaced 10 μm apart were taken from the midpoint of each dorsal and ventral pad, photographed at 10 to 20 X, printed at constant enlargement, and placed on a Ladd graphic digitizer interfaced to a programmable calculator set up for calculating cell number, cell surface (perimeter), and cross-sectional area, from points generated by the stylus of the digitizer.

Transmission Electron Microscopy

Excised AV canals were fixed for 2 hours in 2% glutaraldehyde in Tyrode's solution buffered to pH 7.2 to 7.4, and subsequently rinsed, osmicated for 1 hour, dehydrated, and embedded in Epon 812 by a routine procedure (21). Thin sections were obtained using diamond knives and were stained with uranyl acetate and lead citrate and examined in a Zeiss 10A electron microscope.

Scanning Electron Microscopic X-Ray Energy Dispersive Microanalysis

Excised AV canals fixed for 3 hours in glutaraldehyde/CPCL, as described for light microscopy, were rinsed in buffer, embedded in agar, sectioned at 75 μm in a Smith-Farquhar tissue chopper, reimmersed in buffer, and stained with alcian blue (AB) at pH 2.5 for 3 hours at 37°C, dehydrated in graded ethanols, critical point-dried using CO_2, affixed to carbon stubs, and coated with carbon, using a Denton vacuum evaporator. ^{29}Cu (core of AB dye molecule) and ^{16}S X-ray emissions generated by Hitachi S500 scanning electron microscope using the spot mode (1 μm-diameter spot) were recorded using a Princeton Gamma Tech X-ray detector. The resultant signals were analyzed by a PGT 1000 microanalyzer. All measurements were made at constant specimen tilt, detector take-off angle, and beam current (23).

RESULTS

72 to 76-Hour Control Embryos (Stages 18 to 20)

Cytoplasmic hypertrophy of the endocardium, its reorientation into a closely packed epithelium (high cell density), and endocardial surface phenomena (formation of locomotive appendages on the cardiac jelly border) of sterile water controls were identical to conditions recently reported for non-injected animals (3). Also typical of this stage was the tendency of endocardial cells to overlap or overgrow adjacent cells, resulting in the formation of a loosely knitted epithelium possessing few cell-to-cell contacts and many laterally positioned intercellular spaces (3). As shown in Fig. 1, initiation of cushion cell formation had begun in stage 18 controls. Some newly seeded CT cells remained closely associated with the endocardium, but the majority had moved out into the cardiac jelly. Those free of direct endocardial association were generally stellate in appearance, as the result of acquisition of locomotive processes (Fig. 1).

72- to 76-Hour DON Treated Embryos (Stages 16 to 18)

Only embryos having beating hearts, an intact vitelline circulation, and developed beyond the point at which they were injected were collected. Embryonic death approached 50% at the 50 μg level, but at 10 to 20 μg dosage mortality rate (6%) was identical to saline controls. In general, DON embryos were equivalent to or one stage (9) behind comparably incubated water control embryos.

Cushion development varied with the dosage of DON (Figs. 2 and 7). Hypertrophy and reorientation of the endocardium occurred at all dosages (Fig. 3); the ability to seed CT cells progressively diminished with increasing concentrations of DON. At 50 μg few, if any, CT cells were present in the cardiac jelly of the AV canal (Figs. 2 and 4). Neural crest cell migration and formation were also arrested (Fig. 4). Endocardial cells appeared viable, but processes such as filopodia and pseudopodia were usually absent on the cardiac jelly border (Figs. 3 and 5). Conversely, the luminal border showed increased surface activity reflected in the formation of atypical, elongated microvilli (Figs. 5 and 6).

At 10 μg DON, CT cell seeding occurred, but the number of cells formed normalized to the cross-sectional area of the tissue examined was approximately one-half that of water controls (Table 1). As shown in Fig. 7, many of the seeded cells after DON treatment were spherical and in close contact with the endocardium. Ultrastructurally, the "piled-up" CT cells were viable (no

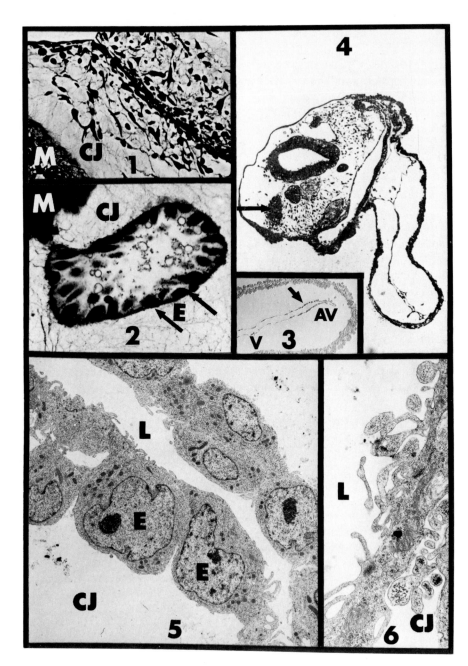

TABLE 1. *DON effects upon cushion cell formation and shape*

Treatment[a]	Cell perimeter (μm)[b]	Cell no./ area sampled (μm²)
48 hr (H₂O)/72 hr	60.08 ± 6.11	0.07 ± 0.02
48 hr (10 μg DON + 50 μg GSA)/72 hr	53.87 ± 7.02	0.08 ± 0.05
48 hr (10 μg DON)/72 hr	38.30 ± 8.31	0.03 ± 0.02
48 hr (H₂O)/90 hr	47.50 ± 5.65	0.21 ± 0.04
48 hr (10 μg DON + 50 μg GSA)/90 hr	49.33 ± 9.30	0.19 ± 0.07
48 hr (10 μg DON)/90 hr	35.37 ± 4.11	0.08 ± 0.05

[a] HOH or DON, etc., given at first hour stated and tissue collected at second hour stated—10 samples/treatment group analyzed.
[b] function of migratory potential (see text).

pyknotic nuclei or cytoplasmic degeneration) and resembled controls, except for the absence of locomotive appendages (Figs. 7 and 8). Some cells at the free edge of the CT cell population formed unusual cytoplasmic protrusions, involving most of the cell's cytoplasm, which were not seen in control CT cells (Fig. 8). The perimeter of CT cells was measured as a function of migratory capacity, since the presence of locomotive appendages increased cell perimeter. Thus, the greater the cell perimeter, the greater the potential for motility. DON treatment decreased this measurement to about one-third of the perimeter of saline controls (Table 1).

The morphological effects of DON (up to 20 μg) observed at 72 hours could be completely overriden with GSA (Table 1). Above this level, only incomplete

---

FIG. 1. Cross-section of the AV canal at 76 hours (stage 18) from a water control. An extensive outgrowth of stellate cushion cells into the cardiac jelly (CJ) has occurred. M, myocardium. Glutaraldehyde/CPCL fixation ($\times$ 450).

FIG. 2. Partial tangential cut through the AV canal from a 72-hour embryo treated with 50 μg DON. No cushion cells have been seeded. Endocardial cells (E, *arrows*) exhibit cytoplasmic hypertrophy but no cytoplasmic processes extend into the cardiac jelly. Glutaraldehyde/CPCL fixation ($\times$ 450).

FIG. 3. Longitudinal section through atrioventricular (AV) canal and ventricular (V) regions of a stage 17 heart from a 50 μg DON-treated embryo. Note *(arrow)* that the endocardium of the AV area has some features of activation, i.e., cells have hypertrophied and become closely packed as compared to ventricular mural endocardium. However, locomotive appendages as in Fig. 2 are absent ($\times$ 150).

FIG. 4. Same as Fig. 3, except showing the embryo. Arrow denotes aggregated neural crest cells leaving behind an enlarged cell-free space ($\times$ 100).

FIG. 5 and 6. AV endocardium from an area comparable to that indicated by the arrow in Fig. 3. Same age and treatment as described for Fig. 3. The cardiac jelly (CJ) border of endocardial cells is mostly devoid of filopodia or pseudopodia. The luminal (L) surface is characterized by numerous elongated microvilli shown at higher magnification in Fig. 6. Figure 5, $\times$ 3,100; Fig. 6, $\times$ 12,000.

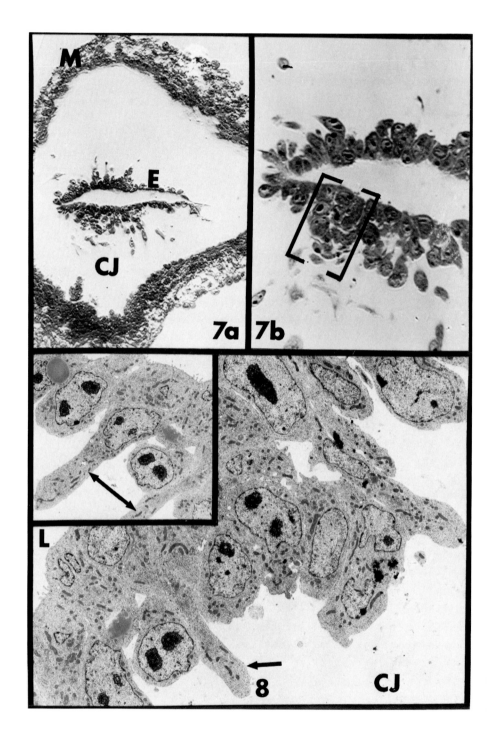

blockage of DON effects could be achieved with concurrent administration of GSA. For this reason, quantitative measurements in this study were restricted to embryos receiving 10 μg DON.

90- to 96-Hour Sterile Water Control Embryos (Stages 22 to 23)

At this stage, the leading edge of the migratory wave of CT cells had reached the myocardium in most areas (Fig. 9). Cardiac jelly was densely and uniformly populated by CT cells, their number having increased threefold since 72 hours (Table 1) (Fig. 9). Some cells still retained a stellate appearance, but many were ovoid or fusiform, reflecting a decrease in cell perimeter (Table 1).

90- to 96 DON Treated Embryos (Stages 21 to 22)

Major effects continued to be a reduction in CT cell number and suppression of locomotive appendages. However, within each dosage group the number of CT cells increased. For example, a few CT cells were seen even in embryos receiving 50 μg DON (Fig. 10). In 10 μg samples, the number of cells increased threefold from 72 hours, but were still threefold fewer than in water controls (Table 1) (Fig. 11). As previously shown, the effects of 10 to 20 μg DON on CT cell seeding and perimeter could be overridden with GSA (Table 1, Fig. 12).

Seeded CT cells, despite the fact that most remained spherical (Table 1), did not remain piled up against the endocardium as in 72 hour embryos (Figs. 11, 13, and 14). Retention of the rounded cell shape was reflected in abnormal migratory behavior. Some areas of the cardiac jelly were completely devoid of cells (Fig. 14). If such areas were contiguous with the myocardium, the latter frequently extended muscular evaginations (trabecula?) into the cell-free matrix (Fig. 14). In other areas of the cardiac jelly, the CT cells coalesced with one another, forming epithelial-like cell islands or aggregates of tightly packed cells (Fig. 15). Ultrastructurally, both free and coalesced cells resembled controls, except for the absence of motility appendages (Fig. 15). The atypical, elongated microvilli initially seen at stages 16 to 17 along the luminal surface of the endocardium were often interdigitated, uniting adjacent cells and creating the impression of a tightly knit epithelium (Fig. 16).

FIG. 7. **(a):** AV canal from a stage 17 (72-hour) embryo treated with 10 μg DON. At lower dosage, cushion cells remain in close proximity to the endocardium (E). As shown in **(b)** many of the cushion cells lack locomotive appendages. An area comparable to that enclosed by the brackets is shown in Figure 8. M, myocardium; CJ, cardiac jelly. Fig. 7a, × 360; Fig. 7b, × 1,040.

FIG. 8. Stage 17, 10 μg DON. Although rounded, seeded cushion cells appear viable without evidence of degeneration. Arrow indicates an unusual cushion cell cytoplasmic projection (× 2,625). Inset: Arrows indicate atypical appendages which contain most of the cytoplasm of cells exhibiting such processes. L, Lumen. × 1,650.

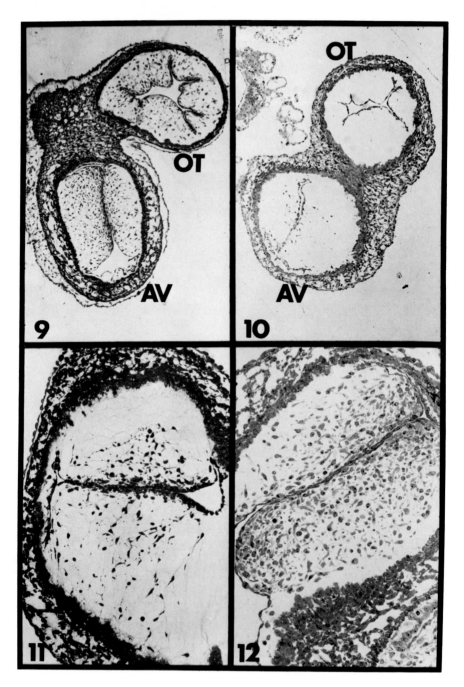

SEM X-Ray Energy Dispersive Microanalysis

Results comparing DON with water controls are shown in Table 2. Emission from ^{29}Cu reflects the molar mass of cardiac jelly polyanionic components reactive with AB at pH 2.5. DON treatment decreased the amount of extracellular AB positive material (^{29}Cu emission) twofold in 72-hour embryos and threefold in 90-hour samples. ^{16}S emission was unchanged in 72-hour tissues, but in the 90-hour group ^{16}S emission in DON embryos did not keep pace with the increase observed in water controls. DON plus GSA controls were not examined in this study because of the limited availability of DON.

TABLE 2. *Semiquantitative X-ray microanalysis or AV cushion extracellular matrix[a] stained with alcian blue[b] at pH 2.5[c]*

Treatment group[d]	Emission ^{29}Cu	Counts/sec.[e] ^{16}S
Control: 48 hr (H$_2$O)/72 hr	535 ± 75	340 ± 68
DON: 48 hr (10 μg)/72 hr	210 ± 70	308 ± 49
Control: 48 hr (H$_2$O)/90 hr	441 ± 53	465 ± 110
DON: 48 hr (10 μg)/90 hr	135 ± 40	311 ± 60

[a] fixed in 2% glutaraldehyde/1% CPCL.
[b] ^{29}Cu core of dye molecule.
[c] affinity for cardiac jelly ionized carboxyl groups (20,23).
[d] DON or saline given at first hour stated and tissue collected at second hour stated.
[e] based on analyzing 3 samples/treatment group with 10 matrix sites per sample, made by moving the spot mode systematically from the endocardium to the myocardium.

DISCUSSION

The basic supposition of this study is that extracellular macromolecules have dynamic functions in development which may serve to mediate genetic expression in tissue interactions. Possibly the best illustration of the importance of the tissue microenvironment is seen with neural crest cells. When young neural crest cells are grafted into progressively older hosts, the distal migration of the cells is arrested (33). In contrast, old neural crest cells grafted to young

---

FIG. 9. Stage 23 (90-hour) water control. Normal cushions from both the AV canal and outflow (OT) tract are shown ($\times$ 100).

FIG. 10. Stage 22 (90 hours). 50 μg DON embryo. Compare with Fig. 9 ($\times$ 100).

FIG. 11. Stage 22 (90 hours), 10 μg DON embryo showing the AV area. Increased seeding occurs at lower doses, but migration of cells is altered ($\times$ 250).

FIG. 12. Stage 23 (90 hours), 10 μg DON + 50 μg GSA. AV canal; compare with Fig. 11 ($\times$ 250).

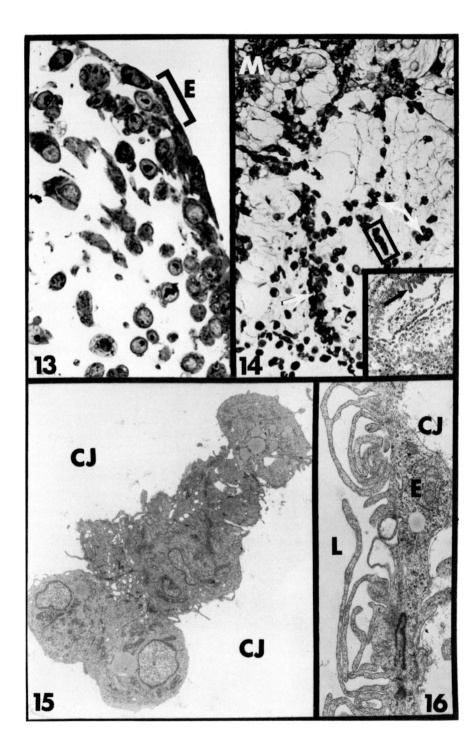

hosts gave rise to the full range of neural crest cell derivatives (13). Noden (25) transplanted brachial neural crest cells to the cranial region and found that the transplanted cells mimicked the migratory pattern of the host region. Here is solid evidence that morphogenetic events, migration and differentiation, were determined not by the cells themselves but by their extracellular environment.

Our own recent studies (23,24) suggest that the properties and composition of normal cardiac jelly (extracellular matrix) can be correlated spatially and temporally with the three major events in CT morphogenesis. The predominant GAG synthesized prior to the seeding of cushion cells was hyaluronate (HA). Lesser but potentially significant amounts of chondroitin sulfate (CHS) were also synthesized. Reduced HA and increased CHS synthesis accompanied cell migration. Structural analyses of the matrix during CT development indicated that these synthetic events represented actual differences in bulk composition and in intermolecular associations. The present study represents our initial attempt to elucidate the meaning of these observations using the inhibitor DON. Admittedly, inhibitors are never totally specific and never shut off all synthesis. However, they afford consideration of the embryo as a whole and provide *in situ* information.

The basic morphological effect produced by DON was suppression of motility characteristics. A major consequence of suppressing AV endocardial motility was reduced cushion cell formation. Virtually identical results were also obtained with cytochalasin B (cyto B). Treatment with 5 μg of this drug, administered just before endocardial activation (55 to 60 hours), blocked formation of endocardial motility appendages and created a very tightly knit epithelium. Formation of the atypical microvilli which interdigitated with those of adjacent cells, as observed after DON administration, may also reflect loss of endocardial mobility characteristics. The close correlation between arrested endocardial motility behavior and reduced formation of CT cells suggests that a principal mechanism for cushion cell formation may be direct translocation of activated endocardium into the adjacent matrix forming mesenchymal progeny. It cannot be concluded

FIG. 13. Stage 22 (90 hours), 10 μg DON. Many AV cushion cells are ovoid to spherical, but most cells appear viable. E, Endocardium. ($\times$ 1,040).

FIG. 14. Same as 13, except cushion cells are shown closer to the myocardium (M). Note tendency of rounded cells to coalesce into aggregates ($\times$ 360). Inset: Arrow denotes myocardial evaginations into unpopulated cardiac jelly at stage 22 after 10 μg DON treatment ($\times$ 100).

FIG. 15. Area showing coalesced cushion cells comparable to that enclosed within the box in Fig. 14. Note that cells are so closely aggregated that they appear almost epithelial. Cardiac jelly (CJ) surrounds the aggregate ($\times$ 2,600).

FIG. 16. AV endocardium (E) from a stage 22 embryo treated with 10 μg DON. Note that the atypical microvilli of the luminal surface (L) interdigitate, creating the appearance of a tightly-knit epithelium ($\times$ 10,000).

that this is the only means of CT cell formation since, at particularly high levels where the effects of DON could not always be overridden with GSA, DON may have directly interfered with additional or alternative seeding mechanisms, e.g., endocardial or CT cell mitotic activity, possibly by an effect on purine metabolism (7,14).

Locomotive appendage formation in seeded mesenchymal cells was also suppressed by DON (as reflected in decreased cell perimeters). Cyto B had a similar effect and, in the case of both drugs, population of the cardiac jelly was abnormal. The jelly was either devoid of cells or populated by aggregates of coalesced CT cells. This provides direct evidence that active cell migration by *in situ* motility mechanisms, i.e., filopodia and pseudopodia (31), is required for normal CT pad formation. Thus, population of cardiac jelly cannot be regarded as a strictly passive process by which progressive endocardial seeding of CT cells displaces or pushes previously seeded CT cells distally towards the myocardium. Based on results obtained with cyto B, the basis for the abnormal pattern of migration may be that CT cells in a rounded condition are unable to integrate randomized collagenous-like microfibrils into polarized matrical tracks normally used as the migratory template (24). Although long-term effects of DON were not studied, the ingrowth of myocardium into unpopulated areas of the cardiac jelly indicate that muscularization of cushion pads may result if population of the cardiac jelly by mesenchymal cells is not complete or uniform.

At 10 to 20 μg amounts, the morphological effects of DON, although less potent than at 50 μg, could be overridden with GSA, indicating that a GSA-containing substance either stimulates or maintains the locomotive activities related to normal CT cell formation and migration. As an inhibitor of GSA formation, DON could potentially minimize the synthesis of HA, CHS (possibly other sulfated GAG), and/or glycoproteins (5,29,32). However, at the time DON was injected, GSA appeared to be preferentially incorporated by the myocardium into HA, with little or none of the precursor utilized for CHS synthesis (19). As shown by Manasek (19), sulfated GAG are produced by the myocardium prior to CT formation but their synthesis does not require GSA. Our X-ray data which reflect molar mass indicated a bulk decrease in matrix material stainable with AB at pH 2.5 following DON treatment. This polyanionic, alcianophilic material was previously identified histochemically as containing HA (20,23). Sulfur-containing components of the matrix were not affected by DON until after the formation of CT cells at 72 hours. These observations confirm Manasek's biochemical identification of a "GSA paradox" and strongly indicate that the GSA-containing substance inhibited by administration of DON at 48 hours is HA. Since GSA can be incorporated into glycoprotein, and since glycoprotein may be covalently or non-covalently interacted with HA (18), it cannot be concluded that only HA is diminished by DON.

The nature of our *in situ* approach inherently precludes the conclusion that morphological effects of DON were solely the result of depleting an extracellular GSA-containing substance that has the potential to initiate motility. However, the administration of DON 24 hours before the initial appearance of CT cells, the absence of cytotoxicity in endocardial and CT cells, and the ability of GSA to override DON effects (at low levels) favor this contention. If this GSA substance is truly HA (or HA + glycoprotein), as suggested above, then the noted correlation of CT seeding with migratory activities within an HA-rich cardiac jelly (23,24) would also be consistent with the conjecture. The studies of Toole and co-workers (30) also strongly implicate HA in coordinating or facilitating migratory behavior. Preliminary results obtained with 3-dimensional cultures, in which the early events of CT formation can be duplicated *in vitro,* indicate that HA can directly promote motility (2). Thus, the similarity of results obtained with DON and cyto B could be interpreted as suggesting that, in the presence of DON, subthreshold amounts of extracellular GSA-containing substances capable of eliciting/maintaining motility in competent cells are formed, whereas cyto B, by virtue of its effect upon cell membranes or microfilaments (15,27,28), directly inhibits the ability of competent cells to respond normally to the stimulus of an extracellular GSA substance.

In summary, DON results suggest that CT development may constitute a tissue interaction in which the capacity of one tissue (the myocardium) to modify the development of an adjacent tissue (AV endocardium) is mediated by extracellular macromolecules (possibly including HA).

ACKNOWLEDGMENTS

The authors wish to express their gratitude to Jayne M. Krook for her excellent technical assistance, Dr. Harry Wood of the Cancer Institute, NIH, for supplying the DON, and Cecile Bishop for typing the manuscript. The work was supported by NIH grant HL-19136 and a NIH Research Career Award to Roger R. Markwald.

REFERENCES

1. Bankl, H. (1977): *Congenital malformations of the heart and great vessels,* Urban and Schwarzenberg, Baltimore, pp. 13-23.
2. Bernanke, D. H., and Markwald, R. R. (1978): Culture model for cardiac cushion morphogenesis. *J. Cell Biol.,* 79:156a.
3. Bolender, D. L., and Markwald, R. R. (1979): Epithelial–mesenchymal transformation in atrioventricular cushion tissue morphogenesis. *Scanning Electron Microscopy/1979,* III. 313-321.
4. Buchanan, J. M. (1973): The aminotransferases. In: *Advances in Enzymology,* vol. 39, pp. 91-183, edited by A. Meister. John Wiley & Sons Inc., New York.
5. DeLuca, S., Heinegard, D., Hascall, V. C., Kimura J. H., and Caplan, A. I. (1977): Chemical and physical changes in proteoglycans during development of chick limb bud chondrocytes grown in vitro. *J. Biol. Chem.,* 252:6600-6608.
6. Ellis, D. B., and Sommar, K. M. (1972): Biosynthesis of respiratory tract mucins. II. Control of hexosamine metabolism by L-glutamine: D-fructose-6-phosphate aminotransferase, *Biochem. Biophys. Acta,* 276:105-112.
7. Ghosh, S., Blumenthal H. J., and Davidson, E. A. (1960): Glucosamine metabolism. V. Enzymatic synthesis of glucosamine-6-phosphate. *J. Biol. Chem.,* 235:1265-1272.
8. Greene, R. M., and Kochhar, D. M. (1975): Limb development in mouse embryos: Protection

against teratogenic effects of 6-diazo-5-oxo-L-norleucine (DON) in vivo and in vitro. *J. Embryol. Exp. Morphol.,* 33:355-370.

9. Hamburger, V., and Hamilton, H. E. (1951): A series of normal stages in the development of the chick embryo. *J. Morph.,* 88:49-92.

10. Hay, D. A. (1978): Development and fusion of the endocardial cushions. In *Birth Defects: Original Article Series,* vol. XIV, No. 7, pp. 69-90, edited by G. C. Rosenquist and D. Bergsma. Alan R. Liss, Inc., New York.

11. Johnson, R. C., Manasek, F. J., Vinson, W. C., and Seyer, J. M. (1974): The biochemical and ultrastructural demonstration of collagen during early heart development. *Dev. Biol.,* 36:252-271.

12. Kochhar, D. M., Adyelotte, M. B., and Vest, T. K. (1976): Altered collagen fibrilogenesis in embryonic mouse limb cartilage deficient in matrix granules. *Exp. Cell Res.,* 102:213-322.

13. Le Douarin, N. M., and Teillet, M. A. M. (1974): Experimental analysis of the migration and differentiation of neuroblasts of the autonomic nervous system and of neuroectodermal mesenchymal derivatives using a biological cell marking technique. *Dev. Biol.,* 41:162-184.

14. Levenberg, B., Melnick, I., and Buchanan, J. M. (1957): Biosynthesis of the purines. XV. The effect of aza-L-serine and 6-diazo-5-oxo-L-norleucine on inosinic acid biosynthesis de novo. *J. Biol. Chem.,* 225:163-176.

15. Lin, S., and Spudich, J. A. (1974): Biochemical studies on the mode of action of cytochalasin B. *J. Biol. Chem.,* 249:5778-5783.

16. Linsenmayer, T. F., and Kochhar, D. M. (1979): In vitro cartilage formation: Effects of 6-diazo-5-oxo-L-norleucine (DON) on glycosaminoglycan and collagen synthesis. *Dev. Biol.,* 69:517-528.

17. Manasek, F. J. (1976): Glycoprotein synthesis and tissue interactions during establishment of the functional embryonic chick heart. *J. Mol. Cell. Cardiol.,* 8:389-402.

18. Manasek, F. J. (1977): Structural glycoproteins of the embryonic cardiac extracellular matrix. *J. Mol. Cell. Cardiol.,* 9:425-429.

19. Manasek, F. M., Reid, M., Vinson, W., Seyer, T., and Johnson, R. (1973): Glycosaminoglycan synthesis by the early embryonic chick heart. *Dev. Biol.,* 35:332-348.

20. Markwald, R. R., and Adams Smith, W. N. (1972): Distribution of mucosubstances in the developing rat heart. *J. Histochem. Cytochem.,* 29:896-907.

21. Markwald, R. R., Fitzharris, T. P., and Adams Smith, W. N. (1975): Structural analysis of endocardial cytodifferentiation. *Dev. Biol.,* 42:160-180.

22. Markwald, R. R., Fitzharris, T. P., and Manasek, F. J. (1977): Structural development of endocardial cushions. *Am. J. Anat.,* 148:85-120.

23. Markwald, R., Fitzharris, T. P., Bank, H., and Bernanke, D. H. (1978): Structural analyses on the matrical organization of glycosaminoglycans in developing endocardial cushion. *Dev. Biol.,* 62:292-316.

24. Markwald, R. R., Fitzharris, T. P., Bolender, D. L., and Bernanke, D. H. (1979): Structural analysis of cell: Matrix association during the morphogenesis of atrioventricular cushion tissue. *Dev. Biol.,* 69:634-654.

25. Noden, D. M. (1975): An analysis of the migratory behavior of avian cephalic neural crest cells. *Dev. Biol.,* 42:106-130.

26. Spooner, B. S., and Conrad, G. W. (1975): The role of extracellular materials in cell movement I. Inhibition of mucopolysaccharide synthesis does not stop ruffling membrane activity or cell movement. *J. Cell Biol.,* 65:286-297.

27. Tannenbaum, J., Tannenbaum, S. W., and Godman, G. C. (1977): The binding sites of cytochalasin D. I. Evidence that they may be peripheral membrane proteins. *J. Cell Physiol.,* 91:225-238.

28. Tannenbaum, J., Tannenbaum, S. W., and Godman, G. C. (1977): The binding sites of cytochalasin D. II. Their relationship to hexose transport and to cytochalasin B. *J. Cell Physiol.,* 91:239-248.

29. Telser, A., Robinson, H. C., and Dorfman, A. (1965): The biosynthesis of chondroitin-sulfate protein complex. *Proc. Natl. Acad. Sci.,* 54:912-919.

30. Toole, B. P., Okayama, M., Orkin, R. W., Yoshimura, M., Muto, M., and Kaji, A. (1977): Developmental roles of hyaluronate and chondroitin sulfate proteoglycans. In: *Cell and Tissue Interactions,* edited by J. W. Lash and M. M. Burger, pp. 139-154. Raven Press, New York.

31. Trinkaus, J. P. (1976): On the mechanisms of metazoan cell movements. In: *The Cell Surface*

in *Animal Embryogenesis and Development,* edited by G. Poste and G. L. Nicolson, pp. 225-329. Elsevier-North Holland, Amsterdam.

32. Trujillo, J. L., and Gan, J. C. (1973): Glycoprotein biosynthesis. VI. Regulation of uridine diphosphate N-acetyl-D-glycosamine metabolism in bovine thyroid gland slices. *Biochim. Biophys. Acta,* 304:32-41.
33. Weston, J. A., and Butler, S. L. (1966): Temporal factors affecting localization of neural crest cells in the chicken embryo. *Dev. Biol.,* 14:246-266.

DISCUSSION

Kulikowski: I would like to ask what you think about the hypothesis that by removing glutamine, using DON as competitive inhibitor, you stop purine biosynthesis and consequently cell division? Is glucosamine the best competitive compound as control, or is glutamine better?

Markwald: The addition of glucosamine did not alter the cell count nor the cell migration. This may indicate that at this stage of development there is a sufficient amount of glutamine. Migration would seem to be more important than cell division in early seeding of the cushion tissue. It is also possible that the two pathways (proliferation and migration) have different degrees of dependence on the amount of glutamine available.

Kulikowski: But Dr. Fitzharris has shown a reasonable mitotic index in the endocardium at that point.

Markwald: Yes, but he has shown it in the outflow tract. I believe that the initial seeding is by locomotive mechanisms that can also be disrupted by cytochalasin B. If we had given DON at a later stage, maybe we would have seen the effect on mitosis.

Kulikowski: Had you tried to add glutamine?

Markwald: No.

Kulikowski: And you know what the mitotic index of the endocardium is at the stages you are looking at?

Markwald: Glutamine can itself be toxic.

Kulikowski: But you have not demonstrated that DON is non-toxic to cell division.

Markwald: The cells did not show signs of arrested mitosis, nor did they show signs of degeneration. They showed only signs of lacking locomotive appendages.

De Haan: We have seen several fairly convincing and even elegant demonstrations of few observations. I think that once we go beyond those observations, a great deal of care has to be taken in making the next step of interpretation. The active interpretation we have been assisting in is perhaps valuable for model building. Embryology in general, and morphogenesis in particular, have already been stricken with problems of model building without model identification.

Cell Surface

Perspectives in Cardiovascular Research, Vol. 5,
Mechanisms of Cardiac Morphogenesis and Teratogenesis,
edited by Tomas Pexieder. Raven Press, New York © 1981

Introduction

Johannes A. Los

Department of Anatomy and Embryology, University of Amsterdam,
1092 AD Amsterdam, The Netherlands

During the past decade, research workers in widely differing fields of biological science have focused their interest on the cell surface, its composition, structure, and function. The endless stream of data and literature from the various disciplines forces me to condense this introduction to keep within the limitations of my competence, the field of descriptive embryology. I will restrict myself to only one aspect of the cell surface in heart morphogenesis, i.e., the morphological behavior of the endocardium during the part of the septation process that, in classical embryology, is known as "fusion."

For a detailed review of the literature regarding the function of cell interaction in cardiac morphogenesis, I may refer to Manasek (16). Poste and Nicolson (24) mention the heart as one of the organs in which research on the cell surface has recently made considerable progress. Trinkaus (30), discussing the mechanisms of metazoan cell movement, states that greatest attention has been given to the question of how cells move in culture, but that the central issue in the study of tissue cell movement is how cells move within the organism. From this point of view, the developing heart is an interesting model for the study of cell action and cell interaction *in vivo.* According to Trinkaus's (30) definition of an epithelium (a tissue that lines a cavity or body surface), Manasek considers the young heart to be an epithelial organ. The outermost epithelium forms the myocardium. The lumen is lined by squamous epithelium, the endocardium. Mesenchymal cells appear in later stages.

The migration of precardiac cells in chick embryos was analyzed by Rosenquist and De Haan (25), by use of labeled transplants. The precardiac cells preserve their original position, and the epithelial cells move as an entire sheet.

Development of the myocardium from epithelioid cells lining the coelomic cavity in the rat was studied by Langemeijer (7). Considering the coelomic cavity and its wall as a hollow organ, comparable to neural tube and foregut, Langemeijer studied the epithelial lining of this organ in successive developmental stages. He found the same interkinetic nuclear migration as described for the neuroepithelium and for a variety of other embryonic epithelia (28). Local mitosis, always taking place at the lumen side of the coelomic organ, is responsible for production of developing myocardium, ventral to the foregut. Ventral bulging and dorsal restriction of epithelioid formation, which encircles a primary endothelial plexus, form the heart tube. Apart from this primary plexus, secondary plexi grow out in later stages, as was shown by Rychter et al. (26) and Schiebler et al. (27). The differentiation of these plexi in coronary arteries, veins, and capillary networks was studied by Heintzberger from our group. The remaining epithelioid cells of the coelomic wall function as a source of radially migrating mesenchymal cells. These cells take part in the formation of mesenchyme (e.g., lung mesenchyme). The origin of the cardiac jelly (2) and particularly the contribution of the endocardium to its formation were discussed by many authors, such as Manasek (16), Markwald et al. (17), and Hay (4,5).

The differing viewpoints are still controversial. The endoderm–mesoderm interaction was reviewed by Manasek (16). He stressed the sandwich character of the splanchnopleura, which consists of two dissimilar cell layers (endoderm and premyocardial mesoderm) separated by extracellular matrix. Markwald et al. (18) pointed out that the mesenchymal cells which gradually replace the endocardial jelly in the truncus arteriosus of the heart are derived from endothelium. In an earlier publication, Markwald et al. (17) came to the conclusion that endocardium appears to lose secretory and other potentials when approached by invaginating myocardial trabeculae.

Nakamura and Manasek (20) analyzed the shape and structure of isolated cardiac jelly. They came to the conclusion that the glucosaminoglycans of this jelly play an important part in its hydration. The stability of its shape is due primarily to the filamentous network interacting with the macromolecules present in the jelly.

To summarize, we might say that at the moment of fusion of endocardium-lined structures, essential step in heart septation, these structures are characterized by a three-layered structure: the epimyocardium, the stabilized cardiac jelly and cells, and the endocardium. Despite the tremendous quantity of descriptive embryologic literature produced during the last century regarding heart septation, the details of development and fusion of the endocardial structures remained obscure until recently. Some of the reasons for this gap in our knowledge of morphogenesis were reviewed by Laane (6) in his study of development of the arterial pole of the chicken heart. The consequences of a "trial-and-error" approach to the study of the fusion of the endocardial truncus ridges and their fusion with the aorticopulmonary septum will be discussed by Laane and Roest-Wagenaar (this volume). This "trial-and-error" approach once again stresses the importance of spatial morphology as a prerequisite for studies in developmental biology, as was pointed out by Los (12). New reconstruction methods have been developed by Los (12) and Schook (29). The latter provided us with a method which makes it possible to study structures from one and the same specimen in space, as well as by light microscopy and transmission electron microscopy. Furthermore, scanning electron microscopy shows the three-dimensional structure of surface elements, which would never have been revealed by reconstruction from histological serial sections. Nevertheless, it should be stressed that SEM can never replace the photographic reconstruction. Rather, these techniques are complementary. The photographic LM and TEM reconstruction restores the spatial structure, with preservation of cellular and subcellular information from transsected structures. The SEM preserves the third dimension of histologically-intact structures even from sections.

Our reconstructions revealed essential differences in shape and structure of the septa of the heart in chick, mouse, rat, and human (6,9,10,11,13). Some septa of the heart, such as the truncus ridges and AV endocardial cushions, are formed from endothelialized cardiac jelly. Others are duplications of the triple-laminated heart wall, such as the interatrial plica, the right venous valve, and perhaps the venous sinus septum in mammals. Finally, some septa arise from massive endothelialized myocardial ridges, such as the left venous valve, part of the interventricular septum, and the septum primum, which is lined with an endocardial rim of varying dimensions in different species, as shown by Los (9,11,13) and Morse (19). Most of these septa grow together and their endocardial linings disappear, creating a single cell mass.

Absence of fusion may give rise to many different types of congenital heart malformations. Some of these can be observed in their primary stage in human embryos (9,10). Restricting ourselves to the atrioventricular endocardial cushions, we wish to stress the fact that, in the chick, these cushions are part of a continuous and complex annular endocardial system (4,5,6,11). This is not the case in rat, mouse, and human. Consequently, the AV endocardial cushions in the chick form the column of an arch, the curved part of which is the endocardial rim of septum primum (Fig. 1A). In mouse, rat, and man, the endocardial rim of septum primum is much smaller and spans the cushion masses as a bridge. These facts are essential to a good understanding of the fusion process.

Fusion is one of those elusive terms, frequently intercalated between invagination or evagination and separation, used to indicate morphogenetic movements in classical descriptive embryology. Recently these terms have gained cellular and subcellular perspective, as has been pointed out by Schook (28). The most frequently used model systems for cellular and subcellular fusion are the inter-branchial clefts, the palatal shelves, the neural walls, the optic cup and lens vesicle, and the optic fissure (1,3,28). From a histological point of view, we must distinguish between coalescence in the sense of "merging" and coalescence in the sense of "fusion." In the case of merging, the cleft between the two limbs of an arch-like structure is filled from below; in the case of fusion, two epithelialized surfaces stick together and, as a consequence of disappearance of their lining cells by degeneration or dedifferentiation, form a single structure.

In our experience, coalescence of the arch-like endocardial AV cushions in the chick, and also of the more isolated endocardial cushions in mouse, rat and man, usually starts from the atrial side and proceeds in the direction of the ventricles. This does not necessarily imply that the process starts from the endocardial rim of septum primum, as appears to be the situation in cases of

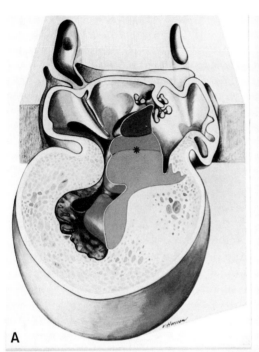

A

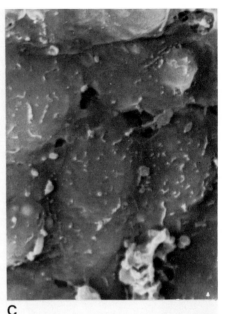

C

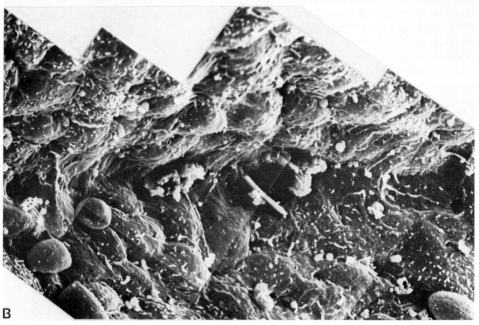

B

persistent subseptal foramen. Neither does the direction of this process imply coalescence in the sense of merging. Starting from the depth of the gap between the cushions, suggesting merging, gradual fusion takes place between the endothelial cells of both cushions (Fig. 1-3)—in other words, a merging-like fusion.

Despite the clinical importance of disturbances in the process of fusion, and therefore of the normal process of fusion itself, only a few investigators have analyzed this process. Hay et al. (4) studied fusion in the chick, using SEM, TEM, mucosubstance histochemistry, and microscopic autoradiography. He suggested that glycoprotein synthesis is not limited to a single cell type. Los et al. (14,15) studied fusion in chick, mouse, and recently in rat, using LM, reconstruction techniques, SEM and TEM. In the region of fusion in chick heart, we found extensive undulating and overlapping cell protrusions. Using the light microscope, we found identical pictures in different species. The TEM and SEM micrographs (Fig. 1,4), however, were quite different. In mouse and to an even lesser extent in rat, small protrusions from the endocardial cells were observed. Some mesenchymal cells were found pouring through interendothelial openings. On the lumenal side of the endothelial cells, only a minor cell coat was observed. Hay (4) stresses the considerable variability in the relationship of endocardial cells to one another at the point of fusion.

All authors agree that the cells adjacent to point of fusion retain their secretory organelles throughout the fusion process, and that no degenerative nuclear changes are observed. (For discussion, see Hay et al. (4), Los et al. (15) and Hay (5). Hay (5) states that, in chick, adjacent endocardial cells appear to maintain cell junctions until the actual edge of cushion matrix continuity is reached. Only at that time do the cells separate. He further states that liberated endocardial cells, no longer subjected to surface stresses, become somewhat rounded, develop pseudopodia and filopodia, and are subsequently undistinguishable from cushion tissue cells.

In this context, a comparison with another extensively studied system seems to clarify the issue. Nelson et al. (21), studying cell movement in corneal endothelium of the avian embryo by SEM, came to the conclusion that ruffling, rather than being a prerequisite for cell movement, might be the result of failure to form new adhesions. Furthermore, these authors state that ruffling ceases abruptly at the point of contact, possibly because a firm adhesion has been made. This can be considered an example of contact inhibition. In their view, the fact that cells do not closely adhere, separated as they are by intercellular

---

FIG. 1. A. Reconstruction of the heart of a chick embryo. Asterisk: fusion of the atrioventricular part of the annular endocardial septal components. **B.** Scanning electron micrograph of the fusion of the atrioventricular part of the septal components in the heart of a 5 e.d. 6 hr chick embryo. Note the lamellipodia and ruffled membranes. **C.** Scanning electron micrograph of the endocardium of the atrioventricular cushions in the heart of a mouse on the 11 e.d. 18 hr. Note the intercellular pores and the mesenchymal cells pouring through one of the pores.

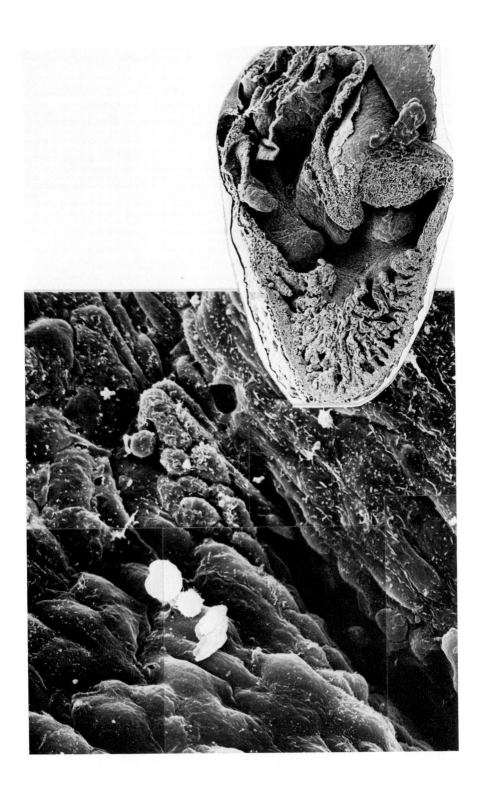

space, might be a way of providing cell–substrate contact rather than cell-to-cell contact.

When Vasiliev and Gelfand (31) analyzed the inverse problem, nonadhesiveness of endothelial and epithelial surfaces, they came to the conclusion that the mechanism involved is an absence of pseudopodial activity. Degrees of adhesiveness differ as a result of varying interactions of membrane components with underlying cortical structures. According to these authors, nonadhesiveness of the luminal surface of endothelia may be a special instance of the nonadhesiveness of the upper surface of epithelial monolayers. In their opinion, the difference between endothelium and epithelium is that the latter has no free active lateral edges, while the former does. Apart from their theories concerning the function of membrane receptors in the adhesiveness or nonadhesiveness of epithelial and endothelial surfaces, this theory, in combination with the observations of Nelson et al. (21), makes the process of fusion of the endocardial AV cushions somewhat less whimsical. The endothelium of the cushions forms a monolayer of firmly interconnected cells, characterized by tight junctions. This monolayer is spread over the primary substrate of mesenchymal cushion cells and is only loosely connected with it. A few filopodia of endothelial cells extend into the cushion mesenchyme. In chick, there are few intercellular pores in the endothelium; there are more in the mouse and rat. In the latter two species, a few mesenchymal cells are found pouring through these pores. This endothelium is a nonadhesive type, and possesses no free lateral edges. From our cinematographic analysis of form and function of the endocardial cushions, we know that they are subjected to considerable intermittent stress during heart action. The influence of hemodynamics on endocardial morphology was discussed by Pexieder (22,23). An even stronger mechanical stress is exerted on the cushions during contraction, which pushes them together. During dilatation, they become separated again. This separation, however, is not instantaneous, because the endothelial cells of both cushions stick together for a moment before loosening. In this way, some endothelial cells may be pulled away from the primary substrate, be torn out during attachment to the opposite side, and, when retracting after separation of the cushions during dilatation, show lamellipodia with ruffled surfaces.

When fusion occurs, the lamellipodia and the ruffles disappear at once, and the endothelial cells become rounded and are transformed into mesenchymal cells (Fig. 5), as was extensively described by Hay et al. (4) and Los et al. (15). The relative scarcity of lamellipodia and ruffles in mouse and rat may be the result of the firmer attachment of the endothelium to the mesenchyme in these species. This seems to be confirmed by the occurrence of mesenchymal cells pouring out through the interendothelial pores. We speculate that this firmer attachment, together with the nature and organization of the membrane

FIG. 2. Scanning electron micrograph of the atrioventricular endocardial cushions in the heart of a rat embryo on the 14 e.d. 6 hr. Note the fusion of opposed endocardial cells, starting from the atrial side.

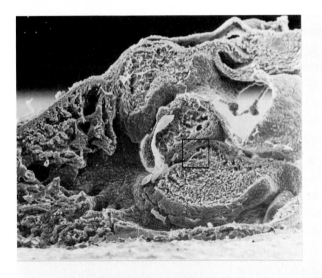

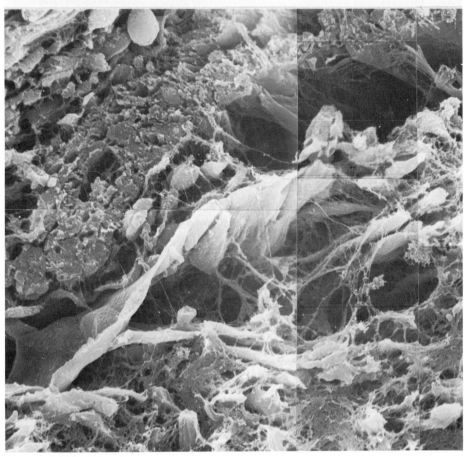

FIG. 3. Scanning electron micrographs of fusing atrioventricular endocardial cushions in the heart of a rat embryo on the 14 e.d. 6 hr. Note the detachment of the endocardial sheet from the dense mesenchyme to which it was loosely attached.

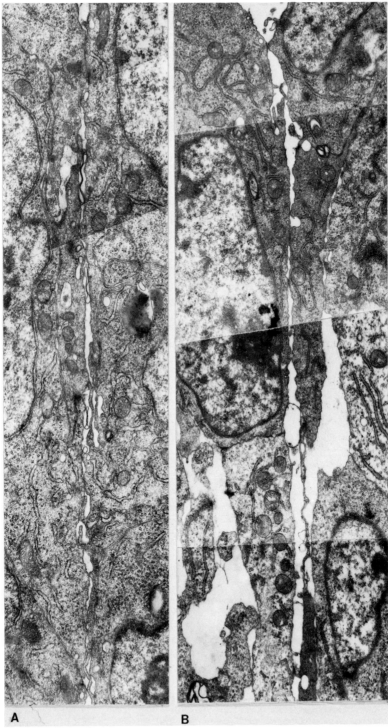

FIG. 4. A. Composite transmission electron micrograph of the fusion of atrioventricular endocardial cushions in the heart of a 5 e.d. 6 hr chick embryo. Note the long, flat protrusions of the opposed endocardial cells. **B.** Composite transmission electron micrograph of the fusion of atrioventricular cushions in the heart of a rat embryo on the 14 e.d. 6 hr. Note the mesenchymal cells below the long flat endocardial cells and the small cell protrusions.

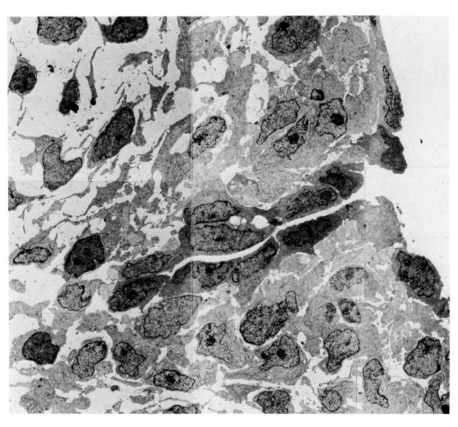

FIG. 5. Fusing endocardia of atrioventricular cushions in the heart of a rat embryo on the 14 e.d. 6 hr.

receptors and the intensity of the mechanical influence (heart contraction in relation to the dimensions of the cushions), may be responsible for a lesser degree of adhesiveness of the cushions in these species. We can extrapolate that this will give rise to the possible occurrence of septal defects. The low adhesiveness may be further decreased during the less active phase of endocardial cytodifferentiation (18), consequent to invagination of myocardial trabeculae. The discussed changes in activity may be responsible for the persistence of primary defects. Some points of this exciting hypothesis remain obscure, however, such as the relative scarcity of junctions between fusing opposite endothelial cells and the organization of microfilaments in the ruffles of the lamellipodia before fusion. Indirect immunofluorescence techniques on detergent-denaturated actin provide further perspective for the study of fusion. However, much work must still be done to confirm our hypothesis or to replace it with a better one.

ACKNOWLEDGMENTS

The author is greatly indebted for scientific and technical contributions to the members of his working group: H.-M. Laane, R. A. Th. M. Langemeijer, P. Schook, C. F. M. Heintzberger, S. C. Tesink-Taekema, and E. Langemeijer van Eyndthoven. Special thanks are due to Dr. J. James, director of the Institute for Histology and Cell Biology, and to Dr. N. Nanninga, director of the Institute for Electron Microscopy and Molecular Cytology, for providing SEM facilities. A special debt is also owed to the medical photographer, C. J. Hersbach, and to the medical artist, A. A. van Horssen, for preparing the figures, and to the secretaries, Mrs. C. K. v.d. Poel-Ras and Mrs. E. M. Prakken-de Wert, for typing the manuscript.

REFERENCES

1. Bancroft, M., and Bellairs, R. (1975): Differentiation of the neural plate and neural tube in the young chick embryo. A study by scanning and transmission electron microscopy. *Anat. Embryol.,* 147:309-335.
2. Davis, C. L. (1924): The cardiac jelly of the chick embryo. *Anat. Rec.,* 27-29.
3. Geeraets, R. (1976): An electron microscopic study of the closure of the optic fissure in the golden hamster. *Am. J. Anat.,* 145:411-431.
4. Hay, D. A. (1978): Development and fusion of the endocardial cushions. In: *Morphogenesis and Malformation of the Cardiovascular System,* edited by G. C. Rosenquist and D. Bergsma, pp. 69-90. *Birth Defects: Original Article Series,* vol. XIV, no. 7. A. R. Liss Inc., New York.
5. Hay, D. A., and Low, F. N. (1972): The fusion of dorsal and ventral endocardial cushions in the embryonic chick heart: A study in fine structure. *Am. J. Anat.,* 133:1-24.
6. Laane, H. M. (1978): The arterial pole of the embryonic heart. *(Thesis.)* Swets and Zeitlinger, Amsterdam.
7. Langemeijer, R. A. T. M. (1976): Le coelome et son revêtement comme organoblastème. *Bull. Assoc. Anat.,* 60:547-558.
8. Lazarides, E. and Revel, J. P. (1979): The molecular basis of cell movement. *Sci. Am.,* 240(5):88-101.
9. Los, J. (1971): A case of heart septum defect in a human embryo of 27 mm C.R. length, as

a helpful record in studying the components participating in heart septation. *Acta Morphol. Neerl.-Scand.,* 8:161-182.

10. Los, J. A. (1972): Analysis of a persistent interventricular communication in a human embryo of 19.8 mm C.R. length. *Acta Morphol. Neerl.-Scand.,* 9:179-206.

11. Los, J. A. (1972): The heart of the 5-day chick embryo during dilatation and contraction. A functional hypothesis based on morphological observation. *Acta Morphol. Neerl.-Scand.,* 9:309-335.

12. Los, J. A. (1973): Reconstructive morphology. Possibilities and limitations. *Acta Morphol. Neerl.-Scand.,* 11:263-278.

13. Los, J. A. (1978): Cardiac septation and development of the aorta, pulmonary trunk and pulmonary veins: Previous work in the light of recent observations. In: *Morphogenesis and Malformation of the Cardiovascular System,* edited by G. C. Rosenquist and D. Bergsma, pp. 109-138. *Birth Defects: Original Article Series,* vol. XIV, No. 7. A. R. Liss Inc., New York.

14. Los, J. A., and Drukker, J. (1969): A light-microscopical study of the process of fusion of the endocardial atrioventricular cushions in the chicken embryo. *Acta Morphol. Neerl.-Scand.,* 7:365.

15. Los, J. A. and van Eyndthoven, E. (1973): The fusion of the endocardial cushions in the heart of the chick embryo. *Z. Anat. Entwickl.-Gesch.,* 141:55-75.

16. Manasek, F. J. (1976): Heart development: Interactions involved in cardiac morphogenesis. In: *The Cell Surface in Animal Embryogenesis and Development,* edited by G. Poste and G. L. Nicolson, pp. 545-598. North-Holland Publishing Company, Amsterdam.

17. Markwald, R. R., Fitzharris, T. P., and Manasek, F. J. (1977): Structural development of endocardial cushions. *Am. J. Anat.,* 148:85-120.

18. Markwald, R. R., Fitzharris, T. P., and Adams Smith, W. N. (1975): Structural analysis of endocardial cytodifferentiation *Dev. Biol.,* 42:160-180.

19. Morse, D. E. (1978): Scanning electron microscopy of the developing septa in the chick heart. In: *Morphogenesis and Malformation of the Cardiovascular System,* edited by G. C. Rosenquist and D. Bergsma, pp. 91-107. *Birth Defects: Original Art Series,* vol. XIV, no. 7. A. R. Liss Inc., New York.

20. Nakamura, A., and Manasek, F. J. (1978): Experimental studies of the shape and structure of isolated cardiac jelly. *J. Embryol. Exp. Morph.,* 43:167-183.

21. Nelson, G. A., and Revel, J. P. (1975): Scanning electron microscopic study of cell movements in the corneal endothelium of the avian embryo. *Dev. Biol.,* 42:315-333.

22. Pexieder, T. (1976): Effects de l'hemodynamique sur la morphologie de l'endocarde embryonnaire. *Bull. Assoc. Anat.,* 60:399-406.

23. Pexieder, T. (1978): Development of the outflow tract of the embryonic heart. In: *Morphogenesis and Malformation of the Cardiovascular System,* edited by G. C. Rosenquist and D. Bergsma, pp. 29-68. *Birth Defects: Original Art Series,* vol. XIV, no. 7. A. R. Liss Inc., New York.

24. Poste, G., and Nicolson, G. L., eds. (1976): *The Cell Surface in Animal Embryogenesis and Development.* North-Holland Publishing Company, Amsterdam.

25. Rosenquist, G. C. and De Haan, R. L. (1966): Migration of precardiac cells in the chick embryo: A radioautographic study. *Carnegie Inst. Wash. Contributions to Embryology,* 38:111-121.

26. Rychter, Z., and Ošťáclal, B. (1971): Mechanism of the development of coronary arteries in chick embryo. *Folia Morphol., (Praha)* 19:113–124.

27. Schiebler, T. H., and Voboǐil, Z. (1969): Zur entwicklung der Gefässe im Herzmuskel. *Experientia,* 25:845.

28. Schook, P. (1978): A review of data on cell actions and cell interactions during the morphogenesis of the embryonic eye. *Acta Morphol. Neerl.-Scand.,* 16:267-286.

29. Schook, P., and Blom, N. (1978): A three-dimensional reconstruction method preserving light microscopic and transmission electron microscopic information. *Acta Morphol. Neerl.-Scand.,* 16:157-170.

30. Trinkaus, J. P. (1976): On the mechanism of metazoan cell movements. In: *The Cell Surface in Animal Embryogenesis and Development,* edited by G. Poste and G. L. Nicolson, pp. 225-329. North-Holland Publishing Company, Amsterdam.

31. Vasiliev, J. M. and Gelfand, I. M. (1978): Mechanism of nonadhesiveness of endothelial and epithelial surfaces. *Nature,* 274:710-711.

Perspectives in Cardiovascular Research, Vol. 5,
Mechanisms of Cardiac Morphogenesis and Teratogenesis,
edited by Tomas Pexieder. Raven Press, New York © 1981

Development and Fusion of Endocardial Structures in the Arterial Pole of the Heart of Chick, Rat and Human Embryos

Henk-Maarten Laane and Jeanette A. Roest-Wagenaar

Department of Anatomy and Embryology, University of Amsterdam,
1092 AD Amsterdam, The Netherlands

During the last decade, there has been a growing interest in the study of the development of the arterial outflow tract (2,3,4,6,8,11,12,14). Some of these studies concerned the development and fusion of the ridges in the outflow tract of the embryonic heart (3,4,13,14,15). An extensive description of the development of the endocardial structures in the arterial pole was published earlier (4). The most important facts, which are essential for a good understanding of the development of the ridges, will shortly be summarized.

MATERIALS AND METHODS

For light microscopic study, the embryos were removed from the egg or the uterus, fixed in Bouin's solution, dehydrated, sectioned at 7 μm, and stained with hematoxylin–azophloxin. Several specimens of each developmental stage were sectioned in frontal, transverse, and sagittal directions. A second procedure was also used: isolated hearts were immersion-fixed in Karnovsky's cacodylate-buffered aldehyde fixative, embedded in Epon, serially sectioned at 5 μm, and stained with iron hematoxylin (16,17).

From the serial sections of some stages, we made three-dimensional reconstructions, using the photographic reconstruction technique (5,7). Finally, glass plate reconstructions were made, enabling small parts of the embryonic heart to be reconstructed very rapidly. For electron microscopy, isolated hearts embedded in Epon were used. Sectioning was performed alternately in 1 μm and 0.06 to 0.09 μm sections. The ultra-thin sections were stained with uranyl acetate and lead citrate. These hearts were also used to make serial sections of 1 μm.

OBSERVATIONS

In the single tube-like heart (chick embryo, 4 e.d.; rat embryo, 12 e.d.; and human embryo, 30 e.d., 5 mm C.R. length), the following parts can be distinguished: the sinus venosus, the atria, the atrioventricular canal, and the primitive ventricle, characterized by its trabeculation. The right part of this ventricle continues into the arterial pole, which can be further subdivided. According to histological criteria, almost the entire arterial pole inside the pericardial cavity consists of an (epi)myocardial and a gelatinous endocardial layer; in the ultimate distal part, both layers are replaced by mesenchyme. Hence, a long proximal myocardial and a short distal mesenchymal arterial trunk can be distinguished. Outside the pericardial cavity, the endothelium of the mesenchymal trunk continues into the mesenchyme ventral to the foregut. Here, the widened endothelial tube, called sinus arteriosus by Los (8), ramifies into the arterial arches in a specific way: the bloodstream from the mesenchymal arterial trunk divides into a cranially-directed aortic stream and a caudally-directed pulmonary stream. The architecture of this bifurcation is such that the wedge-shaped edge of mesenchyme between the origins of both streams acts as a "crista dividens" and is the predecessor of the aorticopulmonary septum.

During the next developmental stage (chick embryo, 40 e.d. 12 h; rat embryo, 12 e.d. 12 h; human embryo 32 e.d., 6 to 7 mm C.R. length), this mesenchymal wedge becomes accentuated, because the angle between the aortic and pulmonary streams decreases. At the same time, the aorta and pulmonary trunk, from their extrapericardial position, become enclosed within the pericardial cavity. During this process, the aorta and pulmonary trunk lengthen considerably and, at the same time, change their relative positions. In the next developmental stage (chick embryo, 5 e.d.; rat embryo, 13 e.d.; human embryo, 34 e.d., 8 mm C.R. length), the aorticopulmonary septum grows out proximally into the truncus to reach the borderline separating the myocardial and mesenchymal arterial trunk. Before the free edge of this septum reaches the distal truncus ridges, it becomes anchored in the endocardial jelly by two proximal extensions. These extensions are well developed, especially in the chick embryo. They can also be distinguished in rat and human embryos. In the 9 mm human embryo, the aorticopulmonary septum has reached the myocardial arterial trunk and grows out into the distal truncus ridges. As a consequence of this ingrowth, the ridges become united. In later stages (chick embryo, 6 e.d.; rat embryo, 13 e.d. 12 hr; human embryo, 11 mm), the truncus ridges fuse proximally to the ingrowing aorticopulmonary septum, thus forming the septum trunci. In the septum trunci, the aorticopulmonary septum extends proximally (Fig. 1). This fusion process is characterized by light microscopy by mutual interdigitation of the endocardial lining cells (Fig. 2B). The aorticopulmonary septum extends

FIG. 1. Parallel cross-sectional diagram of the outflow tract(s) of the 6 days' embryo heart. **A1.** (proximal) left (=septal) ridge; **2:** (proximal) right (=parietal) ridge. **B3.** continuation of the atrioventricular cushion-mass into the truncus endocardial jelly; **4:** lateral-right atrioventricular cushion; **5:** right atrioventricular canal; **6:** left ventricular outflow tract; **7:** right ventricular outlet; **8:** (distal) dorsal (=septal) ridge; **9:** (distal) ventral-right (=parietal) ridge. **C10.** proximal extended cell-columns of the aortico-pulmonary septum; **11:** fusion-line of the truncus ridges. **D12.** aortico-pulmonary septum; **13:** (distal) ventral-left ridge; **14:** (distal) lateral-left ridge. **FIII.** carotid arterial arches; **IV:** (right) aortic arch; **VI:** pulmonary arteries. Reprinted with permission from *Acta Morphol. Neerl.-Scand; Swets en Zeitlinger,* Amsterdam.

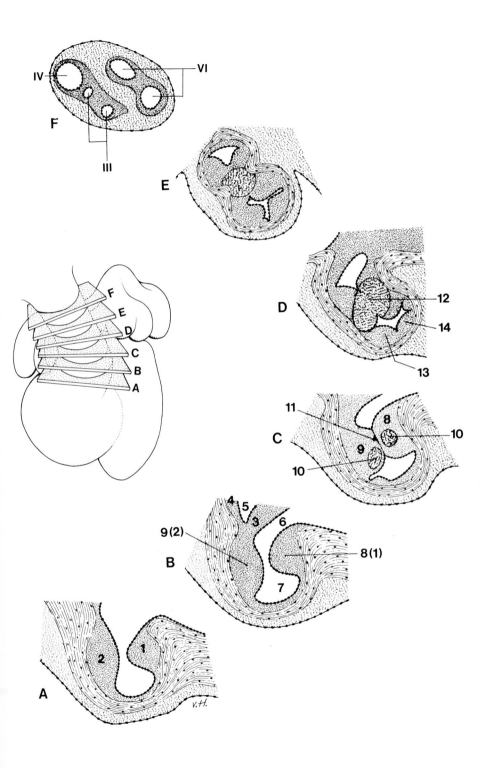

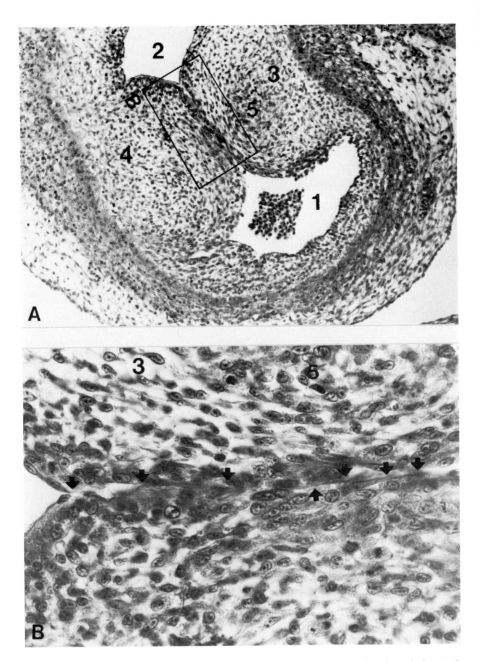

FIG. 2A. Transversal section of the fusing truncus ridges of the 6 days' embryonic heart. **1:** right ventricular outlet; **2:** left ventricular outlet; **3:** (distal) dorsal (septal) ridge; **4:** (distal) ventral-right (=parietal) ridge; **5:** dense mesenchyme of the proximal extension of the aortico-pulmonary septum. **B.** High magnification of the rectangular area marked out by black lines in Fig. 2A. The arrows show the fusion line of the endothelium of both ridges. **C.** A more distal section:

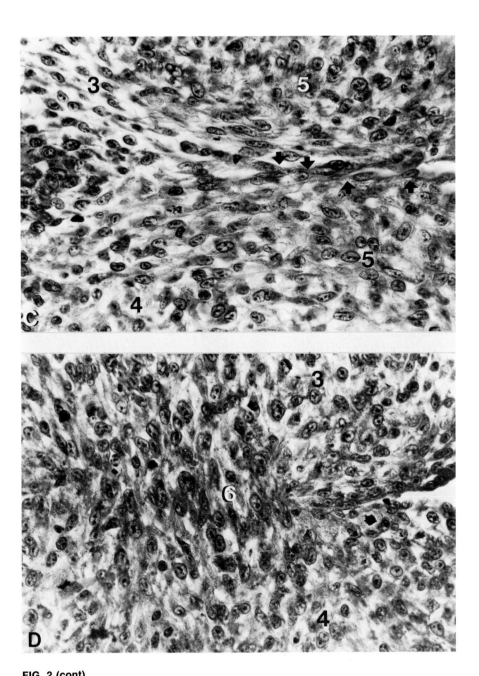

FIG. 2 (cont)
at the right side the fusing endothelia are still recognizable; at the left side the mesenchyme
of both ridges is one continuous endocardial mass. **D.** In a more distal section the dense
mesenchyme of the aortico-pulmonary septum (6) has extended into the fused truncus ridges.
Reprinted with permission from *Acta Morphol. Neerl.-Scand; Swets and Zeitlinger,* Amsterdam.

proximally into the fused ridges (Fig. 2D). This fusion zone extends over an area of about 60 μm in the chick embryo heart. It is much longer in the hearts of rat and human (Fig. 5). With the light microscope, slight differences can be distinguished between the fusion processes of chick and rat. The interdigitation of endocardial cells is most pronounced in the chick embryo. Only in rat and human do we observe that the two endocardia sometimes adhere. The endocardium may even become detached from the truncus ridge on one side.

With the data from the 7 μm sections, the fusion process of the truncus ridges was studied with the electron microscope. This process has already been described for the embryonic chick heart (14). In that study, the heart was sectioned from the arterial arches in the direction of the ventricle, transversally to the truncus. Using the LKB pyramitome, sections of 5 μm were made up to the region of fusion. Serial sections of 1 μm of the whole truncus were made in order to select locations from which, in the next series, ultra-thin sections could be made.

Two series of 1 μm of chick and rat will now be described in the proximo-distal direction. In the chick (Fig. 3), the truncus ridges can be very easily distinguished because of the asymmetrical position of the dense mesenchyme in the spurs of the aorticopulmonary septum. In the septal truncus ridge, the dense mesenchyme is situated very close to the myocardium. In the parietal truncus ridge, the dense mesenchyme lies just below the endocardium at some distance from the myocardium. Fig. 3A shows that the endocardium of the septal truncus ridge consists of very elongated cells which form a continuous layer of endothelium. In the parietal truncus ridge, the endocardial cells intermingle with the cells of the dense mesenchyme. In an earlier publication (14), we described use of the electron microscope to reveal that the cells of the dense mesenchyme of the parietal truncus ridge pass the endocardium and establish the first contact between the truncus ridges (Fig. 4). Fig. 3B shows that, more distally, the continuity of these two rows of endocardium is interrupted on the left side. Here, endocardium-like cells have dispersed in the network of mesenchymal cells. Fig. 3C shows this process, the two truncus ridges forming a continuity. The dense mesenchymal cores of the parietal and septal truncus ridges are still separated. More distally, (Fig. 3D), these mesenchymal cores are forming one continuous aorticopulmonary septum.

Proximally, in the rat, the dense mesenchyme of both truncus ridges lies in the proximity of the myocardium, so that the septal and parietal truncus ridges are identical. The endocardial cover of both ridges consists of a continuous layer of long, flat cells (Fig. 5A). With the electron microscope, the two continuous layers can be distinguished (Fig. 6). No junctions can be observed between cells from opposite sides, but they do occur between cells of the same side.

FIG. 3. Parallel 1-μm cross sections of the outflow tract of the 6 days' embryonic chick heart (arranged like the sequence of Figs. 1 and 2). PR: parietal (distal ventral-right) ridge; SR: septal (distal dorsal) ridge.

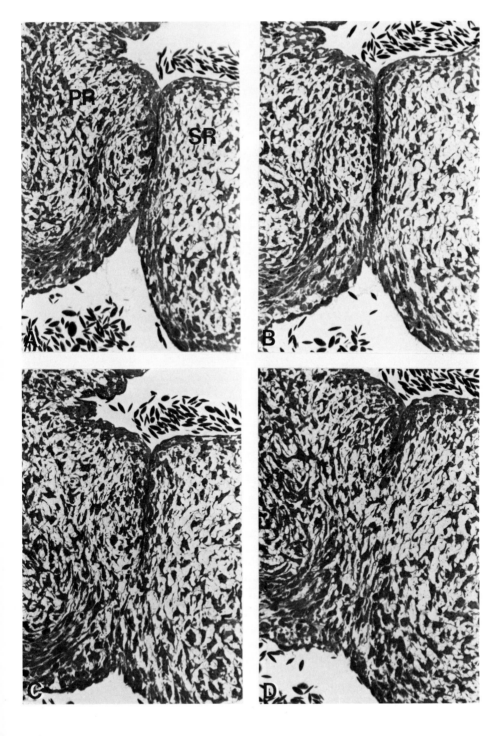

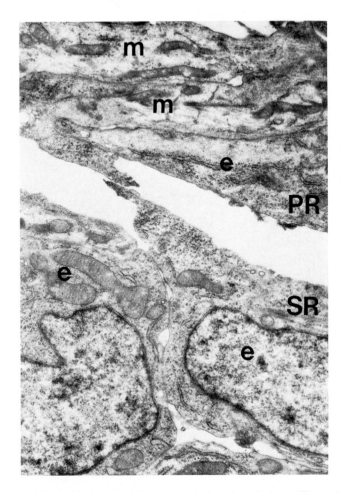

FIG. 4. A part of the fusing truncus ridges in the chick embryonic heart. The endothelium (e) is interrupted by a pseudopodium of a cell of the dense mesenchyme (m).

On a more distal level (Fig. 5B), there are still two rows of endocardial cells. The dense mesenchyme is situated nearer the endocardial cells and is orientated perpendicular to them. Between the layer of endocardial cells and the dense mesenchyme, a few mesenchymal cells remain parallel to the endocardial cells. Fig. 5C shows that the continuity of the two endocardial layers is interrupted by the dense mesenchyme. Several cells, recognizable as endocardial cells, are observed between the dense mesenchyme and the two lumina. Distally

FIG. 5. Parallel 1- and 5-μm cross section of the outflow tract of the 14 days' rat embryonic heart (arranged like the sequence of Figs. 1 and 2). PR: parietal ridge; SR: septal ridge; d: dense mesenchyme; a-p.s.: aortico-pulmonary septum.

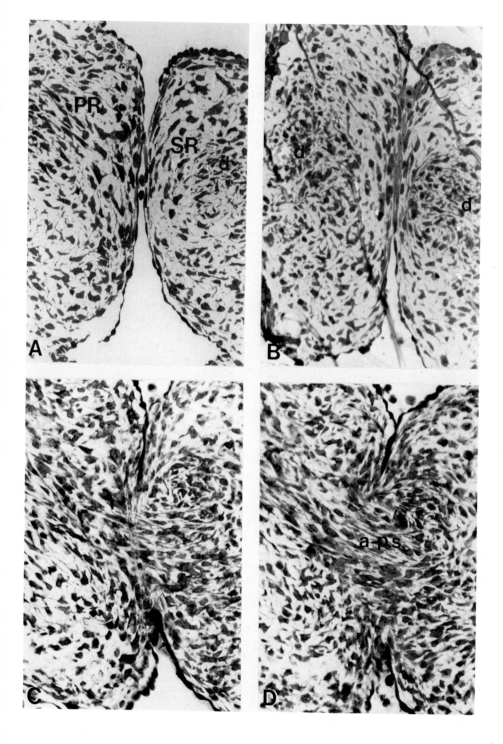

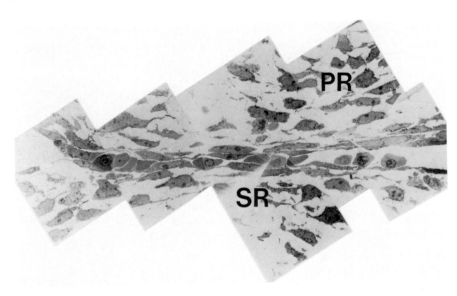

FIG. 6. A survey of the area of fusing ridges in the rat embryonic heart (negative magnification 2,000). PR: parietal ridge; SR: septal ridge.

(Fig. 5D), the dense mesenchyme of both ridges forms one large mass, the so-called aorticopulmonary septum.

DISCUSSION

Descriptions in the literature of the fusion process in the truncus are contradictory, because the characteristics of this process are not precisely defined. The first phase of septation of the myocardial part of the arterial trunk is characterized in chick, rat and human embryonic heart by ingrowth of the dense mesenchyme of the aorticopulmonary septum in the distal truncus ridges. After this ingrowth, the ridges proximal to the septum start to fuse. The light microscope shows the same characteristics of fusion of the ridges, as described by Los et al. (9), for the fusing atrioventricular endocardial cushions. With the electron microscope, it is difficult to distinguish the endocardial from the mesenchymal cells in the fusing ridges of the chick. In the truncus ridges, the mesenchymal cells derive from the endocardial cells by mitosis during an earlier embryonic stage (10). It is therefore not surprising that, when layers of endocardial cells approach each other, the differences between mesenchyme and endocardium gradually disappear.

This dispersion of the endocardial cells in the mesenchyme of the cardiac jelly occurs only in the chick. It is very similar to the process described by Hay and Low in the atrioventricular endocardial cushions (1). These authors also believe that the cushion cells originally derive from the endocardium. However, there are differences between these two processes. Los et al. (9) state that the endocardial cells of the AV endocardial cushions have many interdigitating protrusions, which cannot be detected in the truncus ridges. The dense mesenchyme also cannot be detected in the endocardial cushions. We believe that it is not the endocardial cell that plays the most important role during fusion but rather the dense mesenchyme. In chick and rat, the situation is different. In chick, the dense mesenchyme of the parietal ridge disrupts the endocardium and establishes the first contact with the endocardium of the septal ridge. This process extends over 20 to 60 μm. In rat, dense mesenchyme migrates and penetrates between the endocardial cells, establishing the first contact between the truncus ridges. This process spans no more than 10 to 20 μm, even less than in chick. The fusion of truncus ridges could not be confirmed by TEM using 7 and 5 μm sections. There is no real contact; the junctions between the endocardial cells of both sides cannot be detected in the rat.

REFERENCES

1. Hay, D. A., and Low, F. N. (1972): The fusion of dorsal and ventral endocardial cushions in the embryonic chick. *Am. J. Anat.,* 133:1-24.
2. Jaffee, O. C. (1967): The development of the arterial outflow tract in the chick embryo heart. *Anat. Rec.,* 158:35-42.
3. Laane, H.-M. (1972): Observations concerning the septation process in the truncus arteriosus of the chick embryo. *Acta Morph. Neerl.-Scand.,* 10:376.
4. Laane, H.-M. (1978): The arterial pole of the embryonic heart. *(Thesis.)* Swets and Zeitlinger, Amsterdam.
5. Laane, H.-M., and Bourier, J.: A fast three-dimensional reconstruction method. *Acta Morph. Neerl.-Scand.,* 17 *(in press).*
6. Los, J. A. (1965): Le cloisonnement du tronc artériel chez l'embryon humain. *C.R. Ass. Anat.,* 50:682-686.
7. Los, J. A. (1970/71): A new method of three dimensional reconstruction of microscopic structures based on photographic techniques. *Acta Morph. Neerl.-Scand.,* 8:273-279.
8. Los, J. A. (1978): Cardiac septation and development of aorta, pulmonary trunk and pulmonary veins: previous work in the light of recent observations. In: *Morphogenesis and Malformation of the Cardiovascular System,* edited by A. C. Rosenquist and D. Bergsma, pp. 109-138. *Birth Defects: Original Article Series,* vol XIV, no. 7. A. D. Liss Inc., New York.
9. Los, J. A. and van Eyndthoven, E. (1973): The fusion of endocardial cushions in the heart of the chick embryo. *Z. Anat. Entw.-Gesch.,* 141:55-75.
10. Markwald, R. R., Fitzharris, T. P., and Manasek, F. J. (1977): Structural development of endocardial cushions. *Am. J. Anat.,* 148:85-120.
11. Pexieder, T. (1972): Beobachtungen über den lokalen Zelltod während der Herzbulbusseptierung des Hühnerembryos. Verh. Anat. Ges. 66. *An. Anz.,* 131:279-286.
12. Pexieder, T. (1978): Development of the outflow tract of the embryonic heart. In: *Morphogenesis and Malformation of the Cardiovascular System,* edited by G. C. Rosenquist and D. Bergsma, pp. 29-68. *Birth Defects: Original Art Series,* vol. XIV, no. 7. A. V. Liss Inc., New York.
13. Roest-Wagenaar, J. A. (1972): An electronmicroscopical study of the fusion process in chick embryos. *Acta Morph. Neerl.-Scand.,* 10:337.
14. Roest-Wagenaar, J. A. (1975): An electron-microscopic study of the truncus ridges in chick embryos. *Acta Morph. Neerl.-Scand.,* 13:187-200.
15. Rychter, Z. (1957): The vascular system of the chick embryo. III. On the problem of septation of the heart bulb and trunk in chick embryos. *Cs. Morfol.,* 7:1-20.
16. Schantz, A., and Schechter, A. (1965): Iron hematoxylin and safranin as polychrome stain for Epon sections. *Stain Techn.,* 40:279.

17. Schook, P., and Blom, N. (1978): A three-dimensional reconstruction method preserving light microscopic and transmission electron microscopic information. *Acta Morph. Neerl.-Scand.*, 16:157-170.

DISCUSSION

Pexieder: You have to be very careful in basing the statement on interspecific differences in AV cushion fusion on the approach you have chosen. Fusion is a continuous process, and it may be that what you are considering as species differences are just different phases of essentially the same process. I would like to comment more generally on the application of scanning electron microscopy to the study of heart development. **A.** According to the way the heart is dissected, mounted, and tilted during SEM examination and photography, you may interpret the micrograph in agreement with any particular hypothesis. It will be necessary, in the future, to standardize the SEM micrographs. **B.** At the cellular level, we have to take into account the wide variability of cell morphology as seen with SEM in the developing heart. Ruffling edges mean only that a cell is more active than another cell, but they are not specific for the fusion process.

Laane: There is a histological difference between fusion of AV cushions in the rat and in the chick. Dr. Roest-Waagenaar has standardized the method of sectioning of the region of fusion.

Pexieder: At which interval did you sample your specimens?

Roest-Waagenaar: There is already a wide variability in 6 e.d. chick embryos covering the different phases of the fusion process. We had to modify our method of sectioning for the rat, as the zone of fusion is much greater than in the chick.

Los: On the basis of some references, we consider ruffling a consequence of unsuccessful attachment of a cell to the underlying mesenchyme. In my experience, fusion takes place in a quarter of an hour. It is therefore impossible to stage those embryos. We study some hundreds of embryos, section them all, and can then follow the process of fusion exactly.

Rychter: I would like to suggest another interpretation for the dense mesenchyme replacing myocardium. This may be the ingrowth of the branchial arch mesenchyme into the arterial end of the heart. In relationship to proximal bulbar cushions, I would like to recall our previous work on the frequency of the proximal interstitial bulbar cushion. In experiments, decreasing the space available, and consequently increasing the modeling effect of the bloodstream, decreased the incidence of this small third proximal cushion.

Laane: Myocardium and endocardium are not replaced by dense mesenchyme. It is a gradual and constant transition. I have also observed the temporary third cushion or ridge.

DeHaan: I have seen some mitotic figures subjacent to the endothelium in the region of fusion. Can you generalize that there is a modification of mitotic activity just as the two surfaces come together?

Laane: We did not specifically study the mitotic activity.

Los: In the AV cushions, we usually find mitotic activity in the endothelium just before fusion. We never find degeneration.

Pexieder: Our proliferation studies in the outflow tract (see pps. 79–88) show that there is no increase in proliferation of the endocardium which might accompany the process of cushion fusion. Only between 6 and 7 e.d., during closure of the interventricular communication, is there a general increase in proliferation of all the components and tissue types surrounding the FIV.

Fitzharris: I think that it is very incorrect to use the term "ruffling." Most cell biologists now agree that ruffling has nothing to do with movement. I will suggest the term "microplicae," coined by Keith Porter, for infolding and outpocketing of adjacent cells. These microplicae increase the surface and the contact between the cells and obviously their adhesiveness.

Pexieder: Whatever the correct name may be, my point was that those formations are not specific for the region of fusion. Even if fusion is a very common process in embryonic development, there seem to be some differences, e.g., the epithelial denudation of palatal processes preceeding their contact. This does not seem to happen in the heart. There have also been reports of modifications of the glycocalix during fusion of nasal processes. Do you have any idea what may be the fate of the glycocalix during the fusion of AV cushions?

Los: In my opinion, the term "fusion" is another confusing name. It seems that degeneration, in relationship to fusion, is restricted to epithelia. Endothelium does not seem to be concerned. We did not study the cell coat. In the heart, the cell coat is much less important than in the eye.

Fischman: Is there any evidence that there are biochemical changes in these cells at the point of approximation?

Hay: We have done some basic histochemical studies using ruthenium red and alcian blue at the time of fusion. The cell coat is very dense, but we could not detect any definite change in the pattern of the ruthenium red staining.

DeHaan: The ruffling does really exist in cell cultures, and does not seem to be associated with the loss of contact with a physical substratum.

Los: Does anybody know if the fibronectins have something to do with the process of fusion? My second problem is, how to prevent the fusion of AV cushions?

Hay: One possibility for study of the fibronectins is to obtain fibronectin-specific antibody.

DeHaan: Such antibodies are already available, from Dr. Wartiovaara in Helsinki. The surface glycoprotein may have positive and negative effects on the process of fusion: positive, in recognizing the fusing cells and in their adhesion, and negative, in formation of gap junctions, since the glycoprotein of approaching cell surfaces must somehow be digested or removed in some other way. Did you ever see a junctional complex between these cells?

Los: We have never seen tight or gap junctions.

Markwald: We have seen very strong staining for fibronectin at the luminal surface of the AV pad. If fibronectin is involved, you might have been able to prevent the fusion by using the antibody itself. Since proteoglycans are involved in fibronectin-fibronectin interactions, and hyaluronate is necessary for the fusion, the use of glycosaminoglycan hydrolases may prevent this fusion.

Fischman: There is increasing interest in the role of plasminogen inactivator and its regional disposition in areas of morphogenesis. Since an entire series of very specific protid inhibitors are available, it will be interesting to apply them to the study of the fusion process. Some of these inhibitors are even fluorescent.

Pexieder: You will certainly find a chemical substance that delays the fusion, but the interpretation of your result will be rather difficult because of the complex action of chemical agents. Some of the hemodynamic interventions also will certainly delay this fusion. You may also use a model in which the absence of fusion has a genetic background, as in the keeshond dog. Finally, the easiest and least artifactual way will be organ culture of AV cushions with a mechanical control of fusion or its prevention. The choice of method will depend on the question you want to ask your system.

DeHaan: Taking into account the heart action at that particular moment, the cushions are actually resting together 200 or 300 msec maximum. Yet at a single beat, apparently during that 200 msec period, some cells must adhere tightly enough that they are not blown apart by the next systole!

Los: When analyzing our films of heart action and blood flow in the embryonic chick, we have seen that those cushions stick together for a moment during diastole. Unfortunately, at the very moment of fusion, the heart is no longer transparent to permit a followup of the process.

Hay: The cushions have been progressively blocked together, not only by their own growth but also by their close association and fusion with the basal portion of the interatrial septum. At stage 28, the AV cushions are blocked in contact even during diastole, because they are fused with the bridge of the interatrial septum above.

Cell Physiology and Interactions

Perspectives in Cardiovascular Research, Vol. 5,
Mechanisms of Cardiac Morphogenesis and Teratogenesis,
edited by Tomas Pexieder. Raven Press, New York © 1981

Introduction

R. L. DeHaan

Department of Anatomy, Emory University School of Medicine, Atlanta, Georgia 30322

The cells of the embryonic heart, like those of the adult, are connected by low-resistance junctions (nexuses) that allow passage of ions and small molecules from cell to cell. Even the mesodermal cells from which the cardiac rudiments emerge are joined by such electrotonic coupling junctions long before they differentiate into electrically active membranes and begin their rhythmic discharge of action potentials. Thus, when the heart first starts to beat, the action potentials can be conducted from cell to cell. At this time, however, the heart has different electrophysiological properties than the mature organ; these suggest that spiking activity is based solely on a slow Na^+/Ca^{++} inward conductance mechanism (2). The action potentials of the early heart are small (80 to 100 mV peak-to-peak); they take off from a relatively depolarized threshold (about -40 mV), and they exhibit slow rise-times (5 to 10 V/s). Spontaneous electrical activity of early ventricular cells is suppressed by Mn^{++} or the verapamil derivative D-600, but beating continues in preparations exposed to elevated $[K^+]_o$ or the Na-channel inhibitor tetrodotoxin (TTX). In the mature chick and mammalian ventricle, electrical activity has different characteristics. Action potentials show peak-to-peak amplitudes of 120 to 140 mV, threshold potential is usually at -60 to -70 mV, and the spike upstroke has a fast rise-time (100 to 200 V/s). Spontaneous activity in the well-developed heart is not suppressed by Mn^{++} and is relatively insensitive to D-600, but beating of intact ventricular tissue or reaggregates of ventricle cells is stopped by small elevations in $[K^+]_o$ or low concentrations of TTX. The shift from an I_{si}-like current to an I_{Na}-like mechanism has been directly visualized under voltage clamp in chick embryonic heart cell aggregates when preparations from 3-day embryos were allowed to differentiate *in vitro* (5). In their presentations in these pages, G. H. LeDouarin and D. Renaud *(this volume)* describe the ionic bases for some of these action potential changes during development; Nathan and his colleagues *(this volume)* demonstrate with voltage clamp that pacemaker currents in 7-day chick heart cell aggregates include a background inward current and a time-dependent outward current. These authors also show that pacemaker activity is significantly regulated by cell surface sialic acid residues that control calcium exchange.

During early stages of cardiogenesis, as cells divide, die, and move within the developing heart tissue, new cell contacts are frequently made and broken.

In the intact mouse heart, Gros et al. (3) have recently shown with freeze–cleave technique that the relative membrane area devoted to nexal junctions increases dramatically from 10 days post conception (just after the heart starts to beat) throughout development. In their presentation that follows *(this volume),* they extend this work to describe how the junctions enlarge and become better organized into definitive macular structures with increasing embryonic age. In the closing article in this section (DeHaan et al., *this volume),* my colleagues and I report on recent studies showing that coupling junctions can be formed within minutes between newly apposed heart cells. When two independently beating spheroidal aggregates of ventricle cells are pressed together, the transaggregate resistance falls rapidly as nexal junctions are formed from a long-lived pool of precursors. On the basis of these studies, we have calculated that only a few coupling channels per cell would be sufficient to allow beat synchronization. This may explain how excellent coupling can be maintained even at the earliest stages, when well-formed macular junctions are rare or nonexistent.

The studies described here emphasize the obvious physiological role of coupling junctions in coordinating the beat after the heart begins to function. There can be little doubt, however, that gap junctions are also important during precardiac stages of development, but their role in organ morphogenesis and differentiation is still largely speculative (1,4,6). There are still many questions to be answered in this field by future work.

REFERENCES

1. DeHaan, R. L. (1976): Cell coupling and electrophysiological differentiation of embryonic heart cells. In: *Tests of Teratogenicity in Vitro,* edited by J. D. Ebert and M. Marois, pp. 225-232. North-Holland Publishing Co., Amsterdam.
2. DeHaan, R. L. (1980): Development of rhythmic activity in cardiac cells. In: *Physiology of Atrial Pacemakers and Conductive Tissues,* edited by R. C. Little, pp. 21-53. Futura Press, Mt. Kisco, N.Y.
3. Gros, D., Mocquard, J. P., Challice, C. E., and Schrevel, J. (1979): Formation and growth of gap junctions in mouse myocardium during ontogenesis: Quantitative data and their implications on the development of intercellular communication. *J. Mol. Cell. Cardiol.,* 11:543-554.
4. Loewenstein, W. R. (1975): Permeable junctions. *Cold Spring Harbor Symp. Quant. Biol.,* 40:49-63.
5. Nathan, R. D., and DeHaan, R. O. (1978): *In vitro* differentiation of a fast Na^+ conductance in embryonic heart cell aggregates. *Proc. Nat. Acad. Sci. (USA),* 75:2776-2780.
6. Wolpert, L. (1978): Gap junctions: Channels for communication in development. In: *Intercellular Junctions and Synapses,* edited by J. Feldman, N. B. Gilula, and J. D. Pitts, pp. 61-80. Chapman and Hall, London.

Perspectives in Cardiovascular Research, Vol. 5,
Mechanisms of Cardiac Morphogenesis and Teratogenesis,
edited by Tomas Pexieder. Raven Press, New York © 1981

Assembly of Gap Junctions in Developing Mouse Cardiac Muscle

D. Gros,* J. P. Mocquard,** J. Schrével,* and C. E. Challice†

*Laboratory of Zoology and Cell Biology, (L.A. CNRS 290). U.E.R. Sciences Fondamentales et Appliquées, 86022 Poitiers, France **Laboratory of Crustacean Physiology and Genetics, U.E.R. Sciences Fondamentales et Appliquées, 86022 Poitiers, France †Physics Department, University of Calgary, Calgary, Alberta T2N IN4, Canada*

From the physiological point of view, myocardial cells are electrically coupled by low-resistance pathways which also provide metabolic coupling (7,8,18,36,-37,38). It is now generally accepted that gap junctions or nexuses (or *macula communicans,* 34) are the structures that represent these low-resistance pathways (9,32). Although the ultrastructure of gap junctions in adult cardiac muscle has been the subject of numerous studies (10,22,23,30), little information is available on the structural development of gap junctions in the embryonic and developing heart.

The present results come from a freeze–cleave study of the formation and growth of gap junctions in the ontogenesis of mouse myocardium. In addition, a statistical analysis of the ratio of gap junctional area to plasma membrane area, at each stage studied, is given. The increase of this ratio during maturation of the myocardium is discussed in terms of the development of intercellular communication.

Parts of this study have been previously published (14,15).

MATERIALS AND METHODS

Materials

Embryonic hearts at 10, 12, 14 and 18 e.d. were obtained from pregnant mice by the technique of Gros et al. (14). Adult hearts were taken from 3-month-old female mice.

Preparation of Specimens and Freeze–Cleaving

Samples from the ventricular apex at 12, 14 and 18 e.d. and at the adult stage, or the whole ventricle at 10 e.d., were dissected in a physiological salt solution, pH 7.4 (130 mM NaCl, 2.70 mM KCl, 2.20 mM $CaCl_2$, 1mM NaH_2PO_4,

11.3 mM NaHCO$_3$, 0.24 mM MgCl$_2$, 11.10 mM glucose). Small pieces were immersed for 20 min sequentially in 10, 20 and 30% glycerol in physiological salt solution, at 4°C. Specimens were fixed for 30 min at 4°C in 5% glutaraldehyde solution in 0.1 M cacodylate buffer at pH 7.4, before being infiltrated with glycerol in physiological salt solution. The specimens were mounted on gold disks and frozen in Freon-22 cooled with liquid nitrogen. Freeze-fracturing at −100°C and platinum carbon shadowing were carried out using a Balzers freeze–etch apparatus (25). Cleaned replicas were examined with a Hitachi HU 11 Cs or Siemens Elmiskop 1$_a$ electron microscope.

Surface Measurements

The surface measurements were carried out on 3 unfixed hearts at 10, 14, and 18 e.d., and at the adult stage. The electron microscopes were calibrated using a germanium-shadowed carbon replica (54 864 lines in $^{-1}$). The measurements of the surfaces of the gap junctions (observed both on P and F fracture faces) were all made from micrographs at 90,000 magnification using graph paper. The linear gap junctions observed at the earliest stages (10 and 14 e.d.) were not included in the calculations, because of the difficulty in measuring their surface areas. However, when present, they represent only a small percentage of the total area of gap junctions. The central particle-free zones observed in some nexuses were also excluded from the surface measurements. For the calculation of the ratios : gap junction area/fracture face area, micrographs of all the myocardial cell fracture faces were obtained and measured with a planimeter, in order to calculate the total surface area of plasma membrane cleaved during the freeze–fracture process.

RESULTS

Assembly of Gap Junctions in Developing Cardiac Muscle

Freeze-fracturing cleaves the plasma membrane, producing two fracture faces, the P and E faces (4). Both fracture faces of embryonic and adult fixed myocardial cells are studded with randomly distributed intramembranous particles, whose density (particles/μm^2) ranges from 1,200 to 1,400 and from 200 to 250, respectively (16). Besides these intramembranous particles, diverse arrays of gap particles are also observed, and it is believed that these represent successive steps in the assembly of the gap junctions (see Discussion).

At 10 e.d., the junctions are few in number and their structure varies. For convenience, four types of gap junctions can be categorized (Table 1),

(a) Single chains of 9 nm particles on the PF faces, or linear arrays of pits on the EF faces (Fig. 1). These rows of particles are sometimes associated at their ends to form small areas (see Fig. 6 from a 12 e.d. heart) or loosely organized clusters of particles (Fig. 3).

TABLE 1. *Types of gap junctions found at the stages of development studied in mouse cardiac muscle (for explanation, see text).*

	10 e.d.	12 e.d.	14 e.d.	18 e.d.	Adult
Linear arrays	+	+	+	−	−
Macular gap junctions with "arms"	+	+	+	−	−
Macular gap junctions with particle-free region	+	+	+	−	−
Small gap junctions	+	+	+	+	+
Large gap junctions	−	−	+	+	+

(b) Aggregates of gap particles, on the PF faces, with one, two, or three "arms" which seem to be formed by the successive addition of single gap particles. The latter are observed beside the junction in a kind of stream (Fig. 2 and 3). These aggregates of particles often form hexagonal arrays.

(c) Aggregates of gap particles (observed on the PF faces) with one, two, or three central particle-free zones (Fig. 4). The absence of particles cannot be due to their having been pulled out during the cleaving process, since gap junctions with similar central pit-free areas are also observed on the EF faces (Fig. 5).

(d) Small hexagonal arrays of particles with 9 nm center-to-center spacing, with the corresponding EF faces showing similar arrays of depressions. These structures are characteristic of the classically described gap junctions and they are referred to as "adult-type junctions" (Fig. 12).

The above description applies to both 12 and 14 e.d. hearts, with only slight modification. At 12 e.d. (Fig. 6 and 7) gap junctions are more numerous than at 10 e.d. and the linear arrays of gap particles are abundant. By 14 e.d., (Fig. 8 and 9), the chains of particles have become rarer, whereas the other types of gap junction are relatively numerous. At 18 e.d. (Fig. 10 and 11), and also at the adult stage (Fig. 12), linear gap junctions and gaps with "arms" or central particle-free regions are no longer observed, all the junctions being of the adult type. Some micrographs suggest, especially at 18 e.d., that the large nexuses may have been formed by the fusion of smaller junctions (Fig. 11). At the periphery of completely formed junctions, individual gap particles can still be seen (Fig. 12).

Distribution of Gap Junctions During Development

Fig. 13 shows the distribution of the area S of the gap junctions through the 4 stages studied. At 10 e.d., the area of nexuses observed (n = 83) ranges from 0.1 to $3 \times 10^{-2}\mu m^2$; at 14 e.d. (n = 215) from 0.1 to $15 \times 10^{-2}\mu m^2$; at

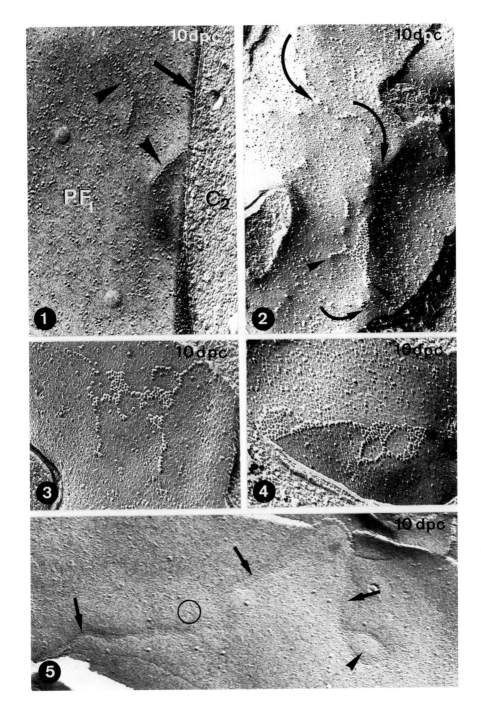

18 e.d. (n = 158) from 0.1 to 26.3 × $10^{-2}\mu m^2$; and at the adult stage (n = 92) from 0.1 to 54 × $10^{-2}\mu m^2$. These results, which demonstrate the growth of the gap junctions, can be expressed in a more significant manner. The junctions measured can be separated into two classes : class I with area (S) < 0.5 × $10^{-2}\mu m^2$ and class II with S > 0.5 × $10^{-2}\mu m^2$, the number 0.5 × 10^{-2} representing the median area of all the gap junctions measured (n = 548). These results are presented in Table II. At 10 e.d. there are 67% in class I, at 14 e.d., 57%, at 18 e.d. 44%, and at the adult stage, 31%.

Estimate of the Junctional Cell Surface

For the calculation, it is assumed that a fracture face is equal to a corresponding area of plasma membrane, and the two terms—fracture face area and plasma membrane area—will be used interchangeably. However, it must be kept in mind that the fracture faces do not necessarily represent a random sampling of the plasma membrane, since a freeze fracture, unlike a thin section, does not occur in a random plane. Gros et al. (14) have discussed the validity of the following statistical analysis.

The proportion of cell surface area that forms gap junctions is represented, at each stage studied, by the ratio of measured gap junction area to plasma membrane area (or fracture face area). The results summarized in Fig. 14 indicate a general tendency of this proportion to increase with age of embryo. The analysis of variance (3) of the ratio of gap junction area to plasma membrane area demonstrates that the results are significant ($P < 0.05$). The geometric means of the ratios, with their confidence intervals, are respectively:

0.014 (0.001 < 0.014 < 0.213) at 10 e.d.
0.153 (0.029 < 0.153 < 0.806) at 14 e.d.

FIG. 1. 10 e.d. heart. Fixed specimen. Arrowheads indicate two linear arrays of particles on the P face of a myocardial cell 1. C_2, cytoplasm of cell 2. The extracellular space separating cell 1 and cell 2 is very narrow *(arrow)* (× 90,000).

FIG. 2. 10 e.d. heart. Fixed specimen. PF face of a myocardial cell with a junction that has two small "arms" *(arrowheads)*. Note the streams of particles *(arrows)* which appear to converge towards the main junction (× 78,000).

FIG. 3. 10 e.d. heart. Unfixed specimen. PF face. Linear arrangements ending in clusters of particles (× 78,000).

FIG. 4. 10 e.d. heart. Unfixed specimen. PF face. Another stage in the formation of gap junctions, characterized by the presence of central particle-free regions (× 90,000).

FIG. 5. 10 e.d. heart. Fixed specimen. EF face. The arrowhead indicates a central pit-free region within the junction. Note the long stream of small depressions *(arrows)*. Some pits can be also identified outside the stream *(circle)* (× 90,000).

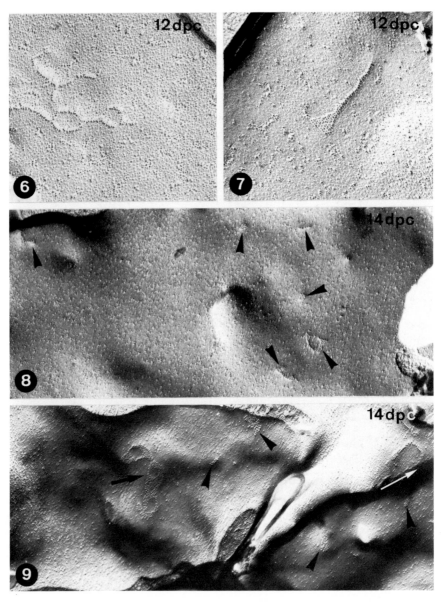

FIGS. 6 and 7. 12 e.d. heart. Unfixed specimens. PF faces. These figures illustrate two steps in the formation of gap junctions: chains of particles (which in the case of the Fig. 6 are anastomosed) and linear arrangements ending in a hexagonal array of particles (× 60,000).

FIGS. 8 and 9. 14 e.d. heart. Unfixed specimens. PF faces. Most of the steps of the formation of gap junctions can be recognized in these two figures: linear arrays of particles (Fig. 9, *right upper part*) and streams of particles *(white arrow)*, small clusters *(arrowheads)*, and a junction with particle-free regions *(black arrow)*. Fig. 8, × 46,000; Fig. 9, × 48,000.

0.346 (0.185 < 0.346 < 0.645) at 18 e.d.
0.816 (0.091 < 0.716 < 5.668) at the adult stage

DISCUSSION

Assembly and Growth of Gap Junctions

In the present study, the structural diversity of gap junctions has been interpreted as representing steps in their ontogenesis. The increase of their surface area with the development of cardiac muscle supports this hypothesis. However, the formation of gap junctions, as schematized in Fig. 15, presupposes two conditions: the mobility of the junctional particles in the plane of the plasma membrane, and a mutual affinity between the particles.

For Johnson et al. (19), Decker and Friend (6), Decker (5), and Griepp and Revel (12), the formation of gap junctions involves, first, the close apposition of adjacent membranes. These areas are characterized in freeze-fracture replicas as "formation plaques" containing 10 to 11 nm particles which are assumed to represent some form of gap junction precursors (Fig. 15-1). Such structures have been identified in 10 e.d. hearts (14), but they are quite rare, and they have not been observed in the later stages of development. The earliest forms of gap junction which can reasonably be categorized as such are rows of particles (Figs. 15-2). These rectilinear or curved arrangements have been described by most of the authors who have investigated the formation of gap junctions (2,5, 6,11,13,21). It is perhaps noteworthy that they are the only type of gap junctions present between myocardial cells of adult *Xenopus* (21). At the next stage of development, the gap particles seem to coil up at one end of a linear row to form structures such as that shown in Fig. 15-3 and are referred to as gap junctions with "arms." As such junctions lengthen, a stream of gap particles is often observed, which is believed to represent the accumulation of particles in the junction corresponding to its growth. Later, the "arms" bend to join the main body of the junction (Fig. 15-4), thereby forming a ring which encloses a particle-free region (Fig. 15-5), which will ultimately disappear to produce an adult-type junction (Fig. 15-6). The junctions grow by incorporation of new gap particles or by fusion with other nexuses.

This hypothesis of the formation of gap junctions in mouse myocardium is consistent with studies on other differentiating tissues and with growing tissue-culture preparations (2,5,6,19). In developing amphibian cardiac muscle, Mazet (21) observed similar steps in the formation of gap junctions, but in adults the junctions never reach a complexity comparable to that in mammals. In regenerating rat liver, many small gap junctions reappear about 40 hours after partial hepatectomy, then increase in size. However, Yee and Revel (39), who investigated the loss and reappearance of gap junctions in this organ, do not mention the presence of linear arrangements. In this instance, reappearance

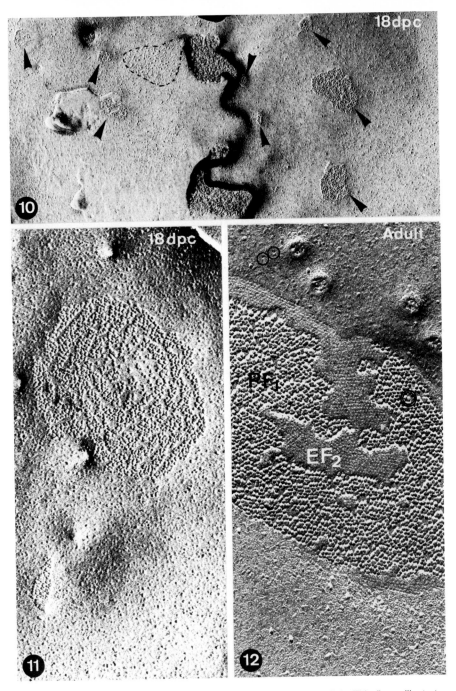

FIG. 10. 18 e.d. heart. Fixed specimen. PF face of an intercalated disk. This figure illustrates typical gap junctions (arrowheads) observed in this age group. The dotted line delimits a desmosome. × 51,000.

FIG. 11. 18 e.d. heart. Fixed specimen. PF face. This junction is probably still developing. Later, the particles will become more closely packed (× 90,000).

FIG. 12. Adult cardiac muscle. Fixed specimen. The cleaving process reveals both the PF and EF faces (PF_1 and EF_2) of a gap junction. The hexagonal arrangement of the junctional structures is well seen on EF_2. At the periphery of such junctions, depressions due to gap particles can be identified *(single circles)*. On the tops of gap particles, small pits are sometimes observed *(double circle)* (× 90,000).

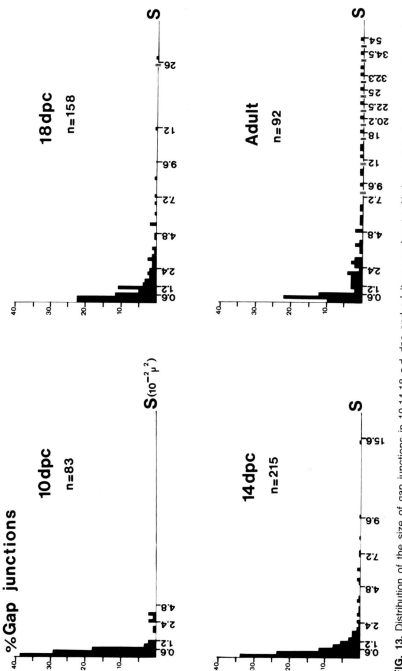

FIG. 13. Distribution of the size of gap junctions in 10,14,18 e.d.-dpc and adult mouse hearts. Abcissa: area, S, of gap junctions; class interval: $3 \times 10^{-2} \mu m^2$. Ordinate: percentage of the ratios, number of gap junctions in class intervals/total number of gap junctions at each stage (n). Three unfixed cardiac muscle preparations used for each stage. (From Gros et al., 1978, *J. Cell Sci.*, 30:45-61, reproduced by permission.)

TABLE 2. *Distribution of junctions between class I (S < 0.5 × 100⁻²μm²) and in class II (S > 0.5 × 10⁻²μm²). Each class contains the same number of gap junctions (for explanation, see text).*

	Area of the gap junctions (μm^2)	
	$S < 0.5 \times 10^{-2}$	$S > 0.5 \times 10^{-2}$
10 e.d.	67%	33%
14 e.d.	57%	43%
18 e.d.	44%	56%
Adult	31%	69%

first takes the form of small aggregates of particles. Thus, in this case, the linear array stage must be of very short duration, or else is bypassed.

Increase of the Junctional Cell Surface During Myocardial Development

Analysis of the ratio of gap junction area to plasma membrane area indicates a significant increase of junctional cell surface during the development of cardiac

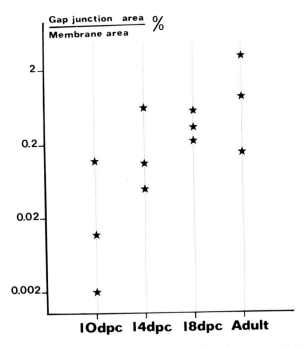

FIG. 14. Estimate of the junctional cell surface in 10,14,18 e.d.-dpc and adult mouse hearts. Abscissa: stages of development. Ordinate (logarithmic scale): percentage of the ratios: gap junction area/plasma membrane (fracture face) area. Each star represents the result of the analysis of the replicas from a single unfixed myocardium. The results are, respectively: 10 e.d., 0.002, 0.117, 0.012; 14 e.d., 0.611, 0.109, 0.054; 18 e.d., 0.233, 0.565, 0.328; adult, 3.94, 0.854, 0.149.

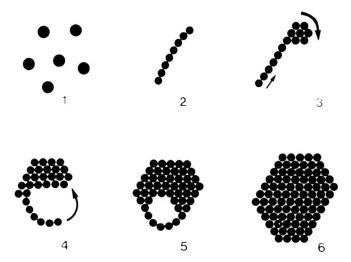

FIG. 15. Successive stages in the formation of gap junctions in developing mouse cardiac muscle. For explanation, see text.

muscle. Hirakow and Gotoh (17) made a similar suggestion after ultra-thin section studies on developing rat heart at later stages. At 10 days post-partum (dpp), they showed $3.9 \pm 2.2\%$ of the intercalated disk area to be occupied by gap junctions. This percentage then increased to $13.4 \pm 8.1\%$ and $17.3 \pm 6\%$, at 20 and 30 dpp, respectively. In addition, Page and his colleagues (27,-28,33) have studied the development of gap junctions in rabbit heart, particularly around the time of parturition. They showed a significant increase in gap junctional area. These studies, together with those of Hirakow and Gotoh (17), appear to represent the only attempts to quantify the development of gap junctions in cardiac muscle. More information is available in the adult, Table 3. However, it is difficult to compare our results with those of Table III, because they refer to different animals.

The increase of junctional cell surface in developing heart has physiological

TABLE 3. *Area of junctional surfaces forming gap junctions in different myocardial cell types. These results were all obtained from ultrathin section studies. LV, left ventricle; RV, right ventricle. From Masson-Pévet et al. (20).*

Tissues studied		Percentage of cell surface occupied by gap junctions	References
Rat	papillary LV	3.7	Page and McCallister (29)
Rat	papillary LV	0.84	Page (27)
Rabbit	papillary RV	3.04	Page (27)
Rabbit	papillary LV	0.75	Nakata, quoted by Page (27)
Calf	bundle RV	3.3	Arluk and Rhodin (1)
Sheep	Purkinje LV	17	Mobley and Page (24)
Rabbit	leading sinus node	0.16–0.22	Masson-Pévet et al. (20)

TABLE 4. *The ratios between cell volume and junctional area characterizing non-electrical communication.*

Age	Characteristics of the cells	Cell volume	Junctional area	Cell volume junctional area
10 e.d.	Spherical with a diameter of 10 μm	520 μm³	0.014%	0.08×10^{-3}
Adult	Cylindrical (100 × 12 μm) with a 9-fold increment of the transverse boundary (26)	11300 μm³	0.72%	4×10^{-3}

implications, particularly for intercellular communication, both electrical and non-electrical. Non-electrical communication (i.e., the intercellular transfer of small regulatory molecules and metabolites) is likely to be at least concomitant with, and probably proportional to, the ratio between gap junction area and cell volume (31). In the present case, calculation of these ratios (Table 4) indicates a 50-fold increase in non-electrical communication between 10 e.d. and the adult stage. Electrical communication refers to the intercellular transmission of electrical transmembrane potentials. The evaluation of this factor for adjacent cells requires a knowledge of both the junctional resistance and the inherent cell membrane resistance (3). The value of input resistance in younger hearts has been reported to be much higher than at maturity (35), and these observations have been interpreted as representing an increase in membrane resistance. However, a high junctional resistance caused by a low junctional area in the younger hearts could give similar results.

ACKNOWLEDGMENTS

The authors are indebted to Mrs. C. Besse (Service Général de Microscopie Electronique Appliquée à la Biologie, Poitiers) and to Mr. J. Rivière for their skillful technical assistance, to Dr. W. Costerton for the generous use of his freeze-fracture equipment in Calgary, and to Miss D. Decourt for the preparation of the manuscript.

This work was supported by D.G.R.S.T. grants, the Alberta Heart Foundation, the National Research Council of Canada, and the C.N.R.S. (France) NRC (Canada) scientific exchange program.

REFERENCES

1. Arluk D. J., and Rhodin, J. A. G. (1974): The ultrastructure of calf heart conducting fibers with special reference to nexuses and their distribution. *J. Ultrastruct. Res.,* 49:11-23.
2. Benedetti, E. L., Dunia I., and Bloemendal, H. (1974): Development of junction during differentiation of lens fibers. *Proc. Natl. Acad. Sci. USA,* 71:5073-5077.
3. Bliss, C. I. (1967): *Statistics in Biology,* McGraw-Hill Book Company, New York.

4. Branton, D., Bullivant, S., Gilula, N. B., Karnovsky, M. J., Moor, H., Mühlethaler, K., North-cote, D. H., Packer, L., Satir, B., Satir, P., Speth, V., Staehlin, L. A., Steere, R. L., and Weinstein, R. S. (1975): Freeze-etching nomenclature. *Science,* 190:54-56.

5. Decker, R. S. (1976): Hormonal regulation of gap junction differentiation. *J. Cell Biol.,* 69:669-686.

6. Decker, R. S., and Friend, A. (1974): Assembly of gap junctions during amphibian neurulation. *J. Cell Biol.,* 62:32-47.

7. Delèze, J. (1976): Passage de cellule à cellule de molécules fluorescentes injectées par pression dans des fibres cardiaques de Mammifères. *J. Physiol. (Paris),* 72:80A-81A.

8. De Mello, W. C. (1975): Effect of intracellular injection of calcium and strontium on cell communication in heart. *J. Physiol. (Lond.),* 250:231-245.

9. Gilula, N. B., Reeves, O. R., and Steinbach A. (1972): Metabolic coupling, ionic coupling and cell contacts. *Nature (Lond.),* 235:262-265.

10. Goodenough, D. A., Paul, D. L., and Culbert, K. E. (1978): Correlative gap junction ultrastructure. In: *Molecular Basis of Cell–Cell Interaction,* edited by R. A. Lerner and D. Bergsma, pp. 83-97. A. R. Liss Inc., New York.

11. Griepp, E. B., Peacock, J. H., Bernfield, M. R., and Revel, I. P. (1978): Morphological and functional correlates of synchronous beating between embryonic heart cell aggregates and layers. *Exp. Cell Res.,* 113:273-282.

12. Griepp, E. B., and Revel, J. P. (1977): Gap junctions in development. In: *Intercellular Communication,* edited by W. C. de Mello, pp. 1-14. Plenum Publishing Corporation, New York.

13. Gros, D., and Challice, C. E. (1976): Early development of gap junctions between the mouse embryonic myocardial cells. A freeze-etching study. *Experientia,* 32:996-997.

14. Gros, D., Mocquard, J. P., Challice, C. E., and Schrével, J. (1978): Formation and growth of gap junctions in mouse myocardium during ontogenesis: a freeze–cleave study. *J. Cell Sci.,* 30:45-61.

15. Gros, D., Mocquard, J. P., Challice, C. E., and Schrével, J. (1979a): Formation and growth of gap junctions in mouse myocardium during ontogenesis: Quantitative data and their implications on the development of intercellular communication. *J. Mol. Cell. Cardiol.,* 11:543-554.

16. Gros, D., Potreau, D., and Mocquard, J. P. (1979b): Myocardial plasma membrane during ontogenesis. Density and size of intramembranous particles. *J. Cell. Sci.,* 43:301-317.

17. Hirakow, R., and Gotoh, T. (1976): A quantitative ultrastructural study on the developing rat heart. In: *Developmental and Physiological Correlates in Cardiac Muscle,* edited by M. Lieberman and T. Sano, pp. 37-50, Raven Press, New York.

18. Imanaga, I. (1974): Cell-to-cell diffusion of Procion Yellow in sheep and calf Purkinje fiber. *J. Membr. Biol.,* 16:381-388.

19. Johnson, R. G., Hammer, M., Sheridan, J., and Revel, J. P. (1974): Gap junctions between reaggregated Novikoff hepatoma cells. *Proc. Natl. Acad. Sci. USA,* 71:4536-4540.

20. Masson-Pévet, M., Bleeker, W. K., and Gros, D. (1979): The plasma membrane of leading pacemaker cells in the rabbit sinus node: A qualitative and quantitative ultrastructural analysis. *Cir. Res.,* 45:621-623.

21. Mazet, F. (1977): Freeze-fracture studies of gap junctions in the developing and adult amphibian cardiac muscle. *Dev. Biol.,* 60:139-152.

22. McNutt, N. S., and Weinstein, R. S. (1970): Ultrastructure of the nexus: A correlated thin-section and freeze–cleave study. *J. Cell Biol.,* 47:666-689.

23. McNutt, N. S., and Weinstein, R. S. (1973): Membrane ultrastructure at mammalian intercellular junctions. *Prog. Biophys. Molec. Biol.,* 26:45-101.

24. Mobley, B. A., and Page, E. (1972): The surface area of sheep cardiac Purkinje fibres. *J. Physiol. (Lond.),* 220:547-564.

25. Moore, H., and Mühlethaler, K. (1963): Fine structure of frozen-etched yeast cells. *J. Cell Biol.,* 17:609-628.

26. Nakata, K., and Page, E. (1978): Morphometry of gap junctional development in rabbit ventricle. *J. Cell Biol.,* 79:330a.

27. Page, E. (1978): Quantitative ultrastructural analysis in cardiac membrane physiology. *Am. J. Physiol.,* 235:C147-C158.

28. Page, E. (1979): Membrane growth and development in myocardial cells. *J. Mol. Cell Cardiol.,* 11:47.

29. Page, E., and McCallister, L. P. (1973): Studies on the intercalated disk of rat left ventricular myocardial cells. *J. Ultrastruct. Res.,* 43:388-411.

30. Revel, J. P., and Karnovsky, M. J. (1967): Hexagonal array of subunits in intercellular junctions of the mouse heart and liver. *J. Cell Biol.,* 33:C$_7$-C$_{12}$.
31. Sheridan, J. D. (1973): Functional evaluation of low resistance junctions: Influence of cell shape and size. *Am. Zool.,* 13:1119-1128.
32. Sheridan, J. D. (1974): Electrical coupling of cells and cell communication. In: *Cell Communication,* edited by R. P. Cox, pp. 31-42. J. Wiley and Sons, New York.
33. Shibata, Y., and Page, E. (1979): Neonatal development of cardiac gap junctions: Freeze-fracture analysis. *J. Mol. Cell. Cardiol.,* 11:57.
34. Simionescu, M., Simionescu, N., and Palade, G. E. (1975): Segmental differentiations of cell junctions in the vascular endothelium. *J. Cell Biol.,* 67:863-885.
35. Sperelakis, N., and Shigenobu, K. (1972): Changes in membrane properties of chick embryonic hearts during development. *J. Gen. Physiol.,* 60:430-453.
36. Weidmann, S. (1969): Electrical coupling between myocardial cells. *Prog. Brain Res.,* 31:275-281.
37. Weingart, P. (1974): The permeability to tetraethylammonium ions on the surface membrane and the intercalated disks of sheep and calf myocardium. *J. Physiol. (Lond.),* 240:741-762.
38. Weingart, P. (1977): The actions of ouabain on intercellular coupling and conduction velocity in mammalian ventricular muscle. *J. Physiol. (Lond.),* 264:341-365.
39. Yee, A. G., and Revel, J. P. (1978): Loss and reappearance of gap junctions in regenerating liver. *J. Cell Biol.,* 78:554-564.

DISCUSSION

Gross: Did you study the contacts between mesenchyme and myocytes?

Challice: No, we did not.

Argello: In earlier stages, we did not see this kind of change in contacts between fibroblasts and myoblasts.

DeHaan: Also, in aggregates we did not see recognizable junctions between myocytes and fibroblasts.

Bogenmann: Did you find different stages of junction formation on the same cell?

Challice: In some cells you can see junctions which we believe represent different stages of development.

Bogenmann: Did you find also different types of junctions on the same cell?

Challice: Yes, we did.

Fischman: Have you looked at gap junctions in dividing muscle cells?

Challice: No, we have not been able to identify dividing cells in this procedure.

Bogenmann: Do you know the nature of the hexagonal particles in gap junctions?

Gros: There is a major polypeptide. The molecular weight of this protein is about 26,000.

Perspectives in Cardiovascular Research, Vol. 5,
Mechanisms of Cardiac Morphogenesis and Teratogenesis,
edited by Tomas Pexieder. Raven Press, New York © 1981

Intercellular Coupling of Embryonic Heart Cells

R. L. DeHaan, E. H. Williams, *D. L. Ypey, and D. E. Clapham

Department of Anatomy, Emory University School of Medicine, Atlanta, Georgia 30322

The cells of many embryonic and adult tissues are connected by communicating channels that permit the direct passage of certain molecules and ions between the cell interiors (for review, see 2,16,20,21,33,37,59). A large body of evidence suggests that the cell-to-cell pathway consists of many parallel channels contained in the clusters of integral membrane proteins (IMP) that comprise the nexuses or gap junctions found between coupled cells (22,31,53,61,81). Each "junctional unit" (36) is formed by a pair of pore-bearing particles or protochannels, one from each membrane, which penetrate the apposed membrane lipid bilayers and abut in the intercellular cleft. The electrical properties of the intercellular channels have been measured in a variety of cell types (7,11,28,61,80). The channels appear to behave like linear (non-rectifying) resistors. The electrical resistance of a simple fluid-filled channel would be

$$r_c = \frac{\rho l}{A}$$

where r_c is the unit channel resistance, ρ is the electrical resistivity of the fluid in the channel, and l and A are its length and cross-sectional area. A tube long enough to span the two apposed membranes of coupled cells, 12 nm long and 2 nm in inside diameter (41), containing fluid with a resistivity of 150 $\Omega \cdot$cm would have a resistance of $10^{10}\Omega$. This is the estimate for unit junctional channel resistance most commonly used (4,5,7,36), in lieu of an accurately measured value. However, recent evidence indicates that junctional resistance is not constant, but is rather a function of local intracellular calcium concentration, pH, and transjunctional voltage. Spray et al. (65) have shown that junctional conductance between pairs of isolated amphibian blastomeres falls exponentially with transjunctional voltage difference. The nexal conductance decreased to about 5% of its maximal value with a voltage gradient of 30 mV between the two apposed cells.

The gap junction is also permeable to molecules larger than the ions that (presumably) act as current carriers. The size limit ascertained for the transjunctional passage of molecules appears to be well over 1000 daltons for certain

---

* Present address: Department of Physiology, University of Leiden, The Netherlands

arthropod junctions (62), but substantially lower for those of vertebrate cells (4,19,50). By this measure of junctional permeability, channels also exhibit voltage dependence (65), and they are apparently reduced in size by Ca^{++} (37,38). Moreover, permeable molecules are limited not only by molecular size but also by their electronegativity (19), suggesting that the channel contains fixed charges.*

COUPLING IN CARDIAC TISSUE

The communicating junctions in the heart represent low-resistance pathways for ionic currents that permit action potentials to be conducted along the multicellular cardiac fibers (16,18,44,47,71). They may also play specific roles during early tissue differentiation (12,36,49,78). The mechanism of cell coupling is thus of great significance in considering the events of cardiac morphogenesis. At early somite stages, the precardiac cells are organized bilaterally within the lateral plate mesoderm (52,56,68). During formation of the tubular heart, this material behaves as a cohesive sheet. It condenses, stretches, folds, and deforms (55), and new cells are added by mitosis at a rapid rate (67). Within a few hours, the primitive heart tube begins to beat rhythmically, and undergoes its characteristic curvature as a result of differential growth and cell movements (66). As cells alter their positions relative to one another during this period of intense morphogenetic activity, they frequently make and break contacts with their immediate neighbors. Nonetheless, even at the earliest stages of cardiogenesis, all embryonic heart cells participate in a common pulsation rhythm, and appear to be electrically coupled with their neighbors (16,69). The implication of these observations is that coupling junctions must be formed rapidly between newly apposed cells of the forming heart.

Support for this idea comes from studies of cells isolated in culture. Gap junctions have never been reported on the surfaces of isolated cells. Moreover, the scattered IMP particles seen in non-junctional membrane could not have patent holes; large numbers of such structures would permit lethal leakage of ions and other molecules across the cell boundary. Nonetheless, when isolated cells make contact, gap junctions appear between the newly apposed surfaces within minutes. From the appearance of freeze-fracture preparations of the contact surfaces of cells immediately after apposition (29,60), and in differentiating (10,40) and regenerating (79) tissues, it is presumed that organized gap junctions form from the IMP particles scattered in the apposed membranes. Common features of the assembly process among a wide variety of embryos and tissue types (9,29,60) include: (a) adhesion of apposed cells and increase in proximity of their contact surfaces; (b) the appearance of flattened regions of membrane in the contact area, 0.1 to 0.6 μm in diameter, termed formation plaques (29,60), which contain a scatter of 8 to 10 nm IMP particles; (c) decrease in width of the intercellular gap to 2 to 4 nm, accompanied or followed by rapid clustering of IMP particles; (d) protrusion of adjacent particles from the apposed surfaces into the intercellular space, and their abutment to form continuous channels (37,47); (e) closer packing of particles into discrete nexal plaques (10,32); and

(f) enlargement of the junctions by recruitment of nearby particles (3,59,79).

From experiments with a variety of tissues other than heart, in which pairs of cells were brought into contact under controlled conditions while the degree of electrical coupling was measured continuously, it is clear that, as gap junctions form, junctional resistance begins to decline from a high initial value ($\sim 10^9 \Omega$) to a steady level three orders of magnitude less in some minutes (28). In newly apposed Novikoff hepatoma cells, electrical coupling (29) and intercellular transfer of fluorescein (58) became detectable at the same time that clusters of particles made their appearance in the formation plaques, between 10 and 30 min after initial contact. Gilula et al. (23) have provided evidence that such particle clusters are associated with metabolic and ionic coupling between cells (reviewed in 49,78). However, Sheridan (60) has recently argued that coupling of Novikoff hepatoma cells in the first minutes after contact may occur across apposed formation plaques, in which particles have not yet aggregated. Moreover, the resistance across apposed cells decreased quantally (39), and the number of particles in the IMP clusters in newly forming gap junctions increased monotonically with time (29). These observations suggest that the definitive low-resistance nexus may form by clustering of single pairs of transgap IMP particles, and that only one or a few such channels are sufficient to allow electrical communication between two cells

Evidence in support of this view also comes from recent observations on coupling and synchronization between spontaneously beating embryonic heart cells, isolated in tissue culture. The development of synchrony is a striking attribute of embryonic cardiac myocytes. Single cells synchronize their visible contractile activity within minutes after initial contact (15). Spheroidal aggregates composed of thousands of cardiac cells (57) also become entrained to a common rhythm when brought together in pairs (13,74,80). It is widely held that cardiac tissue behaves like an electrical syncytium. Signals originating at one point traverse the tissue as if ionic currents can flow freely from cell to cell. Since the discovery of cytoplasmic discontinuity at the intercalated disc (63), the mechanism of this electrical coupling between heart cells has been widely investigated (for early reviews, see 16,17,72). Experiments on adult heart preparations have established their conductive properties (2,18,50,70,73). Moreover, embryonic (11,24,25,34,64) and neonatal heart cell systems (30,31) have been used in a variety of geometries in tissue culture, to investigate the spread of action potentials or other electrical signals from cell to cell. A model for action potential spread that does not depend on low-resistance cell junctions has also been proposed (42,43,64).

ELECTRICAL COUPLING IN EMBRYONIC HEART CELL AGGREGATES

In recent studies (7,80), we have measured directly the decrease in resistance between newly apposed aggregates of embryonic heart cells, and have correlated that decrease with the onset of synchronous beating. From these experiments, we have concluded that pairs of spheroidal aggregates of a few thousand cells become synchronized within as little as 8 min after initial contact, when their adjoining cells contain only 5 junctional channels each (7). We estimate that a pair of single heart cells would require only one functional intercellular channel to synchronize their beats.

For these investigations, we used spheroidal aggregates (Fig. 1) of 7-day embryonic chick ventricle cells (57). Cells within such preparations are in direct electrical communication (11,14), and within strictly defined limits of frequency and amplitude (8), each aggregate approximates an isopotential system. That is, all cells within a single aggregate fire action potentials with not more than a 50 μsec delay (Fig. 2a and ref. 6). They also experience small voltage changes virtually simultaneously and without appreciable decrement (Fig. 2b,c). Replicas prepared from freeze-fractured cells within aggregates exhibit sparse but well-formed gap junctions (Fig. 3). These junctions are composed of 9 to 10 nm subunits arranged in pleomorphic configurations: small macular clusters (Fig. 3b), linear chains, usually 2 to 3 particles in width (Fig. 3d), and partial or closed annuli (Fig. 3c). These structures closely resemble the junctions observed in amphibian embryonic heart by Mazet (45) (For review, see 33.)

When two spontaneously beating aggregates in 1.3 mM K^+ medium were brought into contact, they adhered and gradually increased their shared area of mutual contact (Fig. 4a). Initially, each member of the pair continued to beat at its own rhythm, unaffected by its adhering neighbor. But after 13 to 120 minutes, their rates synchronized. From 19 separate coupling experiments, including 379 self-adhering aggregate pairs, the time between contact and synchrony (t_s) was 40 min. When aggregate pairs were pressed together to increase their area of mutual contact, t_s was reduced to 8 min (75). Twenty or more

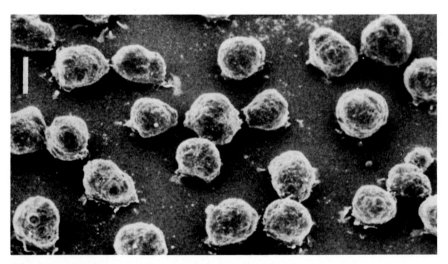

FIG. 1. Field of heart cell aggregates adhering to the surface of a culture dish. Scanning electron micrograph courtesy of Dr. Claudia Baste Adkison. Scale: 100 μm.

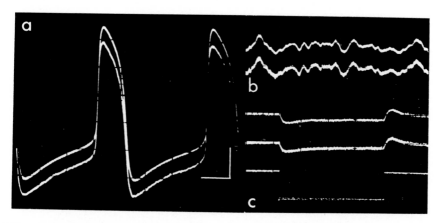

FIG. 2. Demonstration of voltage homogeneity in heart cell aggregates. **a:** Spontaneous action potentials recorded simultaneously through microelectrodes in two cells 223 μm apart at opposite poles of a 260 μm diameter aggregate. The two traces are displaced vertically in order to distinguish them. At a sweep speed of 0.5 msec/div, the upstrokes of the two action potentials can be seen to be separated by approximately 50 μsec (7). Scale: 20 mV, 100 ms. **b:** Voltage noise recorded from two cells 118 μm apart in 154 μm diameter aggregate. Spontaneous action potentials have been suppressed with 3×10^{-6}M tetrodotoxin. Potential fluctuates around a mean resting potential of −51 mV. Scale: 1 mV, 1 sec. **c:** Voltage responses *(upper and middle trace)* to a 2 nA hyperpolarizing current pulse *(lower trace)* recorded from two cells 115 μm apart in a 193 μm diameter aggregate, made quiescent with tetrodotoxin. Resting potential −51 mV. Scale: 20 mV, 2 nA, 1 sec.

aggregates could be stuck together to form long chains (Fig. 4b). Within 1 to 2 hours, all of the aggregates came to beat synchronously, the entire chain behaving essentially as a single cardiac fiber.

The first question to be answered then was, what are the electrical events associated with beat synchronization among aggregates? When aggregates were manipulated into contact under slight pressure (Fig. 5a), the time between contact and synchrony was reduced to a mean of about 8 min (7,75). When each aggregate was impaled with an intracellular electrode within a few minutes after apposition (Fig. 5b), the process of action potential synchronization could be observed (80). After 4 to 5 min of contact, there were no signs of electrical communication between the aggregates; each beat at its own rate, with no apparent effect upon the other (Fig. 5b). After 7 min (Fig. 5c), however, each action potential in the faster (F) aggregate induced a small depolarization in the slower (S), which occasionally reached threshold. Thus, at this early stage, electrotonic impulse transmission had already begun, but failed to cause synchrony of most beats. The action currents flowing from F through the contact area into the cells of S were apparently too small to excite the latter. Although the rate of diastolic depolarization of the slow aggregate might have been altered at this time by currents from F, the most significant feature of this initial stage of weak electric coupling was the occurrence of depolarizations induced by the impulses from

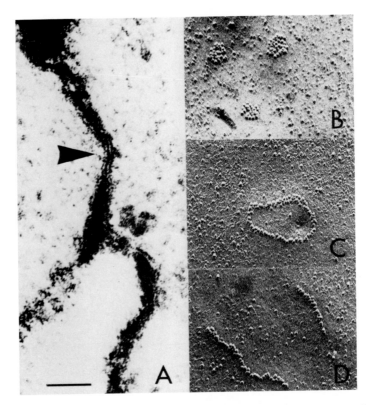

FIG. 3. Gap junctions in embryonic heart cell aggregates. **A:** Transmission electron micrograph of cells within an aggregate stained with ruthenium red. The gap junction *(arrow)* has a characteristic 2 to 4 nm space between the apposed membranes that is filled with dye. **B-D.** Freeze-fracture preparations showing typical configurations of the junctional particles. Shadowing is oriented vertically from bottom to top. Scale: 100 nm, A; 80 nm B-D.

F. At about 10 min (Fig. 5d), one out of every 3 or 4 beats in F, on the average, was followed by an action potential in S (80). This period is equivalent to the stage of "partial synchrony" (15,31) observed during the synchronization of newly apposed pairs of single cardiac myocytes. The coupling between the aggregates increased further with time (Fig. 5e), until every beat in the two aggregates was entrained (Fig. 5f) after a contact period of 15.5 min (in the case illustrated).

The coupling process could be examined in greater detail merely by expanding the time scale on the oscilloscope (Fig. 6) and using the impulse from F to trigger the sweeps (upper beam in all frames). Shortly after contact, the action potentials of the two aggregates were wholly independent (Fig. 6a). Records taken 7 (Fig. 6b) and 10 (Fig. 6c) min after contact showed partial synchrony, in which entrainment of action potentials was variable. But those impulses trig-

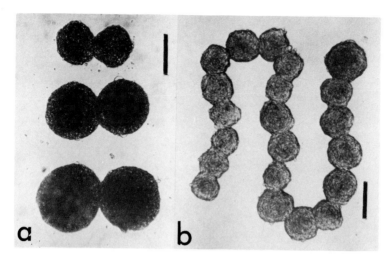

FIG. 4. Linear configurations of spheroidal aggregates for studies of electrical coupling. **a:** Aggregates arranged in equal-sized pairs, photographed 20 minutes after initial adhesion; only the smallest pair had achieved beat synchronization. Scale: 100 μm. **b:** A chain of 21 aggregates, photographed about 90 minutes after construction; all of the aggregates in the chain were beating in synchrony. Scale: 200 μm.

gered in S by F (Fig. 6b) occurred with long variable latencies[1] up to 300 msec. Moreover, some beats in F were missed in S, while F exhibited large fluctuations in its own interbeat interval. As synchronization proceeded (Fig. 6 d-f), both the mean latency ($\overline{L}$) and its variance (V_L) declined. Even when the pair appeared to be well coupled and synchronization was 1:1, both $\overline{L}$ and V_L could still be large (~80 msec; Fig. 6d). But by 20 min after contact, both $\overline{L}$ and V_L reached very low values. With continued time after contact, both parameters continued to decline, reaching values < 10 msec after about an hour.

The next question was whether the rapid decline in $\overline{L}$ and V_L resulted from a decrease in interaggregate coupling resistance (R_c). If the individual aggregate input resistances R_1 and R_2 remain constant during the course of beat synchronization, the coupling process must depend directly on a reduction in R_c. Coupling resistance can be measured directly by injecting pulses of constant current into one aggregate through one microelectrode, while simultaneously recording the transmembrane voltage response to each pulse in both aggregates with two additional electrodes (7). Representative records from one experiment are shown in Fig. 7. When action potential latency and R_c were both measured in the

---

[1] The term latency (L) is used to describe the delay in milliseconds between the fastest parts of the upstrokes of two synchronized action potentials. Synchrony, in this context, means that the action potentials from two aggregates are entrained with a fixed or slowly changing time delay between the leading and following spikes.

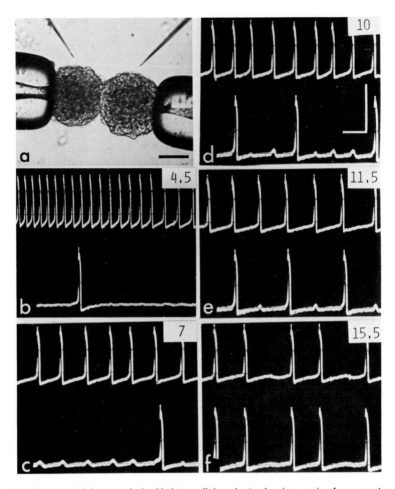

FIG. 5. Action potentials recorded with intracellular electrodes in a pair of aggregates held in contact with suction pipettes. **a:** Each aggregate is held by a suction pipet attached to a micromanipulator. Microelectrodes are seen poised for impalement. Scale: 100 μm. **b-f:** Action potentials recorded from the initially faster (F, upper trace) and slower (S, lower trace) aggregates are totally uncoordinated 4.5 minutes after contact (time shown in upper right corner of each panel) but come progressively into phase with increasing time of apposition. Scales: 100 mV, 1 sec. (From Ypey, Clapham and DeHaan (80), courtesy of *J. Membr. Biol.*)

same pair of synchronizing aggregates (Fig. 8), their rate of decline was almost perfectly parallel, even though the measurement of these parameters was completely independent (R_c is calculated from pulse transfer, and $\overline{L}$ is measured from action potentials). From these data, it is apparent that heart cell aggregates synchronize when R_c is substantially higher than predicted in some model systems (6). Synchrony for the pair measured in Fig. 8 occurred when R_c was about 20 MΩ, about 20 min after the first contact. At first synchrony, when $\overline{L}$ is 100 ms or more, the driven aggregate is in diastolic depolarization with an input resistance of about 1 MΩ, when the lead aggregate initiates an action

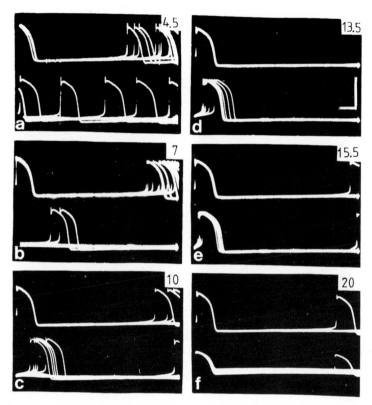

FIG. 6. Changes in latency between the action potentials recorded in the same pair of aggregates as in Fig. 5. Oscilloscope sweeps are triggered by the upper beam. Numbers in the upper corner of each frame are the times since initial contact of the aggregates (min). From the period when impulse transmission first became apparent (7 min), mean latency ($\overline{L}$) and fluctuation in the latency (V_L) both declined steadily as coupling increased. Scales: 100 mV, 100 msec. (From Ypey, Clapham, and DeHaan (80) courtesy of the *J. Membr. Biol.*)

potential. The current required to charge the membrane and shift its voltage from −80 mV to +20 mV at the peak of the action potential upstroke in the lead aggregate is about 2 μA (48). The nexal current is approximately equal to the potential difference between the aggregates during the action potential plateau (~60 mV), divided by R_c (~20 MΩ). Thus about 3 nA of current flows across the coupling junctions into the driven aggregate, producing a small voltage transient (Fig. 5 c-e). This is just sufficient, at time of first synchrony, to entrain the action potentials of the driven aggregate with those of the lead aggregate, but with a long latency and substantial variability in L. As R_c subsequently drops from 20 MΩ to less than 1 MΩ, more and more current flows across the junction into the driven aggregate and both $\overline{L}$ and V_L decrease progressively. These results suggest that low-resistance coupling junctions begin to be formed between aggregates soon after they are brought into contact, and continue to form thereafter.

The synchronization process has been mathematically modeled by treating

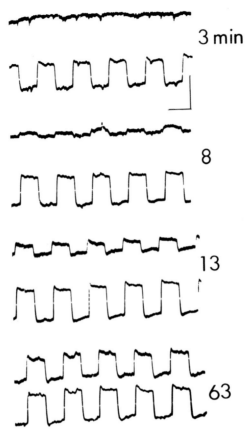

FIG. 7. Representative voltage responses from a pair of coupling aggregates to 5 sec hyperpolarizing pulses of current. Spontaneous action potentials were suppressed with tetrodotoxin. At the times after initial contact shown, current pulses were injected into the aggregate represented by the lower trace (V_1). Coupling resistance fell rapidly to yield a coupling ratio (V_2/V_1) of 0.77 at 63 min. Scales: 5 mV, 5 sec. (Modified from Clapham, Shrier, and DeHaan (7).)

two rhythmically active cells as coupled oscillators (e.g., 35). In such models, cells reach entrainment as resistance is lowered, and achieve a constant "phase shift" (latency) at first synchrony. These models are useful for predicting the effects of action potential parameters and membrane impedance on the time course of coupling. However, they emphasize mechanisms whereby the phase shift can be reduced without changing R_c. Our finding that $\overline{L}$ is related linearly to R_c (Fig. 8) implies that, with heart cell aggregates, the continued addition of junctional channels dominates the synchronization process, rather than entrainment at constant junctional resistance.

As noted above, the resistance of a single putative junctional channel would be about $1 \times 10^{10}\Omega$. When a pair of 150 μm diameter aggregates are pressed together, their shared area of contact (about 8×10^{-5} cm^2) is large enough to

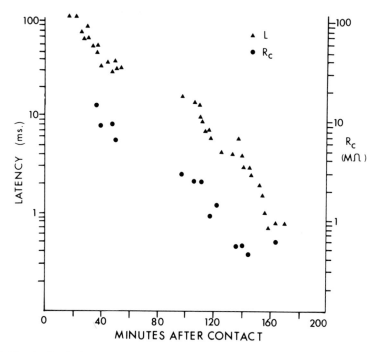

FIG. 8. The decline in latency and coupling resistance as a function of time after contact, in a pair of 160 μm diameter aggregates. During the gap in the data between 50 and 90 minutes after initial contact, the microelectrode came out of the cell in one of the aggregates. Attempts to re-impale the aggregate delayed coupling, but when a new, stable puncture was obtained, the decline in both $\overline{L}$ and R_c resumed at the same slope. (From Clapham, Shrier, and DeHaan (7).)

include about 100 apposed cells. When the first junctional channel forms between any one of these cells in one aggregate and its apposed neighbor in the other member of the pair, only about 10 pA (1×10^{-11}A) of current would flow across the junction with each action potential. On the basis of the kinetics of the decline in R_c, we can make an approximate estimate of the rate of insertion of junctional units between newly apposed aggregates.

It takes 3 to 4 minutes after first contact for the membranes of newly apposed cells to come close enough to form patent junctional channels (Williams and DeHaan, unpublished). If such transaggregate channels were then established among the 100 apposed cells at a constant average rate of about 1 channel/cell/minute, 500 channels would be formed during the first 8 to 9 min of contact, and would yield a junctional resistance of 20 MΩ. As noted above, this is the value of R_c when enough current flows from the lead aggregate across the junction to cause entrainment of its neighbor. That is, an average of only five junctional channels per apposed cell would be enough to permit synchrony between an aggregate pair (7), well before the organized macular or annular nexal junctions that are characteristic of gap junctions in the embryonic chick heart appear (Fig. 3b). At the same continued rate of addition, 10,000 parallel channels (i.e., about 100/cell) would have formed in less than 2 hours, and would result in $R_c = 1$ MΩ, which is the condition in which aggregates are synchronized with short latencies and great beat-to-beat fidelity (7,80). These calculations assume a constant rate of insertion of junctional channels (after an initial delay). The exponential fall in R_c illustrated in Fig. 8, however, implies that junctional units are added at progressively greater rates with time after initial contact. Among nine aggregate pairs, in which junctional conductance was measured continuously for a substantial period after contact (7), the rate of increase was constant in three pairs, approximately exponential in four pairs, and intermediate in the remaining two pairs. We do not know whether a linear or exponential increase in junctional conductance reflects a similar difference in rate of insertion of channels, or reflects other factors, such as rate of increase in appositional area.

These results with experimentally apposed cells seem to mimic the events of coupling during differentiation of the normal embryonic heart. The cells of embryonic mouse heart establish synchrony of contraction at about 8 days after fertilization. At that stage, only single putative junctional particles and a few loose clusters and linear arrays are present in the apposed surfaces. Typical macular gap junctions become apparent only 2 days later, at 10 days of gestation (26,27), and these increase in size and relative area with continued development. Also, in the 5-day chick myocardium prepared for freeze-fracture, Mazet (46) has reported tiny gap junctions with as few as 3 to 17 particles, spanning from the P-face to the E-face at points of close contact. These observations suggest that, at the earliest stages of coupling, heart cells may be electrically synchronized across scattered individual junctional channels. Only later, at more advanced stages of communication, do these channels become organized into definitive macular nexal structures.

We have recently obtained evidence consistent with the idea that embryonic heart cells can be coupled even in the absence of organized gap junctions, by examining aggregates with the freeze-fracture technique (76). Macular and annular gap junctions occupy about 0.3% of the total P-face area of cells within such aggregates, which is similar to the value in the 18-day embryonic mouse heart (27). When aggregates were exposed to 50 μg/ml cycloheximide (CHX), an inhibitor of protein synthesis, they continued beating rhythmically for days, showing no signs of desynchronization of their component cells. Aggregate pairs placed in CHX synchronized normally for the first 12 hr or more, even when amino acid incorporation into protein was reduced to 5% of control levels. However, t_s was prolonged in proportion to time of exposure to the inhibitor, presumably reflecting the gradual disappearance of a pool of preformed channel precursor material (75). Freeze-fracture preparations of the single aggregates in CHX showed that gap junctions between the component cells occupied progressively less of the total P-face area. After 21 hours in CHX, for example, mean junctional area was 0.014% of P-face (76), equivalent to the junctional

area in the 10-day mouse embryo (27). At 27 hours of exposure to CHX, organized gap junctions could no longer be found between the aggregate cells. By
impaling individual aggregates with two electrodes, one of which could be used
for passing current and recording voltage simultaneously through a discontinuous
current injection circuit (77), we could measure input resistance (R_{in}) and coupling ratio of the component cells directly. Coupling ratios of widely separated
cells in control aggregates approached unity, confirming earlier findings (11,14).
However, even after 27 to 30 hours in CHX, although the coupling ratio (V_2/
V_1) declined, substantial current still passed through low-resistance pathways
from cell to cell within the aggregate (Williams and DeHaan, unpublished).
Moreover, the aggregates continued to beat as integrated units, with all cells
firing synchronously. That is, the cells remained well coupled. Since the density
of IMP particles (putative junctional precursor particles) was about $2,100/\mu m^2$
in control aggregates and did not change significantly even after prolonged
exposure to CHX, we suggest that individual particles scattered throughout
the cell membranes are able to come into register across the intercellular space
with similar junctional particles in the apposed cell surface, and to serve as
low-resistance channels, without being organized into recognizable macular or
annular nexal structures.

Cardiac and other cell types tend to decouple (i.e., experience increases in
intercellular resistance) under conditions that lead to increased intracellular
Ca^{++} (18,37,38,54,73). Junctional resistance of amphibian blastomeres increases
markedly when a small voltage gradient is established across their apposed
membranes (65). Furthermore, gap junctions exhibit an altered appearance in
freeze-fracture preparations of infarcted regions of the dog heart (1). It has
recently been suggested that the crystal-like arrays of gap junction particles
often seen in freeze–cleave preparations are caused by fixation artifact and represent an uncoupled or high-resistance state of the nexus (51). If only small numbers
of scattered nexal channels are required to maintain the cells in a cardiac fiber
in a coupled state, it is tempting to speculate that the large number of nexal
particles commonly seen in junctional plaques in the cardiac intercalated disc
may provide a margin of safety, to avoid complete decoupling of mildly damaged
tissue. Alternatively, some nexal channels may serve functions other than ionic
conductance.

CONCLUSIONS

The studies reviewed here clarify certain aspects of intercellular coupling in
cardiac myocytes.

(1) When two spontaneously beating aggregates of embryonic heart cells are
    brought into contact, they synchronize their beats within minutes.
(2) The resistance of the junctional area between the aggregates is at first very
    high (about 250 MΩ), but begins to fall immediately after contact.
(3) Beat synchronization occurs when R_c reaches a value 10 to 20 times the

resting input resistance of the individual aggregates. At that time, however, the latency between the entrained action potentials is long (100 msec or more) and highly variable.

(4) As R_c continues to fall, $\bar{L}$ and V_L also decline apace.

(5) Even when discrete macular and annular gap junctions disappear as a result of prolonged inhibition of protein synthesis, cells within aggregates remain electrically coupled.

These results are consistent with a model that attributes the low-resistance pathway between cells to the pore-bearing IMP particles that normally are organized into defined macular or annular gap junctions. Our studies suggest that, under certain circumstances, heart cells become synchronized when only a small number of isolated junctional channels exist between their apposed surfaces. This occurs at early embryonic stages and at short times after initial cell apposition, before definitive gap junctions appear. It also appears to be the condition of cells exposed for prolonged periods to cycloheximide, when organized gap junctions disappear.

One of the crucial questions still to be answered is, what role is played by the large number of IMP junctional particles normally seen in definitive gap junctions of the heart, if synchrony requires only a few scattered channels per cell?

ACKNOWLEDGMENTS

We express our thanks to Mr. Tom Fisk for his expertise in the preparation and care of the heart cell cultures, to Mrs. Winifred M. Scherer for her cheerful and accurate typing and editorial services, and to Dr. L. J. DeFelice for informative discussions of all parts of this work. This study was supported by Grant # NIH HL16567 (RLD), Medical Scientist Research Training Grant PHS-5-T232-GM-07415 (DEC), and the Netherlands Organization for the Advancement of Pure Research, ZWO (DLY).

REFERENCES

1. Ashraf, M., and Halverson, C. (1978): Ultrastructural modifications of nexuses (gap junctions) during early myocardial ischemia. *J. Mol. Cell. Cardiol.,* 10:263-269.
2. Barr, L., Dewey, M. M., and Berger, W. (1965): Propagation of action potentials and the structure of the nexus in cardiac muscle. *J. Gen. Physiol.,* 48:797-823.
3. Benedetti, E. L., Dunia, I., and Bloemendal, H. (1974): Development of junctions during differentiation of lens fiber. *Proc. Natl. Acad. Sci. USA,* 71:5073-5077.
4. Bennett, M. V. L. (1978): Junctional permeability. In: *Intercellular Junctions and Synapses,* edited by J. Feldman, N. B. Gilula, and J. D. Pitts, pp. 23-36. Chapman and Hall, London.
5. Bennett, M. V. L., Spira, M. E., and Spray, D. C. (1980): Permeability of gap junctions between embryonic cells of Fundulus: A reevaluation. *Dev. Biol.,* 65:114-125.
6. Berkinblit, M. B., Kalinen, D. I., Kovalev, S. A., and Chailakyan, L. M. (1975): Study with the Noble model of synchronization of the spontaneously active myocardial cells bound by a highly permeable contact. *Biofizika,* 20:121-125.
7. Clapham, D. E., Shrier, A., and DeHaan, R. L. (1980): Junctional resistance and action potential delay between embryonic heart cell aggregates. *J. Gen. Physiol.,* 75:633-654.

8. Clay, J. R., DeFelice, L. J., and DeHaan, R. L. (1979): Parameters of current noise derived from voltage noise and impedance in chick embryonic heart cell aggregates. *Biophys. J.,* 28:169-184.

9. Decker, R. S. (1976): Hormonal regulation of gap junction differentiation. *J. Cell Biol.,* 69:669-685.

10. Decker, R. S., and Friend, D. S. (1974): Assembly of gap junctions during amphibian neurulation. *J. Cell Biol.,* 62:32-47.

11. DeFelice, L. J., and DeHaan, R. L. (1977): Membrane noise and intercellular communication. *IEEE Proc.,* 65:796-799.

12. DeHaan, R. L. (1976): Cell coupling and electrophysiological differentiation of embryonic heart cells. In: *Tests of Teratogenicity in Vitro,* edited by J. D. Ebert and M. Marois, pp. 225-232. North Holland Publ. Co., Amsterdam.

13. DeHaan, R. L., Durr, T. E., Krueger, R. C., McDonald, T. F., Moyzis, G., Plitt, C. E., Sachs, H. G., and Springer, M. (1973): Functional differentiation of the embryonic heart. In: *Carnegie Institution of Washington Yearbook 72,* pp. 73-87.

14. DeHaan, R. L., and Fozzard, H. A. (1975): Membrane response to current pulses in spheroidal aggregates of embryonic heart cells. *J. Gen. Physiol.,* 65:207-222.

15. DeHaan, R. L., and Hirakow, R. (1972): Synchronization of pulsation rates in isolated cardiac myocytes. *Exp. Cell Res.,* 70:214-220.

16. DeHaan, R. L., and Sachs, H. G. (1972): Cell coupling in developing systems: The heart cell paradigm. In: *Curr. Top. Dev. Biol.,* 7:193-228.

17. DeMello, W. C. (1972): Intercellular communication in heart muscle. In: *Intercellular Communication,* edited by W. C. DeMello, pp. 87-125. Plenum Press, New York.

18. DeMello, W. C. (1975): Effect of intracellular injection of calcium and strontium on cell communication in heart. *J. Physiol. (Lond.),* 250:231-245.

19. Flagg-Newton, J., Simpson, I., and Loewenstein, W. R. (1979): Permeability of the cell-to-cell membrane channels in mammalian cell junction. *Science,* 205:404-407.

20. Gilula, N. B. (1977): Gap junctions and cell communication. In: *International Cell Biology,* edited by B. R. Brinkley and K. R. Porter, pp. 61-69. Rockefeller University Press, New York.

21. Gilula, N. B. (1980): Cell-to-cell communication and development. In: *The Cell Surface: Mediator of Developmental Processes,* edited by S. Subtelny and N. K. Wessells, pp. 23-41. Academic Press, New York.

22. Gilula, N. B., and Epstein, M. L. (1976): Cell-to-cell communication, gap junctions, and calcium. *Symp. Soc. Exp. Biol.,* 30:257-272.

23. Gilula, N. B., Reeves, O. R., and Steinbach, A. (1972): Metabolic coupling, ionic coupling, and cell contacts. *Nature,* 235:262-265.

24. Goshima, K. (1971): Synchronized beating of myocardial cells mediated by FL cells in monolayer culture and its inhibition by trypsin-treated FL cells. *Exp. Cell Res.,* 65:161-169.

25. Griepp, E. B., and Bernfield, M. R. (1978): Acquisition of synchronous beating between embryonic heart cell aggregates and layers. *Exp. Cell Res.,* 113:263-272.

26. Gros, D., Mocquard, J. P., Challice, C. E., and Schrevel, J. (1978): Formation and growth of gap junctions in mouse myocardium during ontogenesis: A freeze–cleave study. *J. Cell. Sci.,* 30:45-61.

27. Gros, D., Mocquard, J. P., Challice, C. E., and Schrevel, J. (1979): Formation and growth of gap junctions in mouse myocardium during ontogenesis: Quantitative data and their implications on the development of intercellular communication. *J. Mol. Cell. Cardiol.,* 11:543-554.

28. Ito, S., Sato, E., and Loewenstein, W. R. (1974): Studies on the formation of a permeable cell membrane junction. *J. Membr. Biol.,* 19:339-355.

29. Johnson, R., Hammer, J., Hudson, J., and Revel, J.-P. (1974): Gap junction formation between reaggregated Novikoff hepatoma cells. *Proc. Natl. Acad. Sci. USA,* 71:4536-4540.

30. Jongsma, H. J., and van Rijn, H. E. (1972): Electrotonic spread of current in monolayer cultures of neonatal rat heart cells. *J. Membr. Biol.,* 9:341-360.

31. Jongsma, H. J., Masson-Pevet, M., Hollander, C. C., and de Bruyne, J. (1975): Synchronization of the beating frequency of cultured rat heart cells. In: *Developmental and Physiological Correlates of Cardiac Muscle,* edited by M. Lieberman and T. Sano, pp. 185-196. Raven Press, New York.

32. Kalderon, N., Epstein, M. L., and Gilula, N. B. (1977): Cell-to-cell communication and myogenesis. *J. Cell Biol.,* 75:788-806.

33. Larsen, W. J. (1977): Structural diversity of gap junctions: A review. *Tissue Cell,* 9:373-394.

34. Lieberman, M., Kootsey, J. M., Johnson, E. A., and Sawanobori, T. (1973): Slow conduction in cardiac muscle. A biophysical model. *Biophys. J.,* 13:37-55.
35. Linkens, D. A., and Datardina, S. (1977): Frequency entrainment of coupled Hodgkin-Huxley-type oscillators for modeling gastrointestinal and electrical activity. *IEEE Trans. Biomed. Eng.,* 24:362-365.
36. Loewenstein, W. R. (1975): Permeable junctions. *Cold Spring Harbor Symp. Quant. Biol.,* 40:49-63.
37. Loewenstein, W. R. (1977): Permeability of the junctional membrane channel. In: *International Cell Biology,* edited by B. R. Brinkley and K. R. Porter, p. 70-82. Rockefeller University Press, New York.
38. Loewenstein, W. R., and Rose, B. (1978): Calcium in (junctional) intercellular communication and a thought on its behavior in intercellular communication. *Ann. NY Acad. Sci.,* 307:287-309.
39. Loewenstein, W. R., Kanno, Y., and Socolar, S. J. (1978): Quantum jumps of conductance during formation of membrane channels at cell–cell junction. *Nature,* 274:133-136.
40. Magnuson, T., Demsey, A., and Stackpole, C. W. (1977): Characterization of intercellular junctions in the pre-implantantation embryo by freeze-fracture and thin section electron microscopy. *Dev. Biol.,* 61:525-261.
41. Makowski, L., Caspar, D. L. D., Phillips, W. C., and Goodenough, D. A. (1977): Gap junction structure. II. Analysis of the X-ray diffraction data. *J. Cell Biol.,* 74:629-645.
42. Mann, J. E., Jr., Foley, E., and Sperelakis, N. (1977): Resistance and potential profiles in the cleft between two myocardial cells. Electrical analog and computer simulations. *J. Theor. Biol.,* 68:1-15.
43. Mann, J. E., and Sperelakis, N. (1979): Further development of a model for electrical transmission between myocardial cells not connected by low-resistance pathways. *J. Electrocardiol.,* 12:23-33.
44. Matter, A. (1973): A morphometric study on the nexus of rat cardiac muscle. *J. Cell Biol.,* 56:690-696.
45. Mazet, F. (1977): Freeze-fracture studies of gap junctions in the developing and adult amphibian cardiac muscle. *Dev. Biol.,* 60:139-152.
46. Mazet, F. (1979): Etude ultrastructurale des jonctions presente dans la myocarde de le Poulet. *Biol. Cellulaire Francais,* 29:27a.
47. McNutt, N. S., and Weinstein, R. S. (1973): Membrane ultrastructure at mammalian intercellular junctions. *Prog. Biophys. Mol. Biol.,* 26:45-101.
48. Nathan, R., and DeHaan, R. L. (1979): Voltage clamp analysis of embryonic heart cell aggregates. *J. Gen. Physiol.,* 73:175-198.
49. Pitts, J. D. (1978): Junctional communication and cellular growth control. In: *Intercellular Junctions and Synapses,* edited by J. Feldman, N. B. Gilula, and J. D. Pitts, pp. 61-80. Chapman and Hall, London.
50. Pollack, G. H. (1976): Intercellular coupling in the atrioventricular node and other tissues of the rabbit heart. *J. Physiol. (Lond.),* 255:275-298.
51. Raviola, E., Goodenough, D. A., and Raviola, G. (1978): The native structure of gap junctions rapidly frozen at 4°K. *J. Cell Biol.,* 79:229a.
52. Rawles, M. E. (1943): The heart-forming areas of the early chick mesoderm. *Physiol. Zool.,* 16:22-42.
53. Revel, J.-P., Yee, A. G., and Hudspeth, A. J. (1971): Gap junctions between electrotonically coupled cells in tissue culture and in brown fat. *Proc. Natl. Acad. Sci. USA,* 68:2924-2927.
54. Rose, B., and Loewenstein, W. R. (1976): Permeability of a cell junction and the local cytoplasmic free ionized calcium concentration: A study with aequorin. *J. Membr. Biol.,* 28:87-119.
55. Rosenquist, G. C. (1966): A radioautographic study of labeled grafts in the chick blastoderm. Development from primitive streak stages to stage 12. *Carnegie Institution of Washington Contributions to Embryology,* 38:71-110.
56. Rosenquist, G. C., and DeHaan, R. L. (1966): Migration of precardiac cells in the chick embryo: A radioautographic study. *Carnegie Institution of Washington Contributions to Embryology,* 38:111-121.
57. Sachs, H. G., and DeHaan, R. L. (1973): Embryonic myocardial cell aggregates: Volume and pulsation rate. *Dev. Biol.,* 30:233-240.
58. Sheridan, J. D. (1971): Dye movement and low-resistance junctions between reaggregated embryonic cells. *Dev. Biol.,* 26:627-643.
59. Sheridan, J. D. (1976): Cell coupling and cell communication during embryogenesis. In: *The*

Cell Surface and Animal Embryogenesis and Development, edited by G. Poste and G. L. Nicolson, pp. 409-447. Biomedical Press, Elsevier/North Holland.

60. Sheridan, J. D. (1978): Junction formation and experimental modification. In: *Intercellular Junctions and Synapses,* edited by J. Feldman, N. B. Gilula, and J. D. Pitts, pp. 37-60. Chapman and Hall, London.

61. Sheridan, J. D., Hammer-Wilson, M., Preus, D., and Johnson, R. G. (1978): Quantitative analysis of low-resistance junctions between cultured cells and correlation with gap junctional area. *J. Cell Biol.,* 76:532-544.

62. Simpson, I., Rose, B., and Loewenstein, W. R. (1977): Size limit of molecules permeating the junctional membrane channels. *Science,* 195:294-296.

63. Sjostrand, F. S., and Anderson, E. (1954): Electron microscopy of the intercalated discs of cardiac muscle tissue. *Experientia (Basel),* 10:369-370.

64. Sperelakis, N. (1969): Lack of electrical coupling between contiguous myocardial cells in vertebrate heart. In: *Comparative Physiology of the Heart: Current Trends,* edited by F. V. McCann, p. 138. Birhaser-Verlag, Basel.

65. Spray, D. C., Harris, A. L., and Bennett, M. V. L. (1979): Voltage dependence of junctional conductance in early amphibian embryos. *Science,* 204:432-434.

66. Stalsberg, H. (1969a): The origin of heart asymmetry: Right and left contributions to the early chick embryo heart. *Dev. Biol.,* 19:109-127.

67. Stalsberg, H. (1969b): Regional mitotic activity in the precardiac mesoderm and differentiating heart tube in the chick embryo. *Dev. Biol.,* 20:18-45.

68. Stalsberg, H., and DeHaan, R. L. (1969): The precardiac areas and formation of the tubular heart in chick embryo. *Dev. Biol.,* 19:128-159.

69. Van Mierop, L. H. S. (1967): Location of pacemaker in chick embryo heart at the time of initiation of heartbeat. *Am. J. Physiol.,* 212:407-415.

70. Weidmann, S. (1952): The electrical constants of Purkinje fibers. *J. Physiol. (Lond.),* 118:348-360.

71. Weidmann, S. (1966): Cardiac muscle: The functional significance of the intercalated discs. *Ann. NY Acad. Sci.,* 137:540-542.

72. Weidmann, S. (1969): Electrical constants of trabecular muscle from mammalian heart. *J. Physiol. (Lond.),* 210:1041-1054.

73. Weingart, R. (1977): The action of ouabain on intercellular coupling and conduction velocity in mammalian ventricular muscle. *J. Physiol. (Lond.),* 264:341-365.

74. Williams, E. H., and DeHaan, R. L. (1977): Beat synchronization and protein synthesis in spheroidal aggregates of chick heart cells. *VIII Int. Cong. Soc. Devel. Biol. Japan,* (abstract).

75. Williams, E. H., and DeHaan, R. L. (1978): Alterations in synchronization time of newly apposed heart cell aggregates by pretreatment with trypsin and cycloheximide. *J. Cell Biol.,* 79:29a (abstract).

76. Williams, E. H., and DeHaan, R. L. (1979): Changes in IMP particle distribution in gap junctional and non-junctional membrane of heart cells after prolonged inhibition of protein synthesis. *J. Cell Biol.,* 83:81a.

77. Wilson, W. A., and Goldner, M. M. (1975): Voltage clamping with a single microelectrode. *J. Neurobiol.,* 6:411-422.

78. Wolpert, L. (1978): Gap junctions: Channels for communication in development. In: *Intercellular Junctions and Synapses,* edited by J. Feldman, N. B. Gilula, and J. D. Pitts, pp. 61-80. Chapman and Hall, London.

79. Yee, A. G., and Revel, J.-P. (1978): Loss and reappearance of gap junctions in regenerating liver. *J. Cell Biol.,* 78:554-564.

80. Ypey, D. L., Clapham, D. E, and DeHaan, R. L. (1979): The development of electrical coupling and action potential synchrony between paired aggregates of embryonic heart cells. *J. Membr. Biol.,* 51:75-96.

81. Zampighi, G., Corless, J. M., and Robertson, J. D. (1980): On gap junction structure. *J. Cell Biol.,* 86:190-198.

DISCUSSION

Le Douarin: One would expect that coupling of the two aggregates will result in synchronization at faster rhythm. Is that the case? Isolated cells behave in a different way.

DeHaan: The faster aggregate does not merely act as a pacemaker for the second aggregate; the synchronous rate is always intermediate. The rate-setting mechanism has to do with surface-to-volume ratios.

Gros: Do you have fibroblasts around your aggregates?

DeHaan: Yes, the aggregates contain some 15 to 20% of fibroblasts. They tend after 24 to 48 hours to move to the peripheral surface. At 72 hours, we usually pushed the two aggregates together. They formed a 2- to 3-cell-thick layer all around, and they coupled just as well. But we could not see well-formed junctions between myocytes and fibroblasts. Formed gap junctions may not be present in some tissues, and it would still not mean that the cells were not coupled across gap junctions.

Nathan: In the case of potential differences, did you find any difference in coupling duration?

DeHaan: I do not see how you could ever convince yourself that when you have an impalement which showed 40 mV instead of 70 it was not just a bad impalement.

Nathan: Is it possible, when cardiac muscle is damaged, and you have various depolarized areas, that this is one mechanism for cellular decoupling?

DeHaan: Yes, this is the mechanism demonstrated by Spray et al. (65). As soon as the voltage in a given cell depolarizes, that cell is sealed off.

Rosenquist: At what age were the chick hearts disaggregated?

DeHaan: Most of the work was done on 7 e.d. chick ventricles.

Rosenquist: Do you have any cushion, atrial, or sinus tissue involved in your aggregates?

DeHaan: We have been very careful to exclude sinus and atrium. I cannot be so sure about trigone or prospective valvular tissue from which I am sure that many of the fibroblasts come.

Rosenquist: Is there any difference in the percentage or the alignment of the myofibrils in the core cells and those at the outside of your aggregates?

DeHaan: In our Herpes virus studies, we examined cells in a swath across a 100 cell aggregate. I have not looked specifically for myofibrils, but except for the distinction between myocytes and fibroblasts, there was nothing obvious about the cells in different locations.

Rosenquist: But the cells of the periphery of your aggregate are not the cells that you really want to study.

DeHaan: The pictures are indistinguishable in terms of the range of particle numbers, the range of distribution, etc., whether we take two cells deep within an aggregate or a cell at the very periphery.

Rosenquist: I would like to suggest an experiment. Take some 4- or 5-day aggregates and implant them in a host embryo, in the path of the neural crest cells, and observe what will happen as these aggregates become innervated by the host embryo.

Arguello: I was surprised by the number of particles on the P face of the freeze-fractured cells from your aggregate. Did you see any differences from the *in vivo* situation?

DeHaan: The average number of particles per square micron on a P face was 2,100. Your figure from intact heart was not too far off 1,500 or 1,600.

NOTE ADDED IN PROOF*

In two recent studies, J. Flagg-Newton and W. R. Lowenstein have shown that junctional permeability to tracer molecules may be blocked in cells exposed to cyanide and iodoacetate while ionic conductance persists (*J. Membr. Biol.,* 50:65–100, 1979). Moreover, rectifying junctions can be formed when selected cells with dissimilar junctional properties are paired (*Science,* 207:771-773, 1980).

Perspectives in Cardiovascular Research, Vol. 5,
Mechanisms of Cardiac Morphogenesis and Teratogenesis,
edited by Tomas Pexieder. Raven Press, New York © 1981

Differentiation of Cellular Electrical Properties in the Developing Embryonic Chick Heart

Georges H. Le Douarin and Didier Renaud

Laboratory of Animal and Cell Physiology, University of Nantes, Faculty of Sciences, 44072 Nantes Cédex, France

Electrophysiologic studies of developing heart cells have been performed by numerous researchers. It was soon observed that, although maturation of the myocardial tissues occurs very early in some respects, (9), important changes in membrane properties take place during embryonic development of the heart. One of the first evidences for these changes came from the observation of differences between cellular action potentials recorded from embryo and adult rabbit (10).

In the adult vertebrate, the cellular electrogenesis of heart muscle fibers results from complex ionic currents. The rising phase of the action potential (AP) is triggered by a rapid inward current carried by sodium ions. This fast sodium-carrying mechanism can be selectively inhibited by tetrodotoxin (TTX) (4,8,25). Another inward current increases and maintains depolarization; it produces the plateau of the AP. This slow inward current is insensitive to TTX and may be carried by calcium and/or sodium ions (18,19,24,25). It can be blocked by various substances, such as manganese ions or verapamil. Although several outward currents have been described in adult cardiac cells (2,20), the repolarization phase of the AP results from the inactivation of the inward currents and from the occurrence of a delayed outward current.

The cellular electrical activity of the chick embryo heart can be recorded at the initiation of the heart beat (12,21,34). In the first step of cardiac organogenesis, ventricular cells become active. Shortly afterwards, other primitive cardiac chambers differentiate and the characteristic AP of atrial, ventricular, and bulbar cells are observed (Fig. 1). However, in early stages of development the recorded APs differ from APs of the adult heart, indicating that the ionic mechanisms that underlie electrogenesis are markedly different in the two cases. The aim of this work is to summarize the changes in membrane ionic permeabilities of the cardiac cells which occur during embryonic development of the chick.

MATERIALS AND METHODS

Fertilized chicken eggs (White Leghorn) were incubated at 38°C. The embryonic hearts were removed at various stages of development. We focused our attention on the ventricular cells.

In the case of embryos from 2 to 6 e.d., the entire heart was removed, immersed in a Perspex chamber, and perfused by a standard Tyrode solution of the following composition (mM): NaCl, 130; KCl, 2.7; CaCl$_2$, 1.4; MgCl$_2$, 0.5; NaH$_2$PO$_4$, 0.37; NaHCO$_3$, 4; and glucose lg/l), or by modified Tyrode solutions (low K$^+$, Na$^+$, or Ca^{++}). The solution was bubbled with 95% O$_2$ and 5% CO$_2$, and the temperature was maintained at 37°C.

For older hearts, only strips of myocardium from right ventricle were used.

Tetrodotoxin (TTX, Sigma) was injected directly into the Perspex chamber. The volume of drug stock solution added to the medium was 20 to 30 μl. Tetraethylammonium (TEA) (Fluka) in Tyrode solution was also used.

Transmembrane potentials were recorded using conventional glass microelectrodes filled with 3M KCl. The indifferent electrode was an agar-embedded silver–silver chloride electrode placed into the bath fluid.

Current–voltage relations were obtained using a pair of intracellular microelec-

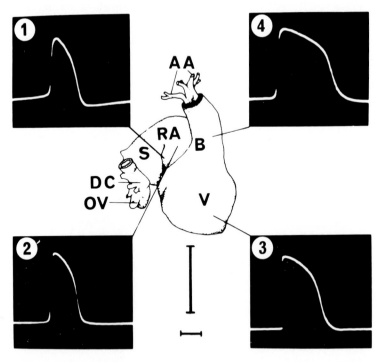

FIG. 1. Action potentials recorded from various regions of 3-day-old chick embryo heart. AA; aortic arches; DC; ductus of Cuvier; OV; omphalomesenteric veins; S; sinus venosus; RA; right atrium; V; ventricle; B; bulbus. Vertical scale: 100 mV; horizontal scale: 100 ms.

trodes according to the technique described by Weidman (35). Depolarizing and hyperpolarizing currents were applied for 1.5 sec.

RESULTS

Effects of Low External Potassium Concentration

The maximum diastolic membrane potential increases with age during embryonic development, from about -35 mV at 2 e.d. to -72 mV at 12 e.d. After this stage, the increase is very small (29). Moreover, the relationship between the resting potential (RP) and $[K^+]_o$ is not quantitatively the same during development: at 15 e.d., RP is nearly equal to the calculated E_K at high $[K^+]_o$, indicating a complete K^+ permeability when $[K^+]_o$ is 10 mM or more. The recorded values deviate from E_K at lower potassium levels and, in younger hearts, the curves of RP plotted as a function of E_K continually bend (29,30). Young hearts are less sensitive to an excess of external potassium than are older hearts (6,29). On the other hand, the diastolic membrane potential of young (2 and 3 e.d.) heart ventricular cells was very sensitive to potassium deprivation. In 0.3 mM $[K^+]_o$ the RP rapidly decreased and a slow diastolic depolarization occurred (Fig. 2). When external potassium was completely suppressed, the electrical activity disappeared within 30 min. Before activity stopped, bursts of APs were frequently recorded (Fig. 3). In older stages of development, the sensitivity of the RP to reduction of external potassium was less important; the electrical activity was not suppressed in 0.3 mM $[K^+]_o$, and RP was much less affected than it was in earlier stages (Fig. 4).

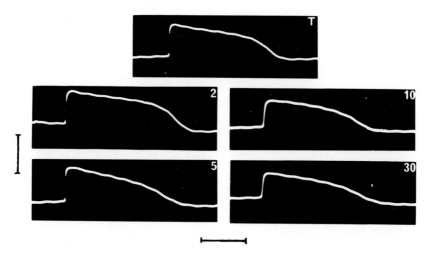

FIG. 2. Effects of low external potassium concentration (0.3 mM) upon ventricular AP of 2-day-old chick embryo heart. All records are from the same cell. T; AP in normal Tyrode solution; 2 to 30: time (min) in low K^+ solution. Vertical scale: 100 mV; horizontal scale: 100 ms.

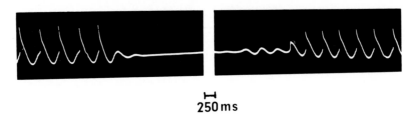

250 ms

FIG. 3. Bursts of activity in 3-day-old chick embryo heart after 60 min in a low external potassium concentration (0.3 mM).

Effects of Low External Sodium Concentration

Normal Tyrode solution was modified by substituting Tris chloride for sodium chloride. A solution containing 10% $[Na^+]_o$ (13.7 mM) produced a negative chronotropic effect in early (12-somite stage) chick embryo heart, and this effect increased with age (Fig. 5).

Ventricular AP was modified by low $[Na^+]_o$. The depolarization phase was slower than in normal Tyrode solution, the plateau was reduced, and the AP duration was shortened (Fig. 6). These effects were observed in hearts at various stages of development (2 to 19 e.d.). However, the loss of electrical activity that occurs in sodium-free solution (18) was observed within a few minutes at day 6 and in older stages, while the excitability of the ventricle cells remained for a longer time (30 min or more) at the 2-day stage. This suggests that sensitivity to sodium deprivation increases after the earliest stages of heart differentiation.

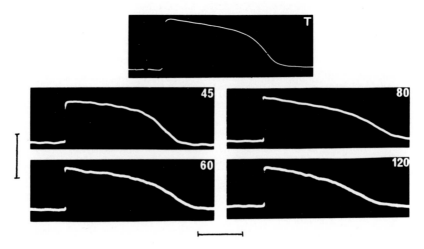

FIG. 4. Effects of low external potassium concentration (0.3 mM) upon ventricular AP at day 19 of embryonic development. All records are from the same cell. T: AP in normal Tyrode solution; 45 to 120: time (min) in low K^+ solution. Vertical scale: 100 mV; horizontal scale: 100 ms.

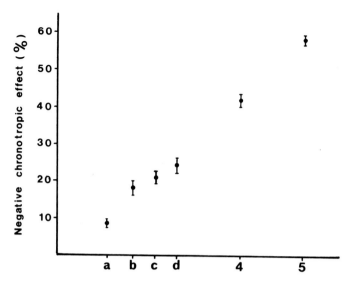

FIG. 5. Negative chronotropic effect (in per cent of the rhythm in normal Tyrode solution) of low concentration of external sodium (13.7 mM) at various stages of development: **a,** 12-16 somites; **b,** 18-23 somites; **c,** 24-29 somites; **d,** 30-35 somites; 4 e.d. and 5 e.d.

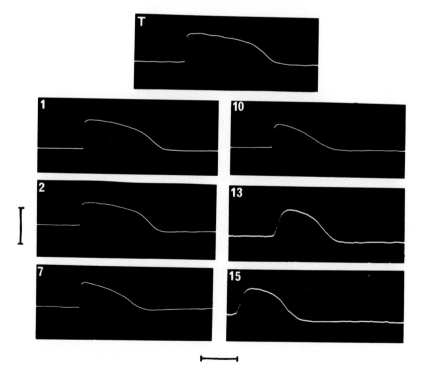

FIG. 6. Effects of low external sodium concentration (13.7 mM) upon ventricular AP in 3-day-old chick embryo heart. All records are from the same cell. T; AP in normal Tyrode solution; 1 to 15: time (min) in low Na+ solution. Vertical scale: 100 mV; horizontal scale: 100 ms.

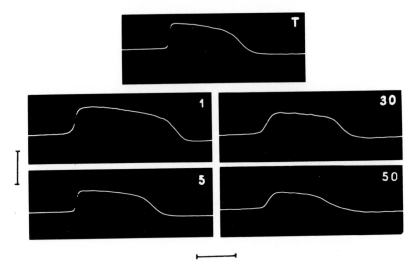

FIG. 7. Effects of low external calcium concentration (0.14 mM) upon ventricular AP in 2-day-old chick embryo heart. All records are from the same cell. T; AP in normal Tyrode solution; 1 to 50: time (min) in low Ca^{++} solution. Vertical scale: 100 mV; horizontal scale: 100 ms.

Effects of Low External Calcium Concentration

The modified Tyrode solution contained 0.14 mM Ca^{++}. In 2-day-old heart, changes in electrical activity occurred rapidly in this solution (Fig. 7). Within the first minutes, the plateau was increased and the AP duration was greater. Afterwards, the AP duration decreased. The rate of rise of the depolarization

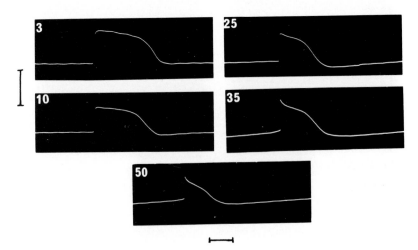

FIG. 8. Effects of low external calcium concentration (0.14 mM) upon ventricular AP in 4-day-old chick embryo heart. All records are from the same cell. 3 to 50: time (min) in low Ca^{++} solution. Vertical scale: 100 mV; horizontal scale: 100 ms.

phase was progressively reduced and the peak amplitude decreased. After 1 h in 0.14 mM $[Ca^{++}]_o$, the rate of rise of the AP depolarization was about 3.5 V/s (versus 5.8 V/s in normal Tyrode solution), and the peak amplitude was reduced to about 45 mV. Moreover, after several minutes in low calcium solution, a slow diastolic depolarization was observed. At 4 e.d. (Fig. 8), the rate of rise of AP depolarization was little or not at all affected, but other changes in electrical activity were observed, i.e., reduction of the plateau, AP duration, and amplitude, and occurrence of a slow diastolic depolarization. Finally, at 19 e.d., the only effects of low calcium solution were a slight reduction of AP amplitude and duration.

Inhibition of the Fast Sodium Inward Current by TTX

Studies of the development of TTX-sensitivity in chick embryonic hearts have shown that, in the first stage of organogenesis, activity is not suppressed by the inhibitor. This has been pointed out by several groups (7,15,27,29). According to these authors, chick embryo heart is insensitive to TTX until 4 or 5 e.d. However, it has been reported that ventricular AP is affected by TTX in the 3-day-old embryonic chick heart (11).

Using a rather high dose of TTX (5.10^{-6} g/ml), we observed that spontaneous activity of the 2-day-old chick embryo heart was not suppressed. However,

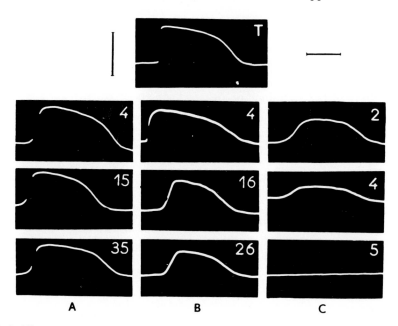

FIG. 9. Effects of inhibitors of ionic permeabilities upon ventricular electrical activity at 26-somite stage. T; AP in normal Tyrode solution; **A:** effects of TTX (5.10^{-6} g/ml); **B:** effects of manganese ions (5 mM); **C:** effects of both inhibitors. Numbers indicate the time (min) of action of inhibitors. Vertical scale: 100 mV; horizontal scale: 100 ms.

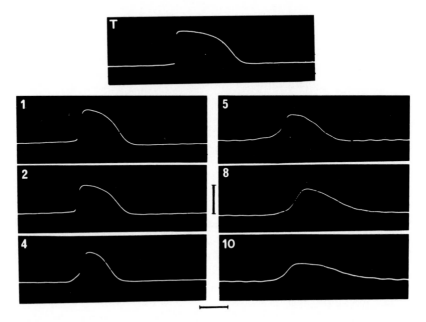

FIG. 10. Effects of TTX (5.10^{-6} g/ml) upon ventricular electrical activity in 4-day-old chick embryo heart. All records are from the same cell. T; AP in normal Tyrode solution; 1 to 10: time (min) of action of TTX. Vertical scale: 100 mV; horizontal scale: 100 ms.

the rate of rise of ventricular AP depolarization was progressively reduced (Fig. 9A). The same effect was observed at the 3-day stage. At 4 e.d., TTX generally suppressed the electrical activity within 30 min after a progressive change in AP shape (Fig. 10). Inhibition of electrical activity produced by TTX was observed within a few minutes in older stages.

Effects of Mn^{++} and La^{+++}

In early stages of cardiac development (2 and 3 e.d.), manganese ions (5 mM) caused a slowing of the rate of AP depolarization, and the AP was progressively shortened (Fig. 9B). However, electrical activity did not stop for an hour or more. Administration of both TTX and manganese ions suppressed electrical activity within a few minutes (Fig. 9C).

The problem of the participation of calcium ions in the development of the slow inward current in chick embryo hearts does not seem to be completely elucidated. It has been suggested that in young hearts, as well as in older stages, the major inward current is carried by sodium (30). However, we observed that La^{+++} (1 mM) caused a decrease in the peak amplitude of ventricular AP of young (3 e.d.) heart, and reduced the rate of rise of depolarization at the terminal phase of the spike. According to this effect of La^{+++} and those of low external calcium concentration, it appears that calcium ions participate in the development of the slow inward current at the early stages of cardiac development in chick embryo. However, this role of calcium ions is much less important than in rat embryo (1). In older stages of development, the spike of the AP becomes insensitive to La^{+++}, and this inhibitor affects only the plateau, which is depressed.

Development of Cardiac Membrane Potassium Rectifications

Permeability of the cardiac cell membrane to potassium increases with age in chick embryo (3,6,29). Sensitivity to TEA also changes with age but, in young (3 e.d.) as well as in older stages, TEA (5 mM) caused an increase in

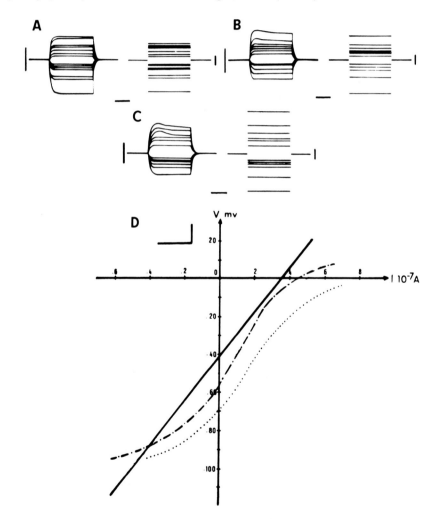

FIG. 11. Current clamp experiments. **A, B,** and **C:** changes in MP produced by transmembrane currents at 2 e.d., 4 e.d., and 19 e.d. Horizontal scale: 500 ms; vertical scale: 50 mV for MP and 2.10^{-7} A for currents. **D:** current–voltage relations observed at 2 (—), 4 (—·—) and 19 (· · · · ·) e.d.

the AP duration. TEA is considered to be a selective inhibitor of delayed potassium current when applied to the internal surface of the cell membrane, but it is not so selective when applied externally. For this reason, the current–clamp technique is very useful for study of the rectification properties of cardiac cell membrane.

Isolated hearts at various stages of development were immersed in Na^+–Ca^{++}-free Tyrode solution and transmembrane currents were applied for 1.5 sec. The relationship between current and membrane potential was determined at 2 e.d., 4 e.d. and 19 e.d. (Fig. 11).

At 2 e.d., for currents ranging from $^-6$ to $+5.10^{-7}$A, the membrane potential (MP) varied from -110 mV to $+20$ mV. After the charge of the membrane when the current was applied, the MP maintained a steady state, and the relationship between current and voltage was linear. In other words, at this stage of embryonic development, the cell membrane behaved as an ohmic resistance.

At 4 e.d., the MP showed a dissymmetrical change for hyperpolarizing and depolarizing currents. For example, the MP was increased by 25 mV with 3.10^{-7}A anodic current, and was decreased by 40 mV with the same value of cathodic current. This result indicates the property of immediate rectification. Moreover, with a depolarization of the membrane greater than 40 mV, the MP progressively increased after maximum depolarization, indicating the property of delayed rectification. At this stage of development, the current–voltage relationship was not linear but S-shaped.

In older stages, the dissymmetry of MPs for anodic and cathodic currents increased, and at 19 days of development the second curvature of the current–voltage relation occurred at about -70 mV.

DISCUSSION

Numerous works have showed that embryonic heart RP and AP change with age (6,7,9,14,15,17,27,29,30). These changes result from maturation of cell membrane properties that underlie the ionic currents responsible for the electrical activity.

It is well established that, in the first stage of cardiac cell differentiation, TTX does not suppress spontaneous activity. However, our results show that, as early as 2 e.d. in the chick, a high dose of TTX decreases the rate of rise of ventricular AP. This suggests that a fast sodium permeability participates in the electrical activity of the ventricular cells prior to the stage at which this permeability becomes indispensable for triggering of the AP (23). It appears that, at this time, cellular electrogenesis can result from one of the two mechanisms of sodium-carried inward current, if the other mechanism is blocked by an inhibitor (Fig. 9). Another support for this hypothesis comes from the observation that, in heart at 3 e.d., hyperpolarizing currents increase the AP amplitude, an effect that is abolished by TTX (unpublished data). Afterwards, the rapid sodium permeability becomes indispensable for the triggering of the AP.

Although the excitability of the embryonic heart in sodium-free solution remains for a longer time at 2 e.d. than in older stages, the effects of sodium deprivation on electrical activity indicate that membrane permeability to sodium ions is important for cellular electrogenesis. This is true in early heart, as well as in later stages of its development. Participation of calcium ions in development of the AP at early stages of cardiac development, as demonstrated by the effects of low external calcium concentrations and by the effects of La^{+++}, becomes less important with age.

The potassium rectification properties of the cardiac cell membrane are observed at 4 e.d. in the chick embryo. The data indicate that the general characteristics of cardiac cellular activity, i.e., the appearance of the major ionic permeabilities that underlie AP, are gained by the cell membrane before establishment of functional cardiac innervation (5,22,32,33).

The chronology of the appearance of ionic permeability mechanisms in chick embryo heart is very different from the sequence of development of these permeabilities in rat embryo (1). In the rat, the first permeability mechanism to appear is the slow inward current which carries calcium ions. The second mechanism is the fast inward current, which appears at 13 e.d. The delayed outward current appears just before birth.

The mechanisms responsible for maturation of the cardiac cell membrane are not yet completely understood. Several experiments have shown that TTX-sensitivity *in vitro* can be affected by inhibitors of protein synthesis (16,26). However, other authors suggest that the changes in membrane characteristics *in vitro* may be independent of protein synthesis (30). In cell culture, sensitivity to TTX in chick cardiomyoblasts is lost within 48 hr (13,15,28). This change can be prevented by insulin (13). Recent results in our laboratory suggest that this effect of insulin may result from a control of protein synthesis (31). Further investigations are required for complete understanding of the functional differentiation of embryonic cardiac cell membrane.

REFERENCES

1. Bernard, C. L. (1975): Establishment of ionic permeabilities of the myocardial membrane during embryonic development of the rat. In: *Developmental and Physiological Correlates of Cardiac Muscle,* edited by M. Lieberman and T. Sano, pp. 169-184. Raven Press, New York.
2. Brown, H. F., and Noble, S. J. (1969): Membrane current underlying delayed rectification and pacemaker activity in frog atrial muscle. *J. Physiol. (Lond.),* 204:717-736.
3. Carmeliet, E. E., Horres, C. R., Lieberman, M., and Vereecke, J. S. (1975): Potassium permeability in the embryonic chick heart: change with age, external K and valinomycin. In: *Developmental and Physiological Correlates of Cardiac Muscle,* edited by M. Lieberman and T. Sano, pp. 103-116. Raven Press, New York.
4. Coraboeuf, E., and Vassort, G. (1968): Effects of some inhibitors of ionic permeabilities on ventricular action potential and contraction of rat and guinea pig hearts. *J. Electrocard.,* 1:19-30.
5. Culver, N. G., and Fischman, D. A. (1977): Pharmacological analysis of sympathetic function in the embryonic chick heart. *Am. J. Physiol.,* 232:R116-R123.
6. DeHaan, R. L. (1970): The potassium sensitivity of isolated heart cells increased with development. *Dev. Biol.,* 23: 226-240.

7. DeHaan, R. L., McDonald, T. F., and Sachs, H. G. (1975): Development of tetrodotoxin sensitivity of embryonic chick heart cells *in vitro*. In: *Developmental and Physiological Correlates of Cardiac Muscle*, edited by M. Lieberman and T. Sano, pp. 155-168. Raven Press, New York.

8. Dudel, J., Peper, K., Rüdel, R., and Trautwein, W. (1967): The effect of tetrodotoxin on the membrane current in cardiac muscle (Purkinje fibres). *Pfluegers Arch.*, 295:215-227.

9. Fingl, E., Woodbury, L. A., and Hecht, H. H. (1952): Effects of innervation and drugs upon direct membrane potentials of embryonic chick myocardium. *J. Pharmacol. Exp. Ther.*, 104:103-114.

10. Gargouïl, Y. M., Coraboeuf, E., Dubois, M., and Strudel, N. (1958): Comparison des électrogrammes cardiaques chez la lapine gravide et le foetus (électrogrammes intracellulaires et ECG). *Bull. Acad. Nat. Méd.*, 23:644-647.

11. Ishima, Y. (1968): The effect of tetrodotoxin and sodium substitution on the action potential in the course of development of the embryonic chick heart. *Proc. Jpn. Acad.*, 44:170-175.

12. Krespi, V., and Sleator, W. W. (1966): A study on the ontogeny of action potentials in chick embryo hearts. *Life Sci.*, 16:1441-1446.

13. Le Douarin, G., Renaud, J. F., Renaud, D., and Coraboeuf, E. (1974): Influence of insulin on sensitivity to tetrodotoxin of isolated chick embryo heart cells in culture. *J. Mol. Cell. Card.*, 6:523-529.

14. McDonald, T. F., and DeHaan, R. L. (1973): Ion levels and membrane potential in chick heart tissue and cultured cells. *J. Gen. Physiol.*, 61:89-109.

15. McDonald, T. F., Sachs, H. G., and DeHaan, R. L. (1972): Development of sensitivity to tetrodotoxin in beating chick embryo hearts, single cells, and aggregates. *Science*, 176:1248-1250.

16. McDonald, T. F., Sachs, H. G., and DeHaan, R. L. (1973): Tetrodotoxin desensitization in aggregates of embryonic chick heart cells. *J. Gen. Physiol.*, 62:286-302.

17. Meda, E. (1960): Potenziali intracellulari in stadi diversi dello sviluppo del cuore embryonale di Pollo. *Bull. Soc. Ital. Biol. Sper.*, 36:249-252.

18. New, W., and Trautwein, W. (1972): The ionic nature of slow inward current and its relation to contraction. *Pfluegers Arch.*, 334:24-38.

19. Niedergerke, R., and Orkand, R. K. (1966): The dual effect of calcium on the action potential of the frog's heart. *J. Physiol. (Lond.)*, 184:291-311.

20. Noble, D., and Tsien, R. W. (1969): Outward membrane currents activated in the plateau range of potentials in cardiac Purkinje fibres. *J. Physiol. (Lond.)*, 200:205-232.

21. Obrecht-Coutris, G., Le Douarin, G., and Coraboeuf, E. (1968): Aspects électrophysiologiques de l'automatisme du myocarde ventriculaire chez l'embryon de poulet. *C. R. Acad. Sc. Sér. D. Nat. (Paris)*, 267:765-768.

22. Papano, A. J. (1975): Development of autonomic neuroeffector transmission in the chick embryo heart. In: *Developmental and Physiological Correlates of Cardiac Muscle*, edited by M. Lieberman and T. Sano, pp. 235-248. Raven Press, New York.

23. Renaud, D., and Le Douarin, G. (1972): Mise en évidence, par l'emploi d'inhibiteurs, d'une évolution des permeabilités membranaires cardiaques aux jeunes stades du développement chez l'embryon de poulet. *C. R. Acad. Sc. Sér. D. Nat. (Paris)*, 274:418-421.

24. Reuter, H. (1967): The dependence of slow inward current in Purkinje fibres on the extracellular calcium concentration. *J. Physiol. (Lond.)*, 192:479-492.

25. Rougier, O., Vassort, G., Garnier, D., Gargouïl, Y. M., and Coraboeuf, E. (1969): Existence and role of a slow inward current during the frog atrial action potential. *Pfluegers Arch.*, 308:91-110.

26. Sachs, H. G., McDonald, T. F., and DeHaan, R. L. (1973): Tetrodotoxin sensitivity of cultured embryonic heart cells depends on cell interactions. *J. Cell Biol.*, 56:255-258.

27. Shigenobu, K., and Sperelakis, N. (1971): Development of sensitivity to tetrodotoxin of chick embryo hearts with age. *J. Mol. Cell. Card.*, 3:271-286.

28. Sperelakis, N., and Lehmkuhl, D. (1965): Insensitivity of cultured chick heart cells to autonomic agents and tetrodotoxin. *Am. J. Physiol.*, 209:693-698.

29. Sperelakis, N., and Shigenobu, K. (1972): Changes in membrane properties of chick embryonic hearts during development. *J. Gen. Physiol.*, 60:430-453.

30. Sperelakis, N., Shigenobu, K., and McLean, M. J. (1975): Membrane cation channels—Changes in developing hearts, in cell culture, and in organ culture. In: *Developmental and Physiological*

Correlates of Cardiac Muscle, edited by M. Lieberman and T. Sano, pp. 209-234. Raven Press, New York.

31. Suignard, G. (1979): Métabolisme protéique et sensibilité à la tétrodotoxine des cardiomyoblastes cultivés *in vitro.* Influence de l'insuline. *J. Physiol. (Paris), (in press).*

32. Szepsenwol, J., and Bron, A. (1935): Le premier contact du système nerveux vagosympathique avec l'appareil cardio-vasculaire chez les embryons d'oiseaux (canard et poulet). *Compt. Rend. Soc. Biol.,* 118:946-948.

33. Szepsenwol, J., and Bron, A. (1936): L'origine et la nature de l'innervation primitive du coeur chez les embryons d'oiseaux (canard et poulet). *Rev. Suisse Zool.,* 43:1-23.

34. Van Mierop, L. S. H. (1967): Location of pacemaker in chick embryo heart at the time of initiation of heart beat. *Am. J. Physiol.,* 212:407-415.

35. Weidman, S. (1951): Effect of current flow on the membrane potential of cardiac muscle. *J. Physiol. (Lond.),* 115:227-236.

DISCUSSION

DeHaan: Are you concerned that the calcium- and sodium-free solutions you have used in your voltage clamping experiments may be strongly modifying the properties of the membrane that you record?

Le Douarin: Of course, it is well known that modified calcium concentrations will interfere with potassium permeabilities, but this was shown for active, not for passive, properties of the cell membrane. The current clamp experiments create artificial conditions, but we asked only the question, does or does not the cell membrane have rectifying properties?

Fischman: Would you please comment on the difference in tetrodotoxin sensitivity of cells in monolayer versus aggregates?

Le Douarin: I believe that the loss of tetrodotoxin sensitivity in cell culture is largely dependent upon culture conditions.

Perspectives in Cardiovascular Research, Vol. 5,
Mechanisms of Cardiac Morphogenesis and Teratogenesis,
edited by Tomas Pexieder. Raven Press, New York © 1981

Role of Fibroblasts in Synchronizing the Beat Rhythm of Isolated Heart Muscle Cells in Culture

W. O. Gross

Institute for Histology and Embryology of the University of Lausanne,
CH 1011 Lausanne, Switzerland

In their film studies of newborn rat heart cells, Mark and Strasser (7) have reported that two neighboring muscle cells first pulsate separately. Within 10 hours, during which time a fibroblast wandered between them, their beating became synchronized. From this and from another example, they concluded that the contraction is led from one muscle cell to the other and that the fibroblast is the conductor.

Nine years ago, the author (4) also filmed a fibroblast that synchronized the rhythm of two pulsating cells in a culture of embryonic chick heart cells. Such a triad of resting fibroblast and two adjacent synchronously pulsating muscle cells could also be electron microscopically examined (5). Nexus-like membrane specializations were found between one muscle cell and the fibroblast, such as are found in muscle cell–muscle cell connections (2).

Working together with the Institute for Scientific Film in Göttingen, the author has filmed further fibroblast–muscle cell connections. The assumption that fibroblasts have the ability to conduct electrical impulses did not hold true during this study. In the precise working out of time-lapse film materials, one could observe the hitherto undiscovered activity of fibroblasts in their relationship to muscle cells. This activity, moreover, makes it clear the reason why fibroblasts seem to be electrical conductors when they are observed in cultures for short periods of time. Further time-lapse-based studies underlined this behavior. When these scenes are assembled, a new concept of the fibroblast appears.

MATERIALS AND METHODS

Culture

White Leghorn chick eggs at 8 e.d. were used. Cell suspensions were prepared by 0.075% trypsin in Minimal Essential Medium (Eagle), with 12% fetal calf serum.

Film

The cell suspension was brought between two coverslips. One of them bore a ring of paraffin. The two coverslips were separated by a frame made from a 1 mm-thick brass sheet. In addition to the main chamber, it comprised two side-chambers for humidification of the gas stream. During the entire period of observation and filming, the chambers were ventilated by 95% O_2 and 5% CO_2. The coverslip without paraffin was covered with a film of 0.3% Parlodion. Cells settled on this coverslip and fixed themselves within a few hours, so that the preparation could be reversed for the usual microscope (Zeiss). The film equipment was that of Zeiss, Oberkochen, constructed by Kurt Michel. Optics consisted of the phase-contrast Planapo 63 objective with aperture 1.4, the Mipro 63 mm ocular, and the Optovar 1.0 to 2.0. Film speeds, with few exceptions, were, for normal speed, 24 pictures/sec, and for time-lapse, one picture/21 min.

RESULTS

As introduction, the film shows the primary difference between the two types of cells: muscle cells usually tend to remain in place, and fibroblasts tend to wander.

The presentation of the topic of the potential power of fibroblasts to conduct electricity begins with a seemingly inexplicable picture: a muscle cell is connected by a fibroblast to a second muscle cell, which beats in the same rhythm as the first but is also attached to a third muscle cell, which beats in a different rhythm. Oddly enough, the contact of the fibroblast with the separately beating cell is significantly wider than that with the cell beating synchronously.

To explain this conflicting picture, the film next shows a few properties of a heart cell culture: a still rounded, completely isolated cell, which, as Burrows (1) discovered in 1912, has a self-contained pulsation stimulus; the continuation of contractile activity during the expansion and pino-cytosis of the cells; two heart muscle cells showing, when separate, a different rhythm and, as Fischer noted in cultured pieces of heart in 1924, when connected, a similar rhythm (3). Besides the extensive connection, as in a monolayer pulsating in the same rhythm, are shown fine muscle cell–muscle cell connections. These isolated connections also lead to synchronization. Among them, one can see the threads, less than 0.5 μm thick, filmed by Gross (4). One cell, connected by such a thread only to a beating heart cell, beats in the same rhythm as this heart cell, and transfers the pulsation over a second thread to another muscle cell.

These well-known properties of a heart cell culture do not suffice to explain the conflicting picture of the fibroblast–muscle cell combination shown. Therefore, an additional expanded scene from a fresh culture of heart cells is introduced. This scene involves 12 still rounded cells. As they expand on the culture floor, they make contacts with one another and pulsate together. One cell is still isolated from the complex. A fibroblast intervenes. It wanders in from beyond the field of vision, passes by the isolated cell, and touches the complex, drawing forth from the latter a process which is attached to the isolated rounded cell. The expansion process continues. The rounded cell also expands and, after a certain period of hesitation, beats together with the complex.

If the film now presents the past history of the cell group already shown, one must studiously observe the activity of a fibroblast in order to understand why the bridge formed later conducts the impulses. This fibroblast first touches a muscle cell, which is still rounded. From the spot that has been touched, the muscle cell, which by this time is also expanded, puts forth a process of about 5 μm diameter. This muscle cell prolongation moves, led by the accompanying fibroblast, towards the second beating muscle cell. When it touches the second cell, it has become more than 50 μm long. Next, this prolongation retreats, leaving behind it a thread of less than 0.5 μm diameter. Cells 1 and 2 are now connected by means of this thread, and normal film speed shows the synchronous beating of these two cells. A fibroblast in mitosis is found above in the field, so that space near cells 1 and 3 is still free. After cell division, the fibroblast covers the total free space, almost entirely hiding the thread (Fig. 1). The synchrony between cells 1 and 2 has come about by means of the muscle cell thread, and this does not support the proposed ability of fibroblasts to conduct electrical current. Furthermore, this impulse transfer is missing between cells 1 and 3 which are broadly connected by the fibroblast. Despite this connection, their beating is not synchronized. In this case, although the fibroblast was not the conductor, it was not without importance in the formation of the impulse-conducting pathway.

Another scene begins by showing a fibroblast that slips into the space between a cell complex and an isolated cell without synchronizing their beating. After it has wandered out of this space, another fibroblast comes forward. It stretches forth a process towards the isolated cell beyond the complex. The prolongation meets the isolated cell. At the same time, when this process of the fibroblast retreats, an extension is put forth from the isolated muscle cell. This extension is pulled by the fibroblast from the complex. After it has torn itself away from the fibroblast, it succeeds in establishing contact with the complex. The connection of the hitherto isolated muscle cell with the muscle cell complex becomes wider, and soon the film shows that the cell is beating synchronously with the complex. In this case, the lead for electrical impulses, which could not be established by the first fibroblast with its own cell constituents, was built by the second fibroblast, using muscle cell material.

In a further expansion scene of 7 cells, 3 such communications are established by fibroblasts. Two cells remain isolated after a certain period of expansion. A fibroblast wanders onto the scene and touches the two cells and the complex. Small outgrowths appear at the points of contact. By these cell processes, one of the cells becomes bound to the complex. The connection continues to develop, until this cell is completely united with the complex. A thread connection with

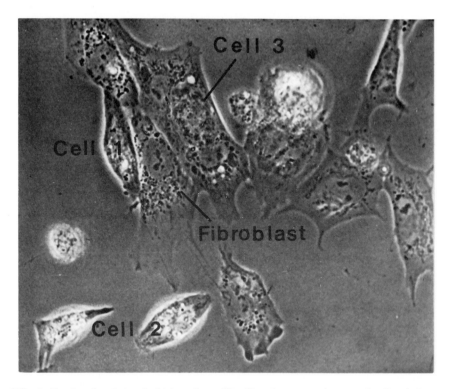

FIG. 1. Heart cell culture of chick embryo. The film shows synchronous beating between cells 1 and 2 and asynchronous beating between cells 1 and 3. Between lies a fibroblast, which connects all 3 cells one to another. The history of the development before this picture is time-lapsed and explains the seeming contradiction (see text).

the farther-lying cell tears away, and this cell becomes isolated again. Later, the same fibroblast returns to the field, bringing a thin thread from outside, with which it wanders around the still isolated cell. Seven hours later, a firm muscle cell–muscle cell connection with a neighboring cell has been established, in the direction from which the fibroblast has brought the thread. Thanks to this outward coupling, the cell has re-established a connection with the complex. The entire complex of 7 cells, including the one formed by cell division, as well as several neighboring cells, now beats synchronously.

The film, in longer sequences, investigates further the capacity of fibroblasts to transmit action potential. Even if a muscle cell pair forms a firm and long-lasting connection with a fibroblast, the rhythm does not become synchronized. In the case of a cell pair, two different fibroblasts wander, one after the other, into the intercellular space, without synchronizing the pulsating rhythm. In a following scene, the same pulsating rhythm is seen to the right and left of a fibroblast. However, when the fibroblast moves away, thin threads are visible: they had been lying under the fibroblast, and had spanned the distance between muscle cells. Synchronized beating continues until these threads break away.

Later, the fibroblast returns. In place of the broken threads it builds another bridge between the two pulsating cells. This illustrates that the fibroblast itself did not take part in the electrical conduction; because, despite its connections with both muscle cells, their rhythms remain different. In two further scenes, in which the space between two muscle cells had been devoid of threads, no synchronized pulsation rhythm was established there by the wandering in of a fibroblast.

DISCUSSION

No concept of purposeful activity can be ascribed to a fibroblast in the culture. This is evident because, in some cases, a fibroblast will not take advantage of the opportunity to establish a communication with the nearest cell. On the other hand, its capacities guarantee that its presence in the culture enables cell complexes to be established more easily. One of these capacities is polymorphic movement, which provides new possibilities for contact with muscle cells. Another capacity is the fibroblast's ability to call forth processes from muscle cells and to fix them onto other muscle cells. Thus, it cannot be denied that the fibroblast takes part in reorganization of trypsin-dissociated muscle cells in culture. By means of this film, a visual impression can be gained as to how mesenchy-matous cells assist in the reorganization of dissociated thyroid cells in follicles during culture (6).

Fibroblasts cannot transfer the electropotential from one heart muscle cell to another. In all cases in which two synchronously beating muscle cells are observed connected by a fibroblast bridge, very fine muscle cell–muscle cell communications can be demonstrated. The presence of electrically conducting threads cannot be excluded in the two figures (7b and 8b) from Mark and Strasser (7). Aside from this, the beat registration in the above-mentioned picture 7b gives a frequency parity, but no time parity. In addition, for the cells in picture 8b, no synchronous rhythm is shown after the tenth second. The presence of impulse synchronizing threads, such as is shown in Gross (4), Fig. 13–16 taken from a film, also cannot be excluded in Fig. 11 of the same author, in which a fibroblast forms a bridge between two synchronously beating muscle cells.

When observing a heart cell culture, it is necessary to find fibroblasts that have just established a thread connection between two muscle cells and are still touching both cells. The position of the fibroblast between two muscle cells, hiding an impulse-conducting thread, is a situation brought about by one of its principal activities and can be thought of as its primary characteristic. Without consideration of the ongoing thread-spinning activity of the fibroblast, every observer who views this "synchronizing" bridge must conclude that the fibroblast possesses conducting power. But in no instance in which a fibroblast wandered into a muscle cell–muscle cell lacuna, previously confirmed as thread-free, did the beating of muscle cells become synchronized. The film shows that, even after several hours' duration, such thread-free fibroblast bridges did not synchronize the beating of the two connected muscle cells. However, the possibility exists that processes extended from the muscle cells may make contact beneath the fibroblast, and thus lead to synchronization.

REFERENCES

1. Burrows, M. T. (1912): Rhythmische Kontraktionen der isolierten Herzmuskelzellen ausserhalb des Organismus. *Münch. Med. Wschr.*, 59:1473-1475.
2. DeHaan, R. L., and Hirakow, R. (1972): Synchronization of pulsation rates in isolated cardiac myocytes. *Exp. Cell Res.*, 70:214-220.
3. Fischer, A. (1924): The interaction of two fragments of pulsating heart tissue. *J. Exp. Med.*, 39:577-583.
4. Gross, W. O. (1970): Reizleitungsphänomene zwischen Herzmuskelzellen in der Kultur (film). *Verh. Anat. Ges.*, 303-310.
5. Gross, W. O. (1971): Die Verbindung zwischen impulsleitenden Fibroblasten in der Kultur mit den Muskelzellen. *Verh. Schweiz. Anat.*, 35. Tagung, Bern.
6. Hilfer, R. (1962): The stability of embryonic chick thyroid cells in vitro as judged by morphological and physiological criteria. *Dev. Biol.*, 4:1-21.
7. Mark, G. E., and Strasser, F. F. (1966): Pacemaker activity and mitosis in culture of newborn rat heart ventricle cells. *Exp. Cell Res.*, 44:217-233.

DISCUSSION

Clark: Is it possible that one of the two different types of fibroblasts represents very primitive conducting tissue?

Gross: I have seen very few examples of fibroblasts bridging two muscle cells. But in no case could a fibroblast synchronize two muscle cells.

Fischman: It looks as though the fibroblast, after it contacted a heart cell, increased the movement of the heart cell, and also directed its migration.

Gross: That is correct. In other cases, the muscle cells followed the fibroblast after an initial contact.

Perspectives in Cardiovascular Research, Vol. 5,
Mechanisms of Cardiac Morphogenesis and Teratogenesis,
edited by Tomas Pexieder. Raven Press, New York © 1981

Mechanisms of Pacemaker Activity in Embryonic Cardiac Muscle

*Richard D. Nathan, *Peter C. Houck, *Simon J. Fung,
**Douglas M. Stocco, and ‡Roger R. Markwald

*Department of Physiology, **Department of Biochemistry, and ‡Department of Anatomy,
Texas Tech University School of Medicine, Lubbock, Texas 79430

Between 3 and 7 days of development in the chick, cardiac myocytes undergo rapid differentiation, in which the action potential upstroke velocity becomes faster and more sensitive to tetrodotoxin (TTX) (23,35,36). At the same time, electrogenesis becomes less dependent upon ionic currents which are blocked by verapamil and D600 (9,34), agents shown to inhibit uptake of ^{45}Ca in cultured rat heart cells (17) and to block the slow inward Ca^{++} current in adult cardiac muscle (15). With the aid of the voltage–clamp technique, these changes have been correlated with transformation from a single TTX-insensitive, slow inward current at 3 days (24) to a two-component system of inward currents at 7 days (25): a fast transient current (i_{Na}) associated with the rapid upstroke of the action potential and abolished by TTX, and a slower component (i_{si}) related to the plateau, which is unaffected by TTX but blocked by D600. The magnitudes, kinetics, and voltage dependence of these two inward currents and a delayed outward current (i_x) agree with those observed in the adult heart (25).

Concomitant with changes in the action potential, automaticity of embryonic hearts, cultured heart cells, and cell aggregates declines during development (5,22,32), in parallel with an increase in sensitivity to external potassium (6, 36,40). These observations can be explained in part by enhanced activity of intracellular K^+ (33), together with a gradual rise (2) in membrane potassium permeability (P_K), which reduces the ratio P_{Na}/P_K (2,21).

In the present study, we seek to describe some of the underlying mechanisms responsible for pacemaker activity in embryonic cardiac muscle and to test the hypothesis that cell surface anions play a role in regulating such properties.

MATERIALS AND METHODS

Tissue Culture

Hearts were removed from 12 to 24 chick embryos after 7 days and the ventricles were dissociated into their component cells by a multiple-cycle trypsinization procedure (5). After plating the cell suspension for 30 min to 1 hr to remove non-myocytes (31), heart cells (0.5 to 1.0 × 10⁶) were added to 3 ml of medium 818A (6) in 25 ml Erlenmeyer flasks. These flasks were gassed with a mixture of 95% air/5% CO_2, sealed, and placed on a gyratory shaker at 75 rpm and 37°C. After 3 to 4 days, the cells formed spheroidal aggregates which ranged between 100 and 250 μm in diameter and were used in electrophysiological, histochemical, or biochemical experiments.

Electrophysiology

During electrophysiological experiments, aggregates attached to the bottom of a plastic culture dish were maintained at 35 to 37°C on the heated stage of a dissecting microscope, and CO_2 was passed through a toroidal gassing ring surrounding the dish to hold the pH at 7.3. The pH and temperature were monitored continuously, and the volume of medium was kept constant at 3 ml by a slow water drip. All experiments were performed in medium 818A (6).

Glass micropipettes (10 to 30 MΩ) were used in conjunction with capacitance-compensated electrometer amplifiers for intracellular recording, and the extracellular medium was coupled to a virtual ground through agar/KCl bridges. The two-microelectrode voltage clamp technique was employed with standard circuitry (25), to record ionic currents directly. One intracellular electrode monitored the "averaged" membrane potential of the aggregate, while the other (in another cell) was used to pass transmembrane current. In previous studies (25), aggregates were found to deviate from isopotentiality by < 3% during voltage steps longer than 10 msec.

Action potentials or membrane currents were amplified and recorded on FM tape. These waveforms were later played back, digitized by a transient waveform recorder, and plotted at reduced speed on a strip chart recorder. Parameters of interest were measured from these expanded traces.

Electron Microscopy

Aggregates were fixed at room temperature (pH 7.2) for 2 hr in 2% glutaraldehyde in 0.065 M cacodylate buffer, and then stained *en bloc* for 1 hr at 37°C with 0.1 to 0.5 mg/ml polycationic ferritin (PCF) (4) in 0.065 M cacodylate buffer. Following staining, specimens were post-fixed in 0.065 M cacodylate-buffered osmium and embedded in Epon-Araldite by routine procedures (20). Thin sections were obtained using a Porter-Blum ultramicrotome, mounted on copper grids, and examined in a Zeiss 10A transmission electron microscope.

⁴⁵Ca Uptake

Aggregates were plated overnight in separate wells of a multi-well culture dish containing medium 818A. The following day, neuraminidase was added to half of the wells; the other half served as controls. After 30 to 100 min incubation at 37°C, the enzyme-containing medium was replaced with 0.5 ml of fresh 818A containing 10 μCi/ml of ^{45}Ca. Uptake (at room temperature) was terminated at 0, 15, 30, 45, 60, and 120 min by removing the medium and washing the aggregates twice with a balanced salt solution (BSS) (27). At the end of 2 hrs, 1% sodium dodecylsulfate was added to each well to disperse the cells, and 0.1 ml aliquots were removed for measurements of protein (19) and radioactivity by scintillation spectrometry (75% efficiency).

Solutions

Medium 818A contained 72.5% modified Earle's BSS (27), 20% medium M199, 4% fetal calf serum, 2% horse serum, 1% glutamine, and 0.5% gentamycin. The final composition (mM/1) was: NaCl 116; NaH$_2$PO$_4$ 0.9; NaHCO$_3$ 22; KCl 1.8; CaCl$_2$ 1.8; MgSO$_4$ 0.8; and dextrose 5.5. Tetrodotoxin (Calbiochem), partially purified neuraminidase (Type NEUP, Worthington; Type VI, Sigma), and purified neuraminidase (Type NEUA, Worthington) were dissolved in distilled water to make stock solutions of 1 mg/ml, 4.1 U/ml, 6.6 U/ml, and 20 U/ml, respectively.

RESULTS

Voltage Clamp Analysis

Both time-dependent and time-independent ionic currents were recorded from 7-day aggregates during 4-sec voltage steps from a holding potential of -59 mV (Fig. 1). Hyperpolarization (A) generated currents which increased with time and exhibited inward-going rectification; depolarization (B) resulted in currents which increased with time and exhibited outward-going rectification.

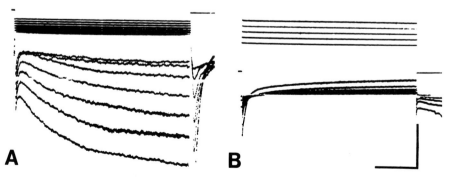

FIG. 1. Voltage clamp steps in two 7-day aggregates incubated in 3 $\times$ 10^{-6}M TTX. Top traces indicate voltage; bottom traces, current. **A:** Hyperpolarizing steps from -67 to -79 mV in 2–mV increments. **B:** Depolarizing steps from -34 to -14 mV in 5–mV increments. Holding potential: -59 mV. Pulse frequency: 0.25 Hz. Horizontal scale: 1.0 sec. Vertical scale: 40 mV and 200 nA **(A)**, 100 nA **(B)**.

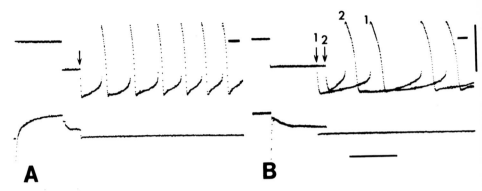

FIG. 2. Relationship of diastolic depolarization to the decay of outward tail current recorded during voltage clamp in a single 7-day aggregate. Top traces indicate voltage; bottom traces, current. **A:** Clamp terminated *(arrow)* 0.4 sec following repolarization to the holding potential, −40 mV. **B:** Clamp terminated 0.40 sec *(arrow # 1)* and 0.48 sec *(arrow # 2)* following repolarization to −40 mV. Voltage step to +3 mV. Vertical scale: 80 mV, 200 nA. Horizontal scale: 1.0 sec **(A)**, 0.4 sec **(B)**. Horizontal lines at upper right in each panel represent 0 mV.

Following periods of spontaneous activity, the net "steady state" current attained during voltage clamp was minimized at a holding potential of −50 mV, which corresponds to the typical resting potential in TTX. This time-independent current was reduced 45% when aggregates were treated with TTX (5.0×10^{-7} M), along with a 67% decline in the slope of diastolic depolarization and beat rate just before action potential blockade.

Diastolic depolarization was also related to the decay of a time-dependent current, as illustrated by the following experiment (Fig. 2). First, outward current was strongly activated by a depolarizing step. Then, if the clamp was turned off *(arrow)* 0.40 sec after return to the holding potential and during the decay of an outward current tail (Fig. 2A), the membrane potential rapidly hyperpolarized; this was followed by a slow diastolic depolarization. Removing this hyperpolarizing influence, by terminating the clamp during later phases of the decaying tail (e.g., at 0.48 sec; *arrow #2*, Fig. 2B), resulted in less hyperpolarization and a steeper pacemaker potential. Note that in this example, a difference of only 80 msec during the decline of outward current was expressed as a 220-msec delay in the timing of action potentials #1 and #2; furthermore, the rate of hyperpolarization following offset of the clamp *(arrow #1)* was almost identical to that during repolarization of the action potential.

Removal of Sialic Acid from the Cell Surface

Treatment of 7-day aggregates with neuraminidase (Type NEUP), an enzyme that specifically cleaves sialic acid from glycoproteins and glycolipids, resulted in dual effects, depending upon the concentration or time of incubation. Following a 3 to 5 min control recording, the addition of .0068 U/ml (Fig. 3 and Table 1) led to hyperpolarization of the maximum diastolic potential (MDP)

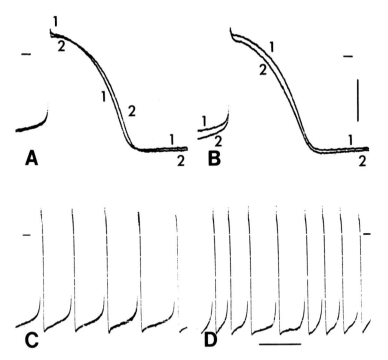

FIG. 3. Intracellular recordings in two aggregates incubated in neuraminidase (.0068 U/ml, Type NEUP). Trace #1 and panel **C**: aggregate #1, control. Trace #2, panel **A**: aggregate #1, 3 min after addition of enzyme. Trace #2, panel **B** and panel **D**: aggregate #2, 60 min after addition of enzyme. Vertical scale: 40 mV. Horizontal scale: 100 ms, **A** and **B**; 2 sec, **C** and **D**. Horizontal lines represent 0 mV.

and action potential threshold (THR), a reduction in the overshoot (OS) of the action potential, and a 25% increase in its maximum rate of rise ($\dot{V}_{max}$). The duration of the action potential (DUR) initially increased (Fig. 3A and 4A) but later declined (Fig. 3B and 4B); these changes might be correlated with a 50% slowing of beat rate (BR) at 3 min and a subsequent acceleration

TABLE 1. *Electrophysiological parameters recorded during incubation in neuraminidase (.0068 U/ml, Type NEUP)[a]*

Time of incubation (min)	MDP (mV)	OS (mV)	THR (mV)	DUR (msec)	$\dot{V}_{max}$ (V/sec)	BR (B/min)
0	−88	+23	−54	151	120	37.1
3	−90	+20	−54	159	120	18.2
60	−91	+23	−56	140	150	70.0

[a] Maximum diastolic potential (MDP), overshoot (OS), threshold (THR), duration measured at −40 mV (DUR), maximum upstroke velocity ($\dot{V}_{max}$), and beat rate (BR) were recorded from two aggregates of equivalent size, the first during the initial 10 min and the second between 48 and 60 min.

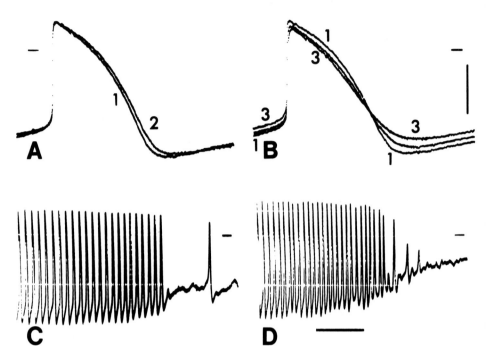

FIG. 4. Intracellular recordings in two aggregates incubated in .068 U/ml **(A, B, C)** and 0.136 U/ml **(D)** neuraminidase (Type NEUP). **A:** Trace #1, control; trace #2, 2 min after addition of enzyme. **B:** Trace #1, same as trace #2 panel **A;** trace #2, 2 min 13 sec after addition; trace #3, 2 min 17 sec after addition. Vertical scale: 40 mV. Horizontal scale: 100 msec, **A** and **B;** 4 sec, **C** and **D.** Horizontal lines represent 0 mV.

TABLE 2. *Changes in electrophysiological parameters recorded during incubation in neuramini-dase (Type VI)[a]*

Concentration (U/ml)	Time of incubation (min)	Δ MDP[b] (mV)	Δ OS[c] (mV)	Δ THR[b] (mV)	Δ DUR (%)	Δ BR (%)
.044	20	+1	−1	+1	+1.7	−7.3
.110	18	+6	−3	0	+5.7	−15.0
.110	30	+5	−1	+1	+8.5	−42.1
.220	50	+3	−6	+2	−8.7	0
Mean ± SE		3.6	−2.8	+1.0	+1.8	−16.1
		±1.1	±1.2	± 0.4	±3.8	±9.2

[a] Changes in maximum diastolic potential (MDP), overshoot (OS), threshold (THR), duration measured at −40 mV (DUR), and beat rate (BR) were determined during continuous recordings from four aggregates. Each value represents the difference in the parameter at the time indicated and the control.
[b] A positive change in MDP or THR represents hyperpolarization.
[c] A negative change in OS represents a decline in absolute value.

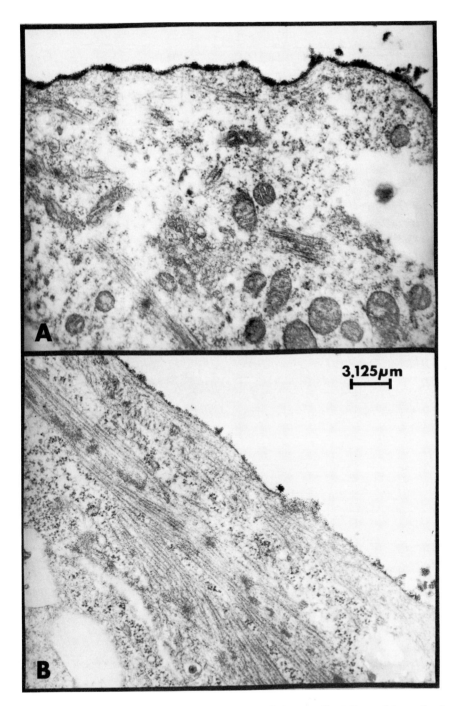

FIG. 5. Transmission electron micrographs of embryonic heart cells at the periphery of a 7-day control aggregate **(A)** and an aggregate incubated 90 min in neuraminidase (0.67 U/ml, Type NEUA; panel **B**). Polycationic ferritin was used to stain the cell surface. Magnification: × 20,000.

of 89% at 1 hr (Table 1). Note that the latter effects were accompanied by loss of rhythmicity (compare Fig. 3C and 3D).

At a tenfold greater dose, the MDP and THR depolarized, $\dot{V}_{max}$ declined, and BR increased significantly (Fig. 4B). Spontaneous activity eventually ceased, and the membrane potential approached a steady state (-30 mV, Fig. 4C; -37 mV, Fig. 4D), which was maintained for more than 45 min. No recovery was observed in such experiments. Since these results were not confirmed in experiments employing even higher concentrations of another neuraminidase preparation (Type VI) (Table 2), they may be due in part to impurities such as proteases or phospholipases.

The removal of sialic acid was confirmed by histochemical and biochemical techniques. Aggregates were incubated in neuraminidase (0.67 U/ml, Type NEUA) at 37°C, pH 7.3 for 90 min. Treated aggregates and controls were then fixed and stained with PCF (0.1 mg/ml). Fig. 5B is typical of enzyme-treated cells in which much of the cationic material had been removed (compare with control, Fig. 5A). Similar results were obtained with myocytes at the periphery of six other aggregates; however, cells within the interior of an aggregate did not stain with PCF. The total sialic acid content of these cells, measured by the thiobarbituric acid technique of Warren (39), was 4.3 ± 0.6 μg/mg

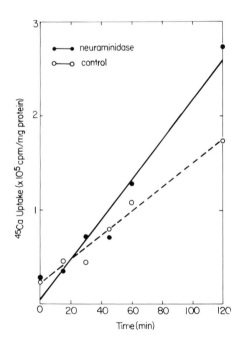

FIG. 6. Uptake of ^{45}Ca in counts/min (cpm) per mg protein in 7-day aggregates following a 40-min incubation in neuraminidase (0.6 U/ml, Type NEUA). The level of membrane binding (time zero) was determined by removing the isotope immediately following its addition. Data points were fitted by linear regression analysis.

protein (mean $\pm$ SE, n $=$ 12). Following a 90-min incubation in neuraminidase (0.67 to 0.75 U/ml, Type NEUA), 49.2 $\pm$ 6.7% (mean $\pm$ SE, n $=$ 6) of this amount was released into the supernatant, as compared with a negligible amount released by controls exposed to medium 818A alone (26).

Increased calcium exchange following the removal of sialic acid from the cell surface was confirmed in three experiments in which ^{45}Ca uptake was measured at various times after incubating 7-day aggregates in neuraminidase (0.2 to 0.6 U/ml, Type NEUA) for 30 to 100 min. Calcium uptake rose 45 to 65% above control levels when measured at the end of 2 hr (26). Fig. 6 is a representative example.

DISCUSSION

Voltage Clamp Analysis

The results of this investigation suggest that pacemaker activity in 7-day chick ventricular cells is generated by the decay of a time-dependent outward current activated during the action potential plateau and by a time-independent inward current flowing through the sodium channel. These mechanisms are supported by the following findings: (a) the rate of diastolic depolarization was strongly dependent upon the amplitude of a decaying outward current tail activated at positive potentials (Fig. 2); (b) application of TTX to spontaneously beating aggregates resulted in reduction of both the slope of diastolic depolarization and the amplitude of a time-independent inward current. The time-dependent outward current recorded in the present study appears to be similar to the pacemaker current (i_p) observed in sinoatrial node cells (30) and the delayed outward current (i_{xI}) activated in Purkinje fibers during the plateau (29). Studies in Purkinje fibers (10), frog atrial trabeculae (1), and adult ventricular myocardium (14) have demonstrated that automaticity in these cell types may be ascribed to the decay of such an outward current in the presence of a background inward current carried by sodium and/or calcium ions.

An additional time- and voltage-dependent current, similar to i_{K2} in Purkinje fibers (28), was recorded in 7-day aggregates at potentials negative to -60 mV (Fig. 1). Using an analysis of outward tail amplitudes following rectangular voltage steps, Clay et al. (3) determined its activation range to lie between -90 and -60 mV. However, experiments in progress (Nathan, unpublished) imply that this current is not essential for automaticity, since the addition of up to 20 mM cesium failed to inhibit pacemaker activity in these cells. This cation has been shown to block the pacemaker current i_{K2} and the instantaneous outward current i_{K1}, but not the delayed outward potassium current i_{xI} in Purkinje fibers (11).

Role of Cell Surface Anions

Intracellular recordings during the removal of sialic acid from the cell surface support the hypothesis that these anions play a role in regulating pacemaker activity in embryonic cardiac muscle. Significant alterations in action potential shape and frequency were correlated with the release of sialic acid and the removal of PCF stain, as determined in biochemical and histochemical experiments.

The marked enhancement of calcium exchange, demonstrated by a 45 to 65% increase in ^{45}Ca uptake after the addition of neuraminidase (Fig. 6), has also been observed in cultured rat heart cells (8,18). In addition to cardiac muscle, sialic acid has been associated with calcium binding and contractility of guinea pig smooth muscle (12), contraction threshold in frog skeletal muscle (7), and synaptic transmission in *Aplysia* neurons (37). Glycophorin, a sialoglycoprotein extracted from human red cell membranes, has been shown to increase the permeability of an artificial membrane following its incorporation into the lipid bilayer (38).

Although sialic acid has been implicated in the binding of external calcium essential to myocardial excitation–contraction coupling (16), the present study is the first to demonstrate its importance in the control of cardiac electrical activity. Experiments in progress are aimed at elucidating the mechanisms involved in such regulation.

Pacemaker Mechanisms During Development

Because sialic acid residues complex strongly and preferentially with free calcium ions in a 1:1 ratio (13), and probably increase in number along with glycoproteins and glycolipids, these anions may help determine the course of electrophysiological changes during myocardial development. In addition to increases in intracellular potassium activity (33) and membrane potassium permeability (2), reduced influx of calcium ions due to greater binding to anions at the cell surface would help to explain the decline in ventricular automaticity and the gradual movement of the maximum diastolic potential toward the potassium equilibrium potential (33) between 3 and 14 days. Additional studies are required to test this hypothesis.

ACKNOWLEDGMENTS

We thank Dr. and Mrs. Marvin R. Shetlar for assisting in the measurements of sialic acid, and Virginia Shelton, Deborah DeHaven, and Jane Krook for their technical help. This study was supported by USPHS grants HL-20708 and HL-19136, and Biomedical Research Support Grant #5-S07-RR 05773 from the NIH.

REFERENCES

1. Brown, H. F., and Noble, S. J. (1969): Membrane currents underlying delayed rectification and pace-maker activity in frog atrial muscle. *J. Physiol. (Lond.),* 204:717-736.
2. Carmeliet, E. E., Horres, C. R., Lieberman, M., and Vereecke, J. S. (1976): Developmental

aspects of potassium flux and permeability of the embryonic chick heart. *J. Physiol. (Lond.),* 254:673-692.

3. Clay, J. R., Shrier, A., and DeHaan, R. L. (1979): Voltage clamp analysis of pacemaker currents in embryonic heart cell aggregates. *Biophys. J.,* 25:301a.

4. Danon, D., Goldstein, L., Marikovsky, Y., and Skutelsky, E. (1972): Use of cationized ferritin as a label of negative charges on cell surfaces. *J. Ultrastruct. Res.,* 38:500-510.

5. DeHaan, R. L. (1967): Regulation of spontaneous activity and growth of embryonic chick heart cells in tissue culture. *Dev. Biol.,* 16:216-249.

6. DeHaan, R. L. (1970): The potassium sensitivity of isolated embryonic heart cells increases with development. *Dev. Biol.,* 23:226-240.

7. Dörrscheidt-Käfer, M. (1977): Release of sialic acids affects contraction threshold in frog sartorius. *J. Physiol. (Lond.),* 273:52-53P.

8. Frank, J. S., Langer, G. A., Nudd, L. M., and Seraydarian, K. (1977): The myocardial cell surface, its histochemistry, and the effect of sialic acid and calcium removal on its structure and cellular ionic exchange. *Circ. Res.,* 41:702-714.

9. Galper, J. B., and Catterall, W. (1978): Developmental changes in the sensitivity of embryonic heart cells to tetrodotoxin and D600. *Dev. Biol.,* 65:216-227.

10. Hauswirth, O., Noble, D., and Tsien, R. W. (1969): The mechanism of oscillatory activity at low membrane potentials in cardiac Purkinje fibres. *J. Physiol. (Lond.),* 200:255-265.

11. Isenberg, G. (1976): Cardiac Purkinje fibres: Cesium as a tool to block inward rectifying potassium currents. *Pfluegers Arch. Eur. J. Physiol.,* 365:99-106.

12. Ishiyama, Y., Yabu, H., and Miyazaki, E. (1975): Changes in contractility and calcium binding of guinea pig taenia coli by treatment with enzymes which hydrolyze sialic acid. *Jpn. J. Physiol.,* 25:719-732.

13. Jaques, L. W., Brown, E. B., Barrett, J. M., Brey, W. S., Jr., and Weltner, W., Jr. (1977): Sialic acid: A calcium-binding carbohydrate. *J. Biol. Chem.,* 252:4533-4538.

14. Katzung, B. G., and Morgenstern, J. A. (1977): Effects of extracellular potassium on ventricular automaticity and evidence for a pacemaker current in mammalian ventricular myocardium. *Circ. Res.,* 40:105-111.

15. Kohlhardt, M., Bauer, B., Krause, H., and Fleckenstein, A. (1972): Differentiation of the transmembrane Na and Ca channels in mammalian cardiac fibres by the use of specific inhibitors. *Pfluegers Arch. Eur. J. Physiol.,* 335:309-322.

16. Langer, G. A. (1978): The structure and function of the myocardial cell surface. *Am. J. Physiol.,* 235:H461-468.

17. Langer, G. A., and Frank, J. S. (1976): Calcium exchange in cultured cardiac cells. In: *Developmental and Physiological Correlates of Cardiac Muscle,* edited by M. Lieberman and T. Sano, pp. 117-126. Raven Press, New York.

18. Langer, G. A., Frank, J. S., Nudd, L. M., and Seraydarian, K. (1976): Sialic acid: Effect of removal on calcium exchangeability of cultured heart cells. *Science,* 193:1013-1015.

19. Lowry, O. H., Rosebrough, N. J., Farr, A. L., and Randall, R. J. (1951): Protein measurement with the folin phenol reagent. *J. Biol. Chem.,* 193:265-275.

20. Markwald, R. (1973): Distribution and relationship of z-line precursor material to organizing myofibrillar bundles in early embryonic rat myocardium: A chemical and ultrastructural study. *J. Mol. Cell. Cardiol.,* 5:341-350.

21. McDonald, T. F., and DeHaan, R. L. (1973): Ion levels and membrane potential in chick heart tissue and cultured cells. *J. Gen. Physiol.,* 61:89-109.

22. McDonald, T. F., and Sachs, H. G. (1975): Electrical activity in embryonic heart cell aggregates: Developmental aspects. *Pfluegers Arch. Eur. J. Physiol.,* 354:151-164.

23. McDonald, T. F., Sachs, H. G., and DeHaan, R. L. (1972): Development of sensitivity to tetrodotoxin in beating chick embryo hearts, single cells, and aggregates. *Science,* 176:1248-1249.

24. Nathan, R. D., and DeHaan, R. L. (1978): *In vitro* differentiation of a fast Na^+ conductance in embryonic heart cell aggregates. *Proc. Natl. Acad. Sci.,* 75:2776-2780.

25. Nathan, R. D., and DeHaan, R. L. (1979): Voltage clamp analysis of embryonic heart cell aggregates. *J. Gen. Physiol.,* 73:175-198.

26. Nathan, R. D., Fung, S. J., Stocco, D. M., Barron, E. A., and Markwald, R. R. (1980): Sialic acid: Regulation of electrogenesis in cultured heart cells. *Am. J. Physiol. (in press).*

27. Nathan, R. D., Pooler, J. P., and DeHaan, R. L. (1976): Ultraviolet-induced alterations of beat rate and electrical properties of embryonic chick heart cell aggregates. *J. Gen. Physiol.,* 67:27-44.

28. Noble, D., and Tsien, R. W. (1968): The kinetics and rectifier properties of the slow potassium current in cardiac Purkinje fibres. *J. Physiol. (Lond.),* 195:185-214.
29. Noble, D., and Tsien, R. W. (1969): Outward membrane currents activated in the plateau range of potentials in cardiac Purkinje fibres. *J. Physiol. (Lond.),* 200:205-231.
30. Noma, A., and Irisawa, H. (1976): A time- and voltage-dependent potassium current in the rabbit sinoatrial node cell. *Pfluegers Arch. Eur. J. Physiol.,* 366:251-258.
31. Polinger, I. S. (1970): Separation of cell types in embryonic heart cell cultures. *Exp. Cell. Res.,* 63:78-82.
32. Sachs, H. G., and DeHaan, R. L. (1973): Embryonic myocardial cell aggregates: Volume and pulsation rate. *Dev. Biol.,* 30:233-240.
33. Sheu, S.-S., and Fozzard, H. A. (1978): Intracellular potassium activity of the chick embryonic heart during development. *Biophys. J.,* 21:55a.
34. Shigenobu, K., Schneider, J., and Sperelakis, N. (1974): Verapamil blockade of slow Na^+ and Ca^{++} responses in myocardial cells. *J. Pharmacol. Exp. Ther.,* 190:280-288.
35. Shigenobu, K., and Sperelakis, N. (1971): Development of sensitivity to tetrodotoxin of chick embryonic hearts with age. *J. Mol. Cell. Cardiol.,* 3:271-286.
36. Sperelakis, N., and Shigenobu, K. (1972): Changes in membrane properties of chick embryonic hearts during development. *J. Gen. Physiol.,* 60:430-453.
37. Tauc, L., and Hinzen, D. (1974): Neuraminidase: Its effect on synaptic transmission. *Brain. Res.,* 80:340-344.
38. Tosteson, M. T. (1978): Interactions between a membrane sialoglycoprotein and planar lipid bilayers. *J. Memb. Biol.,* 38:291-309.
39. Warren, L. (1959): The thiobarbituric acid assay of sialic acids. *J. Biol. Chem.,* 234:1971-1975.
40. Yeh, B. K., and Hoffman, B. F. (1968): The ionic basis of electrical activity in embryonic cardiac muscle. *J. Gen. Physiol.,* 52:666-681.

DISCUSSION

Manasek: How large a molecule is neuraminidase, and does it penetrate into the intercellular regions of the aggregate?

Nathan: I do not know how large the molecule is. From our experiments, we were not able to determine whether it penetrates or not.

Manasek: You can only demonstrate it for the superficial layer?

Nathan: Yes, but this does not mean that it does not happen.

Manasek: But you do not know that it does happen?

Markwald: There is very clearly a problem of getting sialidase into the aggregate.

Markwald: Based on morphological staining, those are the only points to show a change. It may be that the sialidase gets in, but the polycationic ferritin does not.

Perspectives in Cardiovascular Research, Vol. 5,
Mechanisms of Cardiac Morphogenesis and Teratogenesis,
edited by Tomas Pexieder. Raven Press, New York © 1981

Coaggregation of Embryonic Chick Sympathetic Neurons with Cardiac Myocytes: Evidence for Functional Synaptic Development *In Vitro*

*Donald A. Fischman and **Naomi G. Culver

*Department of Anatomy and Cell Biology, State University of New York–Downstate Medical Center, Brooklyn, New York 11203; and **Department of Medicine, University of Chicago, Pritzker School of Medicine, Chicago, Illinois 60637*

The functional implications of sympathetic innervation during cardiac development are poorly understood. It has been considered unlikely that such innervation exerts a significant influence on heart development, because physiological studies have failed to detect function of either sympathetic or parasympathetic systems in the heart until very late in embryogenesis (64). Recently, however, we reinvestigated this question, using a pharmacological approach, and have shown that sympathetic, cardioacceleratory function can be detected by 5 days of embryonic chick development (11), which coincides closely with the stage of nerve fiber entry into the heart *in ovo* (76). To analyze the events of innervation in greater detail, we established an *in vitro* model system, in which sympathetic neurons from paravertebral ganglia can be combined with cardiac myocytes in a semi-organ culture system of spheroidal reaggregates.

Cells differing in origin with respect to age (27), species (26), or tissue type (56,59) can be combined in culture to form aggregates in which the two cell types may "sort out," or segregate, forming identifiable structures which exhibit the histiotypic morphology of the original tissues (58). A particular advantage of aggregate systems is that they permit combination of known ratios of cells from each tissue with reestablishment of characteristic cell–cell contacts, histological structure, and expression of complex tissue functions (12,28,55,57,68).

The value of *in vitro* model systems is evident from previous studies of neuromuscular development. The specificity of interactions between sympathetic neurons and their target cells (54), synaptic localization on skeletal muscle (9), trophic interactions on end organ tissue (10,62), and end organ influence on nerve outgrowth (6,7), or on nerve metabolism (29,30), have been investigated *in vitro*. Synapse formation has been studied between neurons with muscle from either appropriate or inappropriate target tissues, e.g., skeletal muscle with neurons derived from the spinal cord (19,20,72), ciliary ganglion (3,4,39), or sympathetic ganglia (63), smooth muscle with neurons from ciliary and sympathetic ganglia (65), and cardiac muscle with its intrinsic cholinergic innervation (49), or with neurons from superior cervical ganglia (25,46).

In the studies described below, evidence is presented that functional noradrenergic synaptic contacts can be established between sympathetic ganglion and heart cells within coaggregates of the two cell types.

MATERIALS AND METHODS

Culture Procedures

A cell suspension, prepared by dissociation of 7-day-old chick embryonic hearts (22), as modified by Clark (8), or 11-day-old lumbar paravertebral ganglia (77), shown by trypan blue exclusion to contain less than 5% non-viable heart cells or 10% non-viable ganglion cells, was used to establish cultures. Erlenmeyer flasks (25 ml) were seeded with a total of 10^6 cells in 3 ml of aggregation (A) medium, consisting of 47% medium 199, 47% Earle's BSS (K$^+$-free), 3% heat inactivated horse serum, 2% fetal bovine serum, 1% antibiotic solution (50 units/ml penicillin, 50 μg/ml streptomycin) and 5 mg/ml dextrose. To each culture was added 2 units/ml nerve growth factor (NGF), a concentration judged sufficient based on its ability to support outgrowth from sympathetic ganglion explants cultured in monolayer. Coaggregate cultures were seeded with 750,000 heart cells and 250,000 ganglion cells. The flasks were gassed for 1 min with 95% air, 5% CO_2, and then incubated for 24 hr in a rotary shaker waterbath at 37°C and 70 rpm. For subsequent culture, the contents of each flask were transferred to bacteriological 60 mm petri plates (Falcon 1007), which had not been treated for tissue culture and did not sustain attachment or spreading of the aggregates. Incubation was continued in a 37°C incubator under a water-saturated atmosphere containing 5% CO_2. Medium and NGF were replaced on alternate days.

Histological Studies

To identify and localize cardiac myocytes, aggregates fixed for 24 hr in cold formol–alcohol (1 part formalin; 9 parts 95% ethanol) were embedded in paraffin, sectioned, and stained for glycogen, using the PAS technique (40). For silver staining of nerve outgrowth, aggregates were fixed in 10% formalin in 0.1 M phosphate buffer (pH 7.4), embedded in paraffin, and sectioned. Staining was carried out using the technique of Sevier and Munger (69).

Fluorescence studies were carried out on aggregates which had been preincubated in 0.37 mg/ml pargyline for 4 to 6 hr (51), and were then washed in cold Tyrode's solution and affixed to slides treated for 5 min with 0.1 mM poly-l-lysine (MW 3400, Sigma) in 0.1 M phosphate buffer (pH 7.4). The slides were immersed for 5 min in 2% glyoxylic acid made up in 0.15 M phosphate buffer (pH 7.4), according to Bloom and Battenberg (5), drained thoroughly, and allowed to air dry. They were then placed for 10 min in a preheated, covered staining dish in a 100°C oven, coverslipped in paraffin oil, and observed with a Zeiss fluorescence microscope, using BG12 and UG1 excitation and barrier filters with a cutoff at 470 and 510 nm.

Norepinephrine Uptake

Prior to each uptake experiment, 0.37 mg/ml pargyline was added to all cultures for 4 to 6 hr. The cultures of each cell type were then pooled and washed twice in sterile Tyrode's solution to which 1 g/l glucose, 0.2 g/l ascorbic acid, and 0.05 g/l EDTA had been added (MT buffer). Aliquots of each aggregate type, suspended in 1 ml of MT buffer and equilibrated with 95% air, 5% CO_2, were incubated at 37°C on a waterbath shaker for 30 min, during which time cocaine hydrochloride (10^{-4} M) was added to appropriate samples. At the conclusion of the preincubation, 1 μCi of ^{3}H-d,1-NE diluted with unlabeled NE to a final concentration of 1 μM was added to each sample tube. Incubation was continued at 37°C, except for those tubes to be incubated at 0°C, which were exposed to label while immersed in an ice bath. At the end of the appropriate incubation time, samples were washed with 5 ml of Tyrode's solution and resuspended in 0.3 ml volume, sonicated for 30 sec, and two 50 μl aliquots of the suspension distributed onto GF/A filters for scintillation counting. Protein concentrations were measured in 100 μl aliquots of each sample (52).

Pharmacology

To record the contractile activity of individual aggregates, they were first transferred to Falcon tissue culture plates (1008) for adhesion to the substrate. Cardiac aggregates maintained less than 48 hr *in vitro* attached if allowed to sit undisturbed in serum-containing medium for 1 hr at 37°C. For older cardiac (H) aggregates, or for heart-sympathetic ganglion cell (H-SG) coaggregates, it was necessary to pretreat the plates for 5 min with 0.1 mM polylysine. All of the studies on H-SG coaggregates, and most of those on H aggregates, were carried out in 5 ml of A medium from which NGF had been omitted. Light, nontoxic mineral oil (Crestline) was layered over the preparation to prevent evaporation.

Observation was carried out on the stage of an inverted microscope fitted with a water-jacketed chamber maintained at 37°C. An opening in the wall of the chamber permitted the inflow of air–CO_2. After a 15 min equilibration period, pharmacological agents were added in a 3 ml volume of a prewarmed, pregassed medium, aspirated 5 times with a Pasteur pipette to ensure mixing, and the 3 ml of medium was removed to maintain the volume of the culture. Effort was made not disturb the mineral oil layer and cause mixing of oil and medium. Drug effects were measured by clocking the beating rate of several aggregates in a culture; this was done by timing 20 beats with a stopwatch.

Rates were clocked immediately after drug addition and again 5 min later. For time course studies, rate determinations were made every 5 min.

RESULTS

Within 24 hr of establishing the cultures, the aggregates exhibited a characteristic size and shape. H aggregates were spheroids, ranging in diameter from 30 to 250 μm (Fig. 1a), while SG aggregates tended to be larger (250-350 μm) and more ovoid (Fig. 1b). By the second day in culture, H-SG coaggregates exhibited a bilaminar structure, suggesting that "sorting out," the separation of cells of different tissues within a coaggregate, had taken place (Fig. 1c). Up until, but not after, the second day of culture, H aggregates fused with one another, synchronizing their contractile rates in the common cellular mass, while individual SG and H-SG aggregates continued to agglomerate throughout the culture period, forming extended or branching chains, with each individual locus of aggregated myocytes in H-SG aggregates continuing to contract at its own rate.

Periodic acid-Schiff (PAS), which selectively stained the glycogen-containing cardiac myocytes red, showed these cells to be concentrated in the center of the H-SG aggregates (Fig. 2). H aggregates were invested with a thin rim of PAS-negative cells, probably fibroblasts and/or endothelial cells. In H-SG aggregates (Fig. 2), cells with large basophilic nuclei were clustered at the immediate periphery of the heart cell mass. These were identified as sympathetic neurons based on cell size and morphology, because they exhibited green fluorescence when treated with glyoxylic acid (Fig. 3), and they appeared to extend outgrowth around and among the myocytes. Silver stains (results not illustrated) of H-SG aggregates revealed an extensive nerve fiber plexus within the cluster of muscle cells, which was not observed in H aggregates.

Sympathetic neurons take up NE by a high-affinity process characteristic only of catecholaminergic neurons. To determine whether or not reaggregate cultures contained cells capable of carrying out this process, H, H-SG, and SG aggregates were incubated for predetermined periods of time with ^{3}H-NE (total NE concentration of 10^{-6} M) and the accumulated ^{3}H-specific activity measured. The monoamine-oxidase inhibitor pargyline was added to reduce enzymatic degradation of the NE. Aggregates cultured for 7 days were incubated in ^{3}H-NE for 5, 15, 30, 45, and 60 min periods, with uptake times between 5 and 30 min yielding the most reproducible results. SG and H-SG aggregates displayed an apparently linear increase in ^{3}H accumulation over the first 30 min of labeling; this increase was completely blocked by preincubation with 10^{-4} M cocaine or by incubation on ice. In one experiment, preincubation with unlabeled d,1-NE (10^{-5} M) for 30 min reduced ^{3}H uptake by 63%. After labeling periods longer than 30 min, the accumulation of label was unpredictable, either continuing to increase or even decreasing from the 30 min values.

In 3 experiments, ^{3}H-NE uptake levels in 7-day-old H-SG, H, and SG aggre-

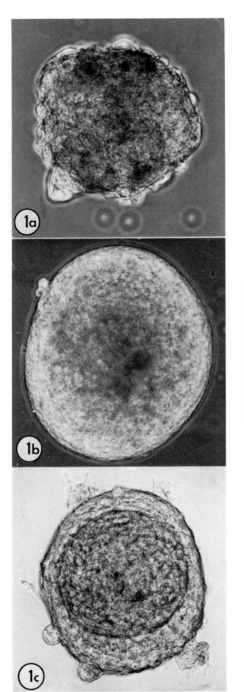

FIG. 1. Light photomicrographs of typical cellular reaggregates in whole mount after 7 days *in vitro*. Heart cells were obtained from 7-day-old chick embryos, sympathetic ganglion cells from 11-day-old embryos. After aggregation for 24 hr in Erlenmeyer flasks, the aggregates were transferred to 60 mm Petri plates and subsequently incubated at 37°C, 95% air–5% CO_2. **a:** Heart cell aggregate; **b:** Sympathetic ganglion cell aggregate; **c:** Coaggregate of heart and sympathetic ganglion cells ($\times$ 200).

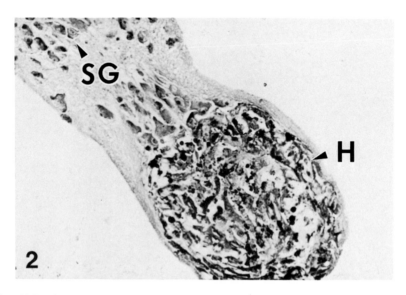

FIG. 2. Light micrograph of a periodic acid-Schiff stained, paraffin-sectioned, H-SG coaggregate after 7 days *in vitro*. Culture conditions as for Fig. 1. H, heart cells; SG, sympathetic ganglion cells (× 320).

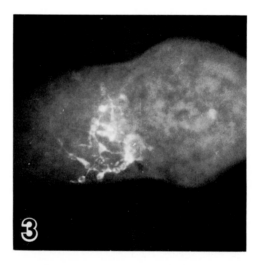

FIG. 3. Whole mount of H-SG coaggregate, reacted with glyoxylic acid after 7 days in culture. Darkfield fluorescence (× 120).

gates were compared. In all 3 experiments, H-SG aggregates contained a higher specific activity than SG aggregates; virtually no significant ³H incorporation was exhibited by H aggregates. A comparative time course from one such experiment is shown in Fig. 4. No systematic analysis has been made of catecholamine uptake as a function of time *in vitro;* most uptake studies utilized aggregates that had been in culture 7 to 14 days. However, significant accumulation of ³H-NE was observed in suspensions of dissociated cells which had been cultured for only 4 hr. No experiments were conducted with 3- or 4-week-old cultures to detect a loss in adrenergic uptake systems with prolonged culture.

Virtually all H and H-SG aggregates contracted spontaneously after the first day in culture, with rates ranging from 50 to 200 bpm for H aggregates (mean ± SEM = 98 ± 7 bpm) and 40 to 150 bpm (86 ± 7) for H-SG aggregates. By the end of the first week in culture, the contraction rate had decreased to 20 to 50 bpm (36 ± 5) for H aggregates. After the second week in culture, most of the H aggregates had ceased to beat; in H-SG cultures, from 30 to 70% of the aggregates contracted spontaneously, usually with rates ranging between 20 and 40 bpm, although some of the smaller aggregates contracted at 50 to 60 bpm.

To establish catecholamine sensitivity, H aggregates composed of atrial, ventricular, or cells released from the whole heart, were exposed to NE (10^{-8} to 10^{-3} M), or d,1-isoproterenol (IPNE; 10^{-10} to 10^{-5} M). A variety of media were tested, but no reproducible positive chronotropic response was observed.

Although most studies were carried out on 24- to 48-hr cultures, aggregates up to one week old were also tested, with similar results in all cases. Since

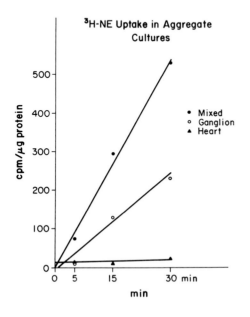

³H-NE Uptake in Aggregate Cultures

• Mixed
○ Ganglion
▲ Heart

FIG. 4. ³H-norepinephrine accumulation in 7-day-old cultures of H, SG, and H-SG aggregates. For each time point in an individual experiment, % H-SG specific activity =

$$\frac{\text{cpm/}\mu\text{g protein} \times 100}{\text{cpm/}\mu\text{g protein of H-SG}}$$

IPNE is not taken up by neurons, this agent was also tested on H-SG aggregates which had been cultured for 13 days, but no reliable chronotropic response was observed.

The absence of catecholamine-induced chronotropy might indicate either that the catecholamines themselves were inactivated *in vitro* or that the adrenergic receptors had degenerated, perhaps from trypsinization. On the other hand, it is possible that reaggregated heart cells were simply incapable of a positive chronotropic response, but that other catecholamine-sensitive processes (e.g., positive inotropy, elevation of cAMP levels, glycogenolysis, etc.) could be induced. To determine whether or not reaggregated cardiac cells were completely unresponsive to catecholamines, we tested the ability of catecholamines to reinitiate contraction in aggregates blocked by TTX. Catecholamines have been demonstrated to restore contraction in TTX-blocked embryonic hearts (70) and, since cardiac aggregates as well as embryonic hearts *in situ* exhibit sensitivity to TTX (55), we examined the response to NE in aggregates cultured for 4 days and then blocked from contraction by the addition of 0.1 μM TTX. Upon addition of 10 to 100 μM NE, H aggregates resumed contraction, and this response could be prevented by preincubation with 1 μM propranolol. We conclude from these results that NE is capable of restoring automaticity in TTX-blocked cardiac aggregates, strongly suggesting that β-adrenergic receptors are present at the cell surface of a significant fraction of the cardiac myocytes.

To investigate the release of intraneuronal catecholamines, we examined the rate of beating of H-SG aggregates in the presence of the nicotinic agonist 1,1-dimethyl-4-phenylpiperazinium iodide (DMPP). In many H-SG aggregates 13 days *in vitro*, DMPP at 0.1 mM elicited a significant increase ($p < 0.001$) in rate. In the presence of DMPP, the contraction rate increased from 28 $\pm$ 1 bpm to 36 $\pm$ 4 bpm, and remained high for at least 30 min (Fig. 5). This apparently modest increase is highly significant, since there was no increase in rate when a diluent blank was added to the cultures. Although very few H aggregates were beating in 13-day-old cultures, it was possible to examine the effect of DMPP on beating aggregates in several cultures. In contrast to the increase observed in the beating rate of H-SG aggregates, the contraction rates of H aggregates did not increase but, in fact, tended to decrease an average of 26% from pre-DMPP rates.

To establish the site of nicotinic action in H-SG coaggregates, DMPP effects were examined in the presence of inhibitors of transmission at the ganglionic and neuroeffector junctions. In 6 H-SG aggregates, prior exposure to the nicotinic antagonist hexamethonium at 10 μM prevented the DMPP-mediated increase in contraction. Of 6 aggregates to which hexamethonium was administered subsequent to DMPP stimulation, 5 decreased their rate substantially, and one remained unchanged.

Preincubation with atropine (2 μM) did not prevent the DMPP-induced positive chronotropy, nor did it cause a rise in beating rate when added alone.

Since TTX prevents propagation of the nerve impulse at a much lower concen-

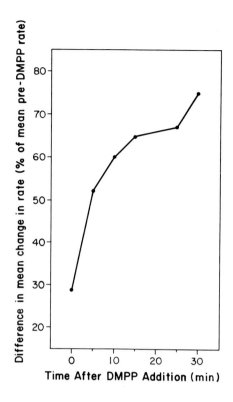

FIG. 5. The time course of the DMPP-induced chronotropic response in H-SG coaggregates. For each time point the data were calculated:

$$\frac{(\text{beats/min})_{\text{DMPP}} - (\text{beats/min})_{\text{Blank}}}{(\text{beats/min})_{\text{pre-DMPP}}} \times 100$$

The rate was determined from five control and five experimental aggregates.

tration than that at which it blocks the action potential in mammalian Purkinje fibers (14), and since we have had some success in using low concentrations of TTX to differentiate between neuronal and cardiac excitability (11), DMPP was administered to H-SG aggregates in the presence of 10 μM TTX, a concentration that did not block contraction in either H or H-SG aggregates. The rate of H-SG aggregates either decreased or remained unchanged when TTX was added, and no increase in rate was observed after subsequent addition of DMPP.

Guanethedine (50 μM) prevented positive chronotropy when administered prior to DMPP. If 10 μM GuE was added to some of the aggregates already accelerated by DMPP, a second increase in rate of beating began immediately. For example, one aggregate, which had increased its rate from 34 bpm to 45 bpm in the presence of DMPP, contracted at 50 bpm after GuE had been added. Subsequent administration of a higher concentration of GuE (0.1 mM) stopped contraction entirely in these aggregates. The TTX and GuE sensitivity of DMPP-induced cardioacceleration argues in favor of a neuronal mechanism for stimulation.

To determine whether the DMPP response required NE binding to β-receptors on the heart cells, DMPP was administered in the presence of 0.1 mM practolol, a β-antagonist highly specific for cardiac receptors (15). When administered prior to DMPP, practolol reduced the contraction rate of aggregates by 44%, and after DMPP addition this lower rate was maintained. The addition of practolol after DMPP administration reduced the beating rate of H-SG aggregates to pre-DMPP levels. Aggregates pre-treated with the α-antagonist phentolamine (1 μM) also failed to respond to DMPP. This effect might be explained by the presynaptic inhibition of the nicotinic cholinergic receptor system by phentolamine (24), or, alternatively, by the required function of both α- and β-receptors in the DMPP-induced acceleration of H-SG aggregates. Further work will be required to clarify this problem.

DISCUSSION

We have established an organ culture system which enables us to study the interactions between embryonic cardiac myocytes and sympathetic neurons. Cardiac cells and cells dissociated from sympathetic ganglia could be cultured as aggregates, either together or separately. When cultured together, the two cell types sorted out, with cardiac cells toward the center and sympathetic neurons located peripherally to the cardiac cell mass. Aggregates containing ganglion cells accumulated tritium when exposed to 1 μM ^{3}H-NE, suggesting a catecholamine uptake process with a K_m in the micromolar range; the time course of this concentration process appeared to be linear over the first 30 min. Aggregates composed only of heart cells accumulated virtually no specific counts. H-SG coaggregates took up more ^{3}H-NE per μg/protein than did aggregates containing only ganglion cells. H aggregates and H-SG coaggregates contracted spontaneously, but H-SG coaggregates continued to contract for the entire culture period (up to three weeks), while, under our culture conditions, H aggregates ceased beating during the second week. No chronotropic response was observed in H aggregates upon addition of NE or IPNE, or in H-SG aggregates exposed to IPNE, but DMPP, a nicotinic agonist, accelerated the contraction rate of 13-day-old H-SG coaggregates. Nicotinic and adrenergic blocking agents, as well as TTX and GuE, prevented DMPP-mediated positive chronotropy. Those few H aggregates that continued to beat did not exhibit an accelerated contraction rate in the presence of DMPP.

Neuromuscular interactions have been studied in tissue culture by many investigators (21,60,71), since the structural simplicity of *in vitro* preparations, as compared with intact tissues, permits easy observation and more accurate control of experimental conditions.

Aggregation and subsequent sorting-out of cells have been described by other researchers (28,58,73,75). The clumping of sympathetic neurons at the periphery of the heart cell mass in our cultures is particularly reminiscent of the clumping of neural retina cells in the heterotypic coaggregates described by Shimada et al. (73).

Exogenous catecholamines induce positive chronotropy in the embryonic chick heart before and after cardiac innervation (2,11,18), and also have been reported to stimulate chick cardiac cells cultured in monolayer (17,37,50,79). However, not all investigators report that the contraction rate of these cultured cells is catecholamine-sensitive (64,74). Despite these conflicting results, a positive chronotropic response to NE might be predicted in aggregates of chick cardiac cells as opposed to single cells, since Lane et al. (48) and Furshpan et al. (25) reported greater sensitivity to autonomic agents in clusters of mouse and rat cardiocytes than in individual cells. A variety of media were used in our studies, and an attempt was made to maximize the concentrations of pacemaker tissue by forming aggregates exclusively from atrial cells; however, exogenous NE or IPNE did not reproducibly stimulate the contraction rate of cardiac aggregates. The inconsistent responses reported by other researchers on chick cells in monolayer, and observed by us in cell aggregates, suggest that the chronotropic response to autonomic agents may be less stable in cultured chick than in mouse cells.

The presence of functional β-receptors in aggregated heart cells is supported by the observation that NE is able to restore automaticity in aggregates blocked by TTX, an agent that prevents excitation and contraction of the heart by blocking the fast inward sodium current responsible for the upstroke of the action potential (14,34) and has also been shown to block contractility of cardiac aggregates (55). Catecholamines have been demonstrated to restore excitability of the TTX-blocked heart, possibly by opening up slow sodium or calcium channels and allowing the inward current to bypass the fast sodium channels (70). This response to NE was sensitive to the β-antagonist propranolol. It is possible that some post-receptor process required for the chronotropic response was lacking, or, alternatively, that pacemaker cells might not survive in culture, that they may be inaccessible to the catecholamines, or that they may possibly require an anatomical arrangement of conducting tissue more analogous to that of the intact heart to exert their chronotropic influence. Since it is possible for NE to elicit a chronotropic response in H-SG aggregates by being taken up into sympathetic neurons and released, the effect of IPNE, which, unlike NE, cannot be taken up by the sympathetic neuron (43), was tested on H-SG aggregates. Both H and H-SG aggregates proved incapable of responding chronotropically to IPNE, suggesting that exogenous catecholamines cannot elicit cardioacceleration in these chick aggregates. It might be fruitful to repeat these experiments during the period required for functional synaptic development. In contrast, the embryonic chick heart *in vivo* exhibits cardioacceleration in the presence of DMPP within one day of nerve entry in to the heart (11). Furthermore, functional cholinergic synapses with skeletal muscle have been observed after 15 hr of culture with ciliary ganglia (3) or 4 days of culture with spinal cord neurons (20). On the other hand, 13-day-old cultures were used by Furshpan et al. (25) to demonstrate synaptic activity between rat sympathetic neurons and cardiac myocytes, and previous studies have shown that the period of greatest catecholamine synthesis occurs during the second week *in vitro* (53).

It is unclear why H aggregates did not beat after the first week in culture, since aggregates of cardiac cells have been observed to beat in monolayer culture for as long as six months (8). However, it is interesting that coaggregation with ganglionic cells prolonged the period during which cardiac cells contracted spontaneously, particularly since Oh and his colleagues have observed that skeletal muscle development (61), and, in particular, cholinesterase activity (62), are enhanced by co-culture with nervous tissue or with spinal cord extract. Medoff and Gross (56) have noted increased nucleic acid synthesis and enzyme activity in kidney cells coaggregated with nervous tissues, as compared to kidney cells coaggregated with liver. The cardiac aggregate system lends itself to studies of "neurotrophic" effects, since it provides a virtual guarantee that all cells of the tissue co-cultured with nerve will be in close proximity to the nerve tissue.

Both H-SG and SG aggregates concentrate ^{3}H-NE in the presence of 1 μM NE, but H aggregates do not. Although no chemical isolation of intracellular NE was performed to confirm that ^{3}H content reflected ^{3}H-NE accumulation, we did include pargyline to inhibit catabolism of NE by monoamine oxidase, and have shown that accumulation was inhibited by cocaine and low temperature, and occurred only in aggregates containing neurons. Similar studies with embryonic chick tissue (66) leave little doubt that such accumulation occurs in the experiments with cardiac aggregates from the embryonic mouse.

A significant increase in beat rate was observed in many H-SG aggregates when DMPP was added to the bath, implying that coaggregates of cardiac cells, like the heart *in vivo* (11), are capable of a positive chronotropic response upon release of endogenous catecholamines. The sensitivity of the DMPP-induced chronotropy to many neuronal junctional antagonists supports the concept that this increase in rate was caused by the release of neurotransmitter. Unlike the embryonic heart *in vivo,* the α-adrenergic antagonist phentolamine, as well as the β-antagonist practolol, blocked the chronotropic response to DMPP, reminiscent of results obtained by Lane et al (48) when studying catecholamine effects on monolayer cultures of mouse heart cells. Hexamethonium, which prevents agonist binding to ganglionic nicotinic receptors, blocked the stimulatory effects of DMPP; the muscarinic antagonist, atropine, neither inhibited nor potentiated the stimulatory effect of DMPP. Potentiation might have been expected if cholinergic neurons derived either from ganglionic or intrinsic cardiac innervation (49) made up a significant proportion of the functional innervation in our system. Previous exposure to GuE, an inhibitor of neuronal release of NE, blocked DMPP stimulation of H-SG aggregates. Subsequent exposure to GuE further stimulated DMPP-accelerated aggregates, presumably reflecting the immediate sympathomimetic effects observed *in vivo* after administration of this agent (1,38). TTX at 10^{-8} M did not prevent cardiac contractility; however, the DMPP-induced cardioacceleration was completely blocked, implying that DMPP acted indirectly upon the heart, most probably via the neurons. The response of H-SG aggregates to DMPP differed when tested after 7 or 13 days of culture. In the 13-day-old H-SG aggregates, DMPP elicited an unabated chronotropic response for at least 30 min (the longest time observed). This response was anticipated, since DMPP is believed not to be metabolized in biological systems (78). However, H-SG aggregates from 7-day-old cultures exhibited only a transient acceleration in beat frequency after exposure to DMPP, suggesting that a maturational period is required for functional synaptic development.

Both H-SG and SG aggregates concentrate ^{3}H-NE in the presence of 1 μM NE, while H aggregates do not. Although no chemical isolation of intracellular NE was performed to confirm that ^{3}H content reflects ^{3}H-NE accumulation, we did include pargyline to inhibit catabolism of NE by monoamine oxidase, and have shown that accumulation was inhibited by cocaine and low temperature, and only occurred in aggregates containing neurons. Similar studies with embryonic chick tissue (Rothman et al., 1978) leave little doubt that such accumulation occurs in form of NE. Autoradiographic studies will be required to localize ^{3}H-NE within intraneuronal sites, perhaps at nerve endings in close contact with the myocytes.

Accumulation of ^{3}H-NE increased in an apparently linear fashion over the first 30 min of incubation; however, results were variable for longer incubation periods. The accumulation of NE by neurons reflects both uptake and intracellular binding. These two sequences may follow independent developmental programs in the postnatal rat heart (32,67) and the embryonic chick heart (41,42). Perhaps insufficient NE binding sites were present in the aggregates, so that leakage obscured uptake.

Although SG cultures were seeded with four times the number of ganglion cells as H-SG cultures, including, presumably, four times the number of sympathetic postganglionic neurons, H-SG aggregates accumulated more specific ^{3}H counts than did SG aggregates. These unexpected data suggest that heart tissue might exert a "trophic influence" upon its innervating sympathetic neurons. The presence of the end organ might increase cell viability, as in the ventral horn (36), spinal ganglia (36), and ciliary ganglia (47), or its presence might permit greater axonal outgrowth, as demonstrated by Chamley et al. (7), thus increasing the axonal surface area and the number of sites available for uptake (16,35). Alternatively, the presence of the heart cells might enhance neuronal metabolic activity, an effect analogous to stimulation of synthetic enzymes in the superior cervical ganglion of the developing rat (13) or in cultured motor neurons (30).

In summary, we have established aggregate culture systems in which heart and sympathetic ganglion cells can be cultured alone or together. Sympathetic neurons, cultured either alone or with heart, take up catecholamines by the characteristic cocaine-sensitive process specific to sympathetic neurons; from this, it can be concluded that sympathetic cells are alive and functional in aggregate culture. Accumulation of label increases linearly over the first 30 min and appears to be enhanced in the presence of cardiac cells. Cardiac cells cultured alone or with sympathetic ganglion cells beat spontaneously, and their beating life is prolonged in ganglion-cell-containing aggregates. Although exogenous catecholamines will not elicit an increase in the beating rate of either cardiac or heterotypic aggregates, DMPP evokes an acceleration in the contraction rate, and pharmacological studies indicate that this acceleration is mediated via release of catecholamines from intra-neuronal stores.

ACKNOWLEDGMENTS

Much of this research was accomplished in the laboratory of Dr. Beatrice Garber. Her encouragement and helpful suggestions, and those of Dr. Harry Fozzard and Suzanne Oparil, are gratefully acknowledged. The authors also express their appreciation for the careful reading and criticism of the manuscript by Drs. Robert Furchgott, Frank Scalia, and Paul Patterson. Excellent technical assistance was provided by Mr. Jerome Schuch, Mrs. Lovenia Williams, Miss Ellie Dimapilis, and Mrs. Sue Lockett. This research was supported by HL 135-05, The New York Heart Association, and the Muscular Dystrophy Association. NGC was supported by PHS 5-01-HD00174-10.

REFERENCES

1. Abercombie, G. G., and Davies, B. N. (1963): The action of guanethidine with particular reference to the sympathetic nervous system. *Br. J. Pharmacol.,* 20:171-177.
2. Barry, A. (1950): The effect of epinephrine on the myocardium of the embryonic chick. *Circulation,* 1:1362-1368.
3. Betz, W. (1976a): The formation of synapses between chick embryo skeletal muscle and ciliary ganglia grown *in vitro. J. Physiol. (Lond.),* 254:63-73.
4. Betz, W. (1976b): Functional and non-functional contacts between ciliary neurons and muscle grown *in vitro. J. Physiol. (Lond.),* 254:75-86.
5. Bloom, F. E., and Battenberg, E. L. F. (1976): A simple and sensitive method for the demonstration of central catecholamine-containing neurons and axons by glyoxylic acid-induced fluorescence. *J. Histochem. Cytochem.,* 24:561-571.
6. Chamley, J. H., and Dowel, J. J. (1975): Specificity of nerve fiber attraction to autonomic effector organs in tissue culture. *Exp. Cell Res.,* 90:1-7.
7. Chamley, J. H., Goller, I., and Burnstock, G. (1972): Selective growth of sympathetic nerve fibers to explants of normally densely innervated autonomic effector organs in tissue culture. *Dev. Biol.,* 31:362-379.
8. Clark, W. A. (1976): Selective control of fibroblast proliferation and its effect on cardiac muscle differentiation *in vitro. Dev. Biol.,* 52:263-282.
9. Cohen, S. A., and Fischbach, G. D. (1977): Clusters of acetylcholine receptors located at identified nerve–muscle synapses *in vitro. Dev. Biol.,* 59:24-38.
10. Crain, S. E., and Peterson, E. R. (1974): Development of neuronal connections in culture. *Ann. NY Acad. Sci.,* 228:6-34.
11. Culver, N. G., and Fischman, D. A. (1977): Pharmacological analysis of sympathetic function in the embryonic chick heart. *Am. J. Physiol.,* 232:R116-R123.
12. DeHaan, R. L., and Sachs, H. G. (1972): Cell coupling in developing systems: The heart cell paradigm. *Curr. Top. Dev. Biol.,* 7:193-228.
13. Dibner, M. D., and Black, I. B. (1976): The effect of target organ removal on the development of sympathetic neurons. *Brain Res.,* 103:93-102.
14. Dudel, J., Peper, K., Rüdel, R., and Trautwein, W. (1967): Effect of tetrodotoxin on membrane currents in mammalian cardiac fibers. *Nature (Lond.),* 213:296-297.
15. Dunlop, D., and Shanks, R. G. (1968): Selective blockade of adrenoreceptive beta receptors in the heart. *Br. J. Pharmacol.,* 32:201-208.

16. England, J. M., Kadin, M. E., and Goldstein, M. M. (1973): The effect of vincristine sulfate on the axoplasmic flow of proteins in cultured sympathetic neurons. *J. Cell Sci.,* 12:549-565.

17. Ertel, R. J., Clarke, D. E., Chao, J. C., and Franke, F. R. (1971): Autonomic receptor mechanisms in embryonic chick myocardial cell cultures. *J. Pharmacol. Exp. Ther.,* 178:73-80.

18. Fingl, E., Woodbury, L. A., and Hecht, H. H. (1952): Effects of innervation and drugs upon direct membrane potentials of embryonic chick myocardium. *J. Pharmacol. Exp. Ther.,* 104:103-114.

19. Fischbach, G. D. (1970): Synaptic potentials recorded in cell cultures of nerve and muscle. *Science,* 169:1331-1333.

20. Fischbach, G. D. (1972): Synapse formation between dissociated nerve and muscle cells in low-density cell cultures. *Dev. Biol.,* 28:407-429.

21. Fischbach, G. D., Fambrough, D., and Nelson, P. G. (1973): A discussion of neuron and muscle cell cultures. *Fed. Proc.,* 32:1636-1642.

22. Fischman, D. A., and Moscona, A. A. (1969): An electron microscope study of *in vitro* dissociation and reaggregation of embryonic chick and mouse heart cells. *J. Cell Biol.,* 43:37a.

23. Fischman, D. A., and Moscona, A. A. (1971): Reconstruction of heart tissue from suspensions of embryonic myocardial cells: Ultrastructural studies of dispersed and reaggregated cells. In: *Cardiac Hypertrophy,* edited by N. R. Alpert, pp. 125-140. Academic Press, N.Y.

24. Furchgott, R. F., Steinland, O. S., and Wakade, T. D. (1975): Studies on prejunctional muscarinic and nicotinic receptors. In: *Chemical Trends in Catecholamine Research,* edited by O. Almgren, A. Carlsson, and J. Engel, pp. 167-174. North Holland Publishing Co., Amsterdam.

25. Furshpan, E. J., MacLeish, P. R., O'Lague, P. H., and Potter, D. D. (1976): Chemical transmission between rat sympathetic neurons and cardiac myocytes developing in microcultures: evidence for cholinergic, adrenergic and dual-function neurons. *Proc. Nat. Acad. Sci. USA,* 73:4225-4229.

26. Garber, B. B., Kollar, E. J., and Moscona, A. A. (1968): Aggregation *in vitro* of dissociated cells. III. Effect of state of differentiation of cells on feather development in hybrid aggregates of embryonic mouse and chick skin cells. *J. Exp. Zool.,* 168:455-472.

27. Garber, B., and Moscona, A. A. (1967): Suppression of feather morphogenesis in co-aggregates of skin cells from embryos of different ages. *J. Exp. Zool.,* 164:351-361.

28. Garber, B. B., and Moscona, A. A. (1972): Reconstruction of brain tissue cell from suspension. 1. Aggregation patterns of cells dissociated from different regions of the developing brain. *Dev. Biol.,* 27:217-234.

29. Giller, E. L., Jr., Schrier, B. K., Shainberg, A., Risk, H. R., and Nelson, P. G. (1973): Choline acetyltransferase activity is increased in combined cultures of spinal cord and muscle cells from mice. *Science,* 182:588-589.

30. Giller, E. L., Jr., Neal, J. H., Bullock, P. N., Schrier, B. K., and Nelson, P. G. (1977): Choline acetyltransferase activity of spinal cord cell cultures increased by co-culture with muscle and by muscle conditioned medium. *J. Cell Biol.,* 74:16-29.

31. Giotti, A., Ledda, F., and Mannaioni, P. F. (1973): Effects of noradrenaline and isoprenaline in combination with α- and β-receptor blocking substances on the action potential of cardiac Purkinje fibers. *J. Physiol.,* 229:99-113.

32. Glowinski, J., Axelrod, J., Kopin, I. J., and Wurtman, R. J. (1964): Physiological disposition of ³H-norepinephrine in the developing rat. *J. Pharmacol. Exp. Ther.,* 146:48-53.

33. Govier, W. C. (1968): Myocardial alpha adrenergic receptors and their role in production of a positive inotropic effect by sympathomimetic agents. *J. Pharmacol. Exp. Ther.,* 159:82–90.

34. Hagiwara, S., and Nakajima, S. (1965): Tetrodotoxin and manganese ion: Effects on action potential of the frog heart. *Science,* 149:1254-1255.

35. Hamberger, B., Malmfors, T., Norberg, K. A., and Sachs, C. (1964): Uptake and accumulation of catecholamines in peripheral adrenergic neurons of reserpinized animals studied with a histochemical method. *Biochem. Pharmacol.,* 13:841-844.

36. Hamburger, V. (1934): The effects of wing bud extirpation on the development of the central nervous system in chick embryos. *J. Exp. Zool.,* 68:449-494.

37. Harrison, D. C., Kleiger, R. E., and Merigan, T. C. (1967): Action of isoproterenol on heart cells in tissue culture. *Proc. Soc. Exp. Biol. Med.,* 124:122-126.

38. Hertting, G., Axelrod, J., and Patrick, R. W. (1962): Actions of bretylium and guanethedine on the uptake and release of ³H-noradrenaline. *Br. J. Pharmacol.,* 18:161-166.

39. Hooisma, J., Shaaf, D. W., Meeter, E., and Stevens, W. F. (1975): The innervation of chick striated muscle fibers by the chick ciliary ganglion in tissue culture. *Brain Res.,* 85:79-85.

40. Humason, G. L. (1967): *Animal Tissue Techniques,* 2nd ed. W. H. Freeman, San Francisco.
41. Ignarro, L. J., and Shideman, F. E. (1968a): Norepinephrine and epinephrine in the embryo and embryonic heart of the chick: uptake and subcellular distribution. *J. Pharmacol. Exp. Ther.,* 159:49-58.
42. Ignarro, L. J., and Shideman, F. E. (1968b): The requirement of sympathetic innervation for the active transport of norepinephrine by the heart. *J. Pharmacol. Exp. Ther.,* 159:59-65.
43. Iversen, L. L. (1967): *The Uptake and Storage of Noradrenaline in Sympathetic Nerves,* p. 211. Cambridge University Press, Cambridge.
44. Kaufman, R., Tritthart, H., Rodenroth, S., and Rost, B. (1969): Das mechanische und elektrische Verhalten isolierter embryonale Herzmuskellen in Zellkulturen. *Pflügers Arch.,* 311:25-49.
46. Landis, S. C. (1976): Rat sympathetic neurons and cardiac myotubes developing in microcultures: correlation of the fine structure of endings with neurotransmitter function in single neurons. *Proc. Natl. Acad. Sci. USA,* 73:4220-4224.
47. Landmesser, L., and Pilar, G. (1974): Synapse formation during embryogenesis on ganglion cells lacking a periphery. *J. Physiol. (Lond.),* 241:715-736.
48. Lane, M. A., Sastre, A., Law, M., and Salpeter, M. (1977): Cholinergic and adrenergic receptors on mouse cardiocytes *in vitro. Dev. Biol.,* 57:254-269.
49. Lane, M. A., Sastre, A., and Salpeter, M. M. (1976): Innervation of heart cells in culture by endogeneous source of cholinergic neurons. *Proc. Natl. Acad. Sci. USA,* 73:4506-4510.
50. Le Douarin, G., Suignard, G., Khaskyie, A., and Renaud, D. (1974): Sensibilite aux catecholamines des cardiomyoblasts embryonnaires de poulet isoles en culture *in vitro. C.R. Hebd. Acad. Sci. Paris,* 278:2943.
51. Levitt, P., Moore, R. Y., and Garber, B. B. (1976): Selective cell association in catecholamine-containing neurons in brain aggregates *in vitro. Brain Res.,* 111:311-320.
52. Lowry, O. H., Rosebrough, N. J., Farr, A. L., and Randall, R. J. (1951): Protein measurement with the Folin phenol reagent. *J. Biol. Chem.,* 193:265-275.
53. Mains, R. E., and Patterson, P. H. (1973): Primary cultures of dissociated sympathetic neurons. III. Changes in metabolism with age in culture. *J. Cell Biol.,* 59:361-366.
54. Mark, G. E., Chamley, J. H., and Burnstock, G. (1973): Interaction between autonomic nerves and smooth and cardiac muscle in culture. *Dev. Biol.,* 32:194-200.
55. McDonald, T. F., Sachs, H. G., and DeHaan, R. L. (1972): Development of sensitivity to tetrodotoxin in beating chick embryo hearts, single cells and aggregates. *Science,* 176:1248.
56. Medoff, J., and Gross, J. (1971): *In vitro* aggregation of mixed embryonic kidney and nerve cells. Influence on macromolecular synthesis. *J. Cell Biol.,* 50:457-468.
57. Morris, J. E., and Moscona, A. A. (1971): The induction of glutamine synthetase in cell aggregates of embryonic neural retina: Correlations with differentiation and multicellular organization. *Dev. Biol.,* 25:420-444.
58. Moscona, A. (1962): Analysis of cell recombinations in experimental synthesis of tissues *in vitro. J. Cell Comp. Physiol.,* 60:65-80.
59. Moscona, M. H., and Moscona, A. A. (1965): Control of differentiation in aggregates of embryonic skin cells: Suppression of feather morphogenesis by cells from other tissues. *Dev. Biol.,* 11:402-423.
60. Nelson, P. G. (1975): Nerve and cells in culture. *Physiol. Rev.,* 55:1-61.
61. Oh, T. H. (1975): Neurotrophic effects: Characterization of the nerve extract that stimulates muscle development in culture. *Exp. Neurol.,* 46:432-438.
62. Oh, T. H., Johnson, D. D., and Kim, S. U. (1972): Neurotrophic effect on isolated chick embryo muscle in culture. *Science,* 178:1298-1300.
63. O'Lague, P. H., MacLeish, P. R., Nurse, C. A., Claude, P., Furshpan, E. J., and Potter, D. D. (1974): Evidence for cholinergic synapses between dissociated rat sympathetic neurons in cell culture. *Proc. Natl. Acad. Sci. USA,* 71:3602-3606.
64. Pappano, A. J., and Loffelhölz, K. (1974): Ontogenesis of adrenergic and cholinergic neuroeffector transmission in chick embryo heart. *J. Pharmacol. Exp. Ther.,* 191:468-478.
65. Purves, R. D., Hill, C. E., Chamley, J. H., Mark, G. E., Frey, D. M., and Burnstock, G. (1974): Functional autonomic neuromuscular junctions in tissue culture. *Pflügers Arch.,* 350: 1-7.
66. Rothman, T. P., Gershon, M. D., and Holtzer, H. (1978): The relationship of cell division to the acquisition of adrenergic characteristics by developing sympathetic ganglion cell precursors. *Dev. Biol.,* 65:322-341.

67. Sachs, C. H., De Champlain, J., Malmfors, T., and Olson, L. (1970): The postnatal development of noradrenaline uptake in the adrenergic nerves of different tissues from the rat. *Eur. J. Pharmacol.,* 9:67-79.
68. Seeds, N. W. (1971): Biochemical differentiation in reaggregating brain culture. *Proc. Natl. Acad. Sci. USA,* 68:1858-1861.
69. Sevier, A. C., and Munger, B. L. (1965): A silver method for paraffin section of neural tissue. *J. Neuropathol. Exp. Neurol.,* 24:130-135.
70. Shigenobu, K., Schneider, J. A., and Sperelakis, N. (1974): Verapamil blockade of slow Na^+ and Ca^{+++} current in myocardial cells. *J. Pharmacol. Exp. Ther.,* 190:280-288.
71. Shimada, Y., and Fischman, D. A. (1973): Morphological and physiological evidence for the development of functional neuromuscular junctions *in vitro. Dev. Biol.,* 31:200-225.
72. Shimada, Y., Fischman, D. A., and Moscona, A. A. (1969): Formation of neuromuscular junctions in embryonic cell cultures. *Proc. Natl. Acad. Sci. USA,* 62:715-721.
73. Shimada, Y., Moscona, A. A., and Fischman, D. A. (1974): Scanning electron microscopy of cell aggregation. Cardiac and mixed retina–cardiac cell suspensions. *Dev. Biol.,* 36:428-446.
74. Sperelakis, N., and Lehmkuhl, D. (1965): Insensitivity of cultured chick heart cells to autonomic agents and tetrodotoxin. *Am. J. Physiol.,* 209:693-698.
75. Steinberg, M. S. (1963): Reconstruction of tissues by dissociated cells. *Science,* 141:401-408.
76. Szepsenwol, J., and Bron, A. (1936): L'origine et la nature de l'innervation primitive du coeur chez les embryons d'oiseaux (canard et poulet). *Rev. Suisse Zool.,* 43:1-23.
77. Varon, S., and Raiborn, D. (1972): Dissociation, fractionation, and culture of chick embryo sympathetic ganglion cells. *J. Neurocytol.,* 1:211-221.
78. Volle, R. L., and Koelle, G. B. (1970): Ganglionic stimulation and blocking agents. In: *The Pharmacological Basis of Therapeutics,* 4th ed., edited by Goodman and Gilman, p. 590. Macmillan, New York.
79. Wollenberger, A. (1964): Rhythmic and arrhythmic contractile activity of single myocardial cells cultured *in vitro. Circ. Res.,* 14-15, Suppl. II:184-201.

DISCUSSION

De Vries: Did you find any evidence of neuromuscular junctions?

Fischman: We have not yet studied the structure of the junctions. Nerve–muscle junctions in the embryonic chick heart are rather primitive, and they do not look like the skeletal neuromuscular junctions. We intend to apply the chromic acid fixation procedure for the TEM, since it gives pretty good catecholamine preservation and reasonable ultrastructure.

Perspectives in Cardiovascular Research, Vol. 5,
Mechanisms of Cardiac Morphogenesis and Teratogenesis,
edited by Tomas Pexieder. Raven Press, New York © 1981

Myofibrillogenesis *In Vitro:* Implications for Early Cardiac Morphogenesis

Robert R. Kulikowski

Department of Anatomy, The University of Chicago, Chicago, Illinois 60637

Shortly after rudimentary heart formation in the chick embryo begins (at 7 to 8 somites), the relatively straight tubular heart undergoes a major morphological change, acquiring a distinctly C-shaped bulge toward the embryonic right side. This process is called looping. During the period of looping, the heart is composed of three layers: the endocardium, the middle connective tissue layer of cardiac jelly, and the outermost myocardium. Concomitant with looping, nascent myofibrils are first observed in the myocardium and the heart begins to beat (8). Myofibrils, at this stage of cardiac development, may be crucial to morphogenesis. It has been demonstrated that protein synthesis (9), and probably that of muscle-specific proteins (2), are required for normal looping to occur. Moreover, formation of fibrillar elements, myofibrils or otherwise, is also essential to normal development (10). Because myofibrillar assembly and growth appear to be as important to looping as the production of myocardial-specific proteins, it is important to consider not only how fibrillogenesis occurs, but also how it is regulated.

During looping, the cells of the myocardium are experiencing significant changes in shape—those on the prospective right side become spread out and flattened, and those on the prospective left side remain columnar. Since myofibrils are forming at this time, it has been postulated (11) that myofibrillar growth could provide the forces responsible for the cell deformations observed in the myocytes. Collectively, these cell shape changes could result in formation of the looped heart. Conversely, the shape changes experienced by the myocytes may be the passive result of forces originating outside the myocardium, but still within the heart. Recent evidence gathered in this laboratory (6) indicates that shape change in cultured embryonic cardiac myocytes temporally precedes myofibrillar formation. Such results effectively rule out myofibrillogenesis as a mechanism of active cell deformation. However, it is still impossible to decide whether the shape changes occurring in cells of the myocardium are the active forces of looping or the passive responses to it.

Whenever a morphological deformation occurs, such as that experienced by the cells of the myocardium during looping, strain is introduced and stress is the result. It has long been believed that strain influences the pattern of fibrillar structures in muscle cells (1). More recently, stress has been recognized to play a role in the development of filament systems of Purkinje fibers (13). These authors have observed that Purkinje fibers and their component myofibrils run parallel to the direction of the calculated tension forces. Accordingly, there appears to be a relationship between myofibril orientation and stress. This interaction may be important in regulating early cardiac morphogenesis (12). In order to explore this proposed regulatory system more fully, we have begun to examine myofibrillogenesis in cultured cells. In the present report, myofibrillogenesis is examined in regions of embryonic cardiac myocyte cytoplasm that are virtually stress-free, and the effects of such an environment on the formation and orientation of myofibrils are probed.

MATERIALS AND METHODS

Cell Cultures

The ventricular portions of hearts from 7-day-old chick embryos were removed aseptically, minced, and washed with Ca^{2+}, Mg^{2+}-free Earle's balanced salt solution (CMF). Subsequent incubation of the ventricular mince in 0.1% trypsin in CMF at 37°C yielded a cell suspension which was filtered through 20 μm mesh nylon cloth and washed with complete medium (Eagle's minimal essential medium without L-glutamine, with Earle's salts, 10% fetal bovine serum, 50 μg/ml streptomycin, 50 U/ml penicillin). Cell density was determined by hemacytometer count in 0.1% trypan blue, and cells were plated at an initial density of 5×10^5 viable cells per ml into Falcon Multiwell tissue culture dishes containing 12 mm round glass coverslips. Cultures were incubated at 37°C in a humid atmosphere of 5% CO_2 in air.

Preparation of Antibody

The preparation and characterization of myosin from adult chicken pectoralis muscle (antigen), as well as the antibody which was subsequently raised against this antigen, have been described elsewhere (6). Briefly, the antibody was shown to react with embryonic cardiac myosin, but not with non-muscle (human platelet) myosin or myofibrillar thin filament proteins.

Localization of Myosin-Containing Structures

Cells adherent to coverslips were washed with phosphate buffered saline (PBS) and then fixed by rapid immersion of the coverslip in absolute acetone at −20°C. Subsequent to washing with PBS, the cells were reacted with the IgG fraction (containing the anti-skeletal muscle myosin antibody) of rabbit immune serum for 30 min at 37°C. Cells were washed copiously with PBS and exposed to rhodamine-conjugated antibody to rabbit IgG prepared in goats (Cappel Laboratories, Cochranville, Pa.). After extensive washing with PBS, cells were mounted in glycerol and examined with a Leitz Orthoplan microscope equipped with epifluorescence optics using a 63x oil-immersion objective (NA = 1.3) and an excitation-barrier filter combination for rhodamine. Images were photographed using Plus-X film (Kodak, Rochester, N.Y.), which was developed in Diafine (Accufine, Inc., Chicago, Ill.) according to the manufacturer's instructions.

RESULTS

When disaggregated by trypsin in divalent cation-depleted medium, embryonic chick cardiac myocytes suffer a reversible disruption of their myofibrils. Subsequent growth in culture results in attachment of the cells to the substrate, their assumption of a typical shape, and the reassembly of their myofibrils. Most myocytes tend to form bipolar cells that have myofibrils aligned parallel to the long axis of the cell (Fig. 1). In these myofibrils, staining with anti-myosin antibody is confined to the A-band region. These mature myofibrils are frequently seen against a cytoplasmic background of extrafibrillar forms of myosin. In some instances, myofibrils are fixed in a contracted state, which results in the appearance of very narrow I-bands.

Some cultured cells, however, do not acquire the typical bipolar shape. Instead, they spread out extremely thinly upon the substrate (Fig. 2A), with no apparent preferred long axis. Before the appearance of definitive myofibrils, the myosin may appear in a variety of morphological forms, such as coarse clumps. Myofibrils that are observed in the interiors of such thinly spread cells appear to lack a preferential orientation (Fig. 2B) and are interspersed among non-fibrillar forms of myosin. Myofibrils that are located at the periphery of such cells do follow the cell outline rather closely.

Other well-spread cells (Fig. 3) exhibit a more extensive array of myofibrils. In the interiors of these cells, myofibrils are not aligned in any apparent pattern. Over a cytoplasmic distribution of non-fibrillar forms of myosin, myofibrils branch and anastomose in nonpredictable patterns. Associated with the myofibrils are short, myosin-containing bars which are approximately the length of the A-band of mature myofibrils. These A-band-sized bars are present at multiple loci along the length of the myofibril (at the level of the I-band), as well as at the free termini. No preferential orientation of these bars is observed. Frequently, several bars are associated with the same I-band, forming varying angles to the main fibrillar axis. Well-developed reticular structures, formed by A-band-sized bars, are often seen connecting adjacent myofibrils.

These points are dramatically illustrated in Fig. 4. The myofibrils in this cell are oriented virtually at right angles to each other, and A-band-sized bars have formed a cross-shaped aggregate around a non-staining area, presumably Z-substance.

Similar observations are made when the fibrillar structures present in the

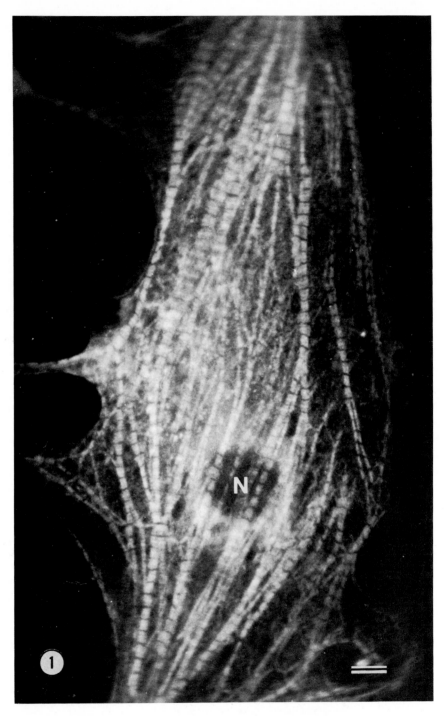

FIG. 1. A cultured embryonic cardiac myocyte stained with anti-muscle myosin antibody. Note the typical bipolar shape of the cell and the alignment of the myofibrils in the long axis. N, nucleus. The calibration bar in this and in Figs. 2-6 all represent 5 μm.

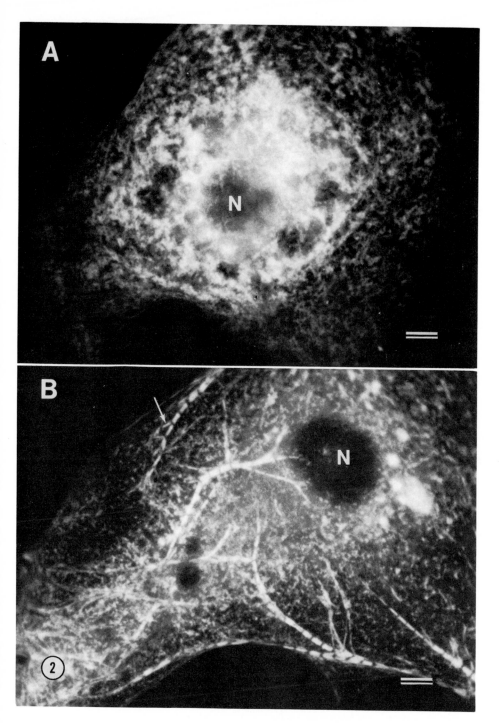

FIG. 2. A: This spreading myocyte exhibits its myosin in predominantly non-fibrillar forms. **B:** In this cell, myofibrils are recognizable over a background of non-fibrillar forms. The fibrils branch and A-band-sized rods are closely associated with them *(arrow)*. N, nucleus.

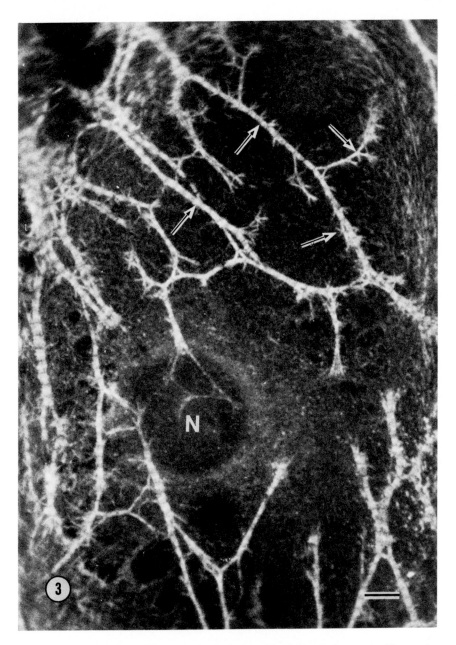

FIG. 3. This micrograph shows the central portion of a well-spread myocyte. The nucleus (N) is apparent as a non-staining circular area. The myofibrils are arranged in a crystalline-like manner throughout the cytoplasm, and have A-band-sized rods associated with them at multiple sites *(arrows)* along their lengths.

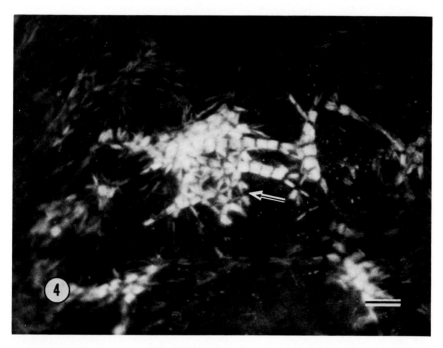

FIG. 4. This portion of a well-spread cell depicts a cluster of myofibrils. Note that the long axes of two myofibrils are oriented at nearly right angles to each other, and A-band-sized segments form a reticular pattern *(arrow)*.

cytoplasm of thinly spread cells do not yet have the form of mature myofibrils. Fig. 5 depicts fibrillar structures that do not exhibit the typical A-band staining pattern seen in mature myofibrils. However, these fibrillar structures do branch and anastomose in a manner similar to the myofibrils shown in Fig. 3. Again, A-band-sized bars are seen in the cytoplasm and at various positions along fibrillar structures, although perhaps not to as great a degree as seen in Fig. 3. The bars do not appear to be localized at specific loci on the fibrillar structures, as is true in the case of mature myofibrils.

Some flattened cells display extreme examples of packing disorder of myofibrils (Fig. 6). These fibrils form a three-dimensional web, interconnected with myosin-containing structures of varying lengths and diameters.

DISCUSSION

Myofibrillogenesis in a Stress-Free Environment

The deformation of cytoplasm results in the production of strain, defined by the equation

$$\sigma = \frac{\Delta l}{l_0}$$

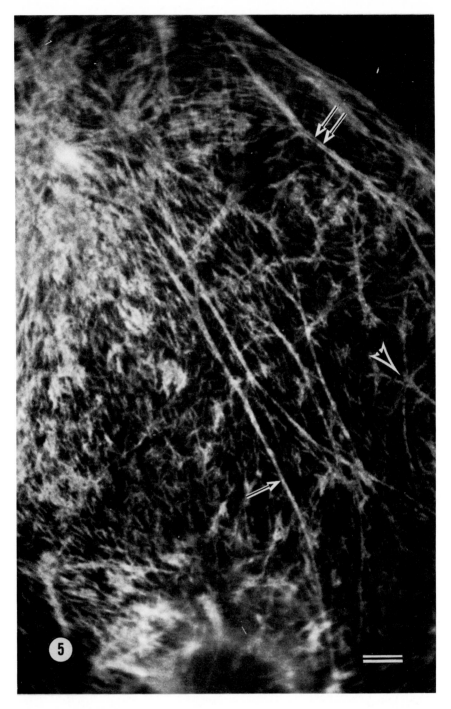

FIG. 5. This well-spread myocyte exhibits many myosin-containing rods, in addition to single *(arrow)* and double *(double arrow)* filamentous structures. The fibers branch and may form stellate structures *(arrowhead)*.

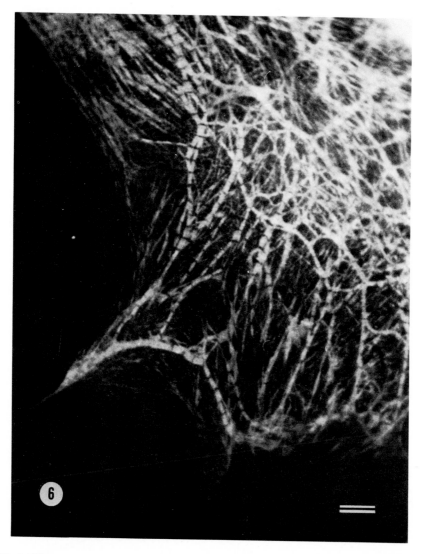

FIG. 6. This portion of a well-spread myocyte demonstrates the elaborate network of myosin-containing structures which may form. Mature myofibrils are seen interconnected by such reticular structures.

where $\Delta 1$ = change in length and 1_0 = original length (15). The force which accompanies strain is stress. When a cultured cell attaches to a substrate and spreads out, it generally does so in a predictable manner, with most of the cytoplasmic deformation occurring at the periphery of the cells, in such specialized structures as lamellopodia (14). If the spreading cell is round, stress will be radially oriented. Because the peripheral cytoplasm is undergoing the greatest amount of deformation and the interior cytoplasm the least (14), a decreasing gradient of strain, and hence of stress, will be set up from the edge to the center of the cell. In the very thin, well-spread myocytes considered here, the central portions of the cells are experiencing little, if any, deformation at the time of examination. Hence, stress in the central portions of these cells will be minimal.

When myofibrils that have formed under relatively stress-free conditions are examined, they appear morphologically normal, but their orientation within the cytoplasm is not predictable. Moreover, fibrillar growth appears to occur in a manner reminiscent of crystal growth. Although the growth of myofibrils in these cells appears to be different from that reported by Legato (7) for cultured cardiac myocytes under similar conditions, other work (6) indicates that myofibrillogenesis is indeed a complex phenomenon. Although our results do not preclude fibril growth by Z-substance hypertrophy (7), fibrils can clearly grow both terminally and laterally by the addition of A-band-sized segments.

It is now germane to consider how stress, or lack thereof, may influence the orientation of such A-band-sized bars. Any linear structures embedded in a viscous medium will tend to be aligned in the direction of stress. Diagrammatically, if the cell depicted in Fig. 7A is deformed in the direction of the arrows, the result would be the cell in Fig. 7B; the rod-shaped structures are oriented parallel to the principal axis of stress. If no stress were introduced, the orientation of the bars would remain as in Fig. 7A. Fibrillogenesis in a stress-free environment could then be viewed as occurring in a pseudocrystalline fashion, with no preferred orientation being indicated by stress patterns.

Implications for Cardiac Morphogenesis

It is important to consider the implications of these results for the *in vivo* event of cardiac looping. We have previously postulated a model of heart looping in which physical forces play an important role (12). This model assumes the embryonic heart to be a hydrostatically supported cylinder, and, as such, myocardial hoop (circumferential) stress is twice myocardial longitudinal stress (15). Further, during looping, the cells of the bulging side of the myocardium undergo the greatest deformation and, therefore, experience the greatest stress in an anterior–posterior dimension. One would then predict, based on the assumption that stress is important for fibrillar orientation, that myofibrils in the pre-looped heart would be predominantly in a circumferential orientation, and that, during looping, myofibrils would be formed along the greater curvature of the heart. This is indeed what is observed (12). Hence, a specific pattern of myofibrils is associated with normal looping, and it coincides with the predicted pattern of stress in the developing organ. The importance of fibrillar patterns in early heart development is reinforced by results obtained with the so-called cardiac lethal mutant of *Ambystoma* (4). The hearts of the mutant embryos do not beat *in situ* and do not contain cross-banded myofibrils. The hearts from *c/c*

A

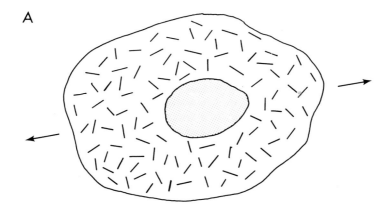

B

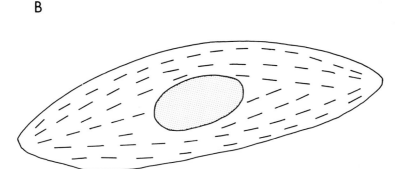

FIG. 7. This figure depicts diagrammatically what happens to rod-shaped structures embedded in a viscous medium when stress is applied in the direction of the arrows. **A.** Before stress; **B.** after stress.

embryos do, however, loop in a relatively normal fashion. Polarized light microscopic examination of these hearts reveals a fibrillar pattern which is very similar to the pattern of myofibrils in a heart from a comparably staged normal sibling (5).

Based on results presented here on myofibrillogenesis in a stress-free environment, as well as on the demonstrated relationship between stress and fibril orientation (3,13), it is tempting to predict that the absence of stress or a significant deviation from the normal stress pattern in the developing heart could result in aberrant patterns of myofibrils. If myofibrils are indeed an underlying regulatory mechanism of early cardiac morphogenesis, it can easily be visualized that abnormal myofibrillar patterns could mediate aberrant looping patterns which, in turn, result in cardiac anomalies.

ACKNOWLEDGMENT

This work was supported by grant HL 13831 from the National Institutes of Health. The author is a Research Fellow of the Chicago Heart Association.

REFERENCES

1. Carey, E. J. (1920): Studies in the dynamics of histogenesis. I. Tension of differential growth as a stimulus to myogenesis. *J. Gen. Physiol.,* 2:357-372.
2. Chacko, S., and Joseph, X. (1974): The effect of 5-bromodeoxyuridine (BrdU) on cardiac muscle differentiation. *Dev. Biol.,* 40:340-354.
3. Gross, W. O., and Müller, C. (1977): A mechanical momentum in ultrastructural development of the heart. *Cell Tiss. Res.,* 178:483-494.
4. Humphrey, R. R. (1972): Genetic and experimental studies on a mutant gene (c) determining absence of heart action in embryos of the Mexican axolotl *(Ambystoma mexicanum). Dev. Biol.,* 27:365-375.
5. Kulikowski, R. R., and Manasek, F. J. (1977): Cardiac mutant salamanders: Evidence for heart induction. *J. Exp. Zool.,* 201:485-490.
6. Kulikowski, R. R., and Manasek, F. J. (1979): Immunofluorescent localization of myosin during myofibril reformation in cultured embryonic cardiac myocytes *(submitted for publication).*
7. Legato, M. J. (1972): Ultrastructural characteristics of the rat ventricular cell grown in tissue culture, with special reference to sarcomerogenesis. *J. Mol. Cell. Cardiol.,* 4:299-317.
8. Manasek, F. J. (1968): Embryonic development of the heart. I. A light and electronmicroscopic study of myocardial development in the early chick embryo. *J. Morphol.,* 125:329-366.
9. Manasek, F. J. (1976): Heart development: interactions involved in cardiac morphogenesis. In: *The Cell Surface in Animal Embryogenesis and Development,* edited by G. Poste and G. Nicholson, pp. 545-598. North-Holland Publishing Co., Amsterdam.
10. Manasek, F. J., Burnside, M. B., and Stroman, J. (1972): The sensitivity of developing cardiac myofibrils to cytochalasin B. *Proc. Natl. Acad. Sci. USA,* 69:308-312.
11. Manasek, F. J., Burnside, M. B., and Waterman, R. E. (1972): Myocardial cell shape change as a mechanism of embryonic heart looping. *Dev. Biol.,* 29:349-371.
12. Nakamura, A., Kulikowski, R. R., Lacktis, J. W., and Manasek, F. J. (1979): Heart looping: A regulated response to deforming forces. In: *Etiology and Morphogenesis of Congenital Heart Disease,* edited by R. Van Praagh and A. Takao. Futura Publ. Co., New York *(in press).*
13. Thornell, L.-E., Sjöström, M., and Andersson, K.-E. (1976): The relationship between mechanical stress and myofibrillar organization in heart Purkinje fibers. *J. Mol. Cell. Cardiol.,* 8:689-695.
14. Vasiliev, J. M., and Gelfand, I. M. (1977): Mechanisms of morphogenesis in cell cultures. In: *Int. Rev. Cytol.,* edited by G. H. Bourne and J. F. Danielli, pp. 159-274. Academic Press, Inc., New York.
15. Wainwright, S. A., Biggs, W. D., Currey, J. D., and Gosline, J. M. (1976): *Mechanical Design in Organisms.* John Wiley and Sons, New York.

DISCUSSION

De Vries: Did you bring cells under stress and watch the realignment of the myofibrils?
Kulikowski: Not yet. We have just finished constructing a device that will do this.
Fischman: Why do you think it is not a prior orientation of other cytoplasmic structures (microtubules, intermediate filaments, and microfilaments), rather than strain itself, that is causing the myofibril orientation?
Kulikowski: I did not try to indicate any mechanisms here. All I wanted to say is

that you get fibrillar deposition or alignment along the predictable principal axes of stress.

De Vries: Can you connect the stress-related myofibril orientation with the looping of the heart?

Kulikowski: During cardiac looping, you get a deformation of the cell, which may then set up a pattern of strain. Resulting stress then allows fibrillar alignment along that direction. That further limits any deformation in that dimension. In that sense, these fibrils act as a cytoskeleton.

Fitzharris: I cannot believe that the stress forces are zero. I think the net effect is zero. Right around the nuclei, you have radial orientation of a fair number of fibrils taking stress in all directions.

DeHaan: If you consider the way cells spread in culture, this is all very circular.

Manasek: I think that Dr. DeHaan is talking now about strain. If you want to deform the cell, you introduce strain. The resulting stress will be directed. It can be predicted that the linear elements, microtubules, myofibrils, or any such elements, will direct the forces. The molecules that interact to form these structures are asymmetric. If one has a stress gradient in an elastic medium, asymmetric structures within will line up along the lines of stress.

Rosenquist: I want to point out another type of strain. In an 11-somite embryo, the cells in the somatic mesoderm would be stretched away from an area in the zona pellucida down towards the heart. This set of stretch relationships is related to the separation of splanchnic and somatic mesoderm. Another set is related to the elongation of the gut, or to the separating dorsal mesocardium.

Genetic Control

Perspectives in Cardiovascular Research, Vol. 5,
Mechanisms of Cardiac Morphogenesis and Teratogenesis,
edited by Tomas Pexieder. Raven Press, New York © 1981

Genetic Aspects of Congenital Heart Disease

Tomas Pexieder

Institut d'Histologie et d'Embryologie, Université de Lausanne, Lausanne, Suisse

Congenital heart disease (CHD) belongs to the category of rather frequent congenital malformations. It is present in 5 to 8.6% of all live births (10,12,18, 26,28,29,33,42) and in 1 to 8% of autopsies (18,49). Of the different structural abnormalities of the heart, ventricular septal defect (VSD) is most frequent (incidence 1.6 to 3.13 per thousand), followed by tetralogy of Fallot (TOF) (incidence 0.3 to 0.8 per thousand), transposition of great vessels (TGV) (incidence 0.2 to 0.8 per thousand), and double-outlet right ventricle (DORV) (incidence 0.04 to 0.1 per thousand) (2,4,23,26,33). This sequence is slightly different in autopsy statistics, in which VSD accounts for 44.3% of all CHD, patent ductus arteriosus (PDA) for 29.3%, atrial septal defect (ASD) for 29.6%, TGV for 17.6%, and pulmonary artery stenosis (PS) for 16.9% (49).

What do we know about the etiology of malformations of the cardiovascular system? As suggested by Mitchell (33), the etiology of CHD may be approached by epidemiologic, genetic, embryologic, and teratological studies. This combination of approaches produces the following distribution of causes of CHD (Fig. 1): 5% are due to pure environmental factors (alcohol, trimethadione, lithium, thalidomide, estrogen and progesterone, hydantoin, amphetamine, hypervitaminosis D, maternal diabetes, viral infections, hypoxia) (9,20,22,24,34,37,45). Hypotheses relevant to the genetic bases of CHD were tested in 1968 by Nora (35). The possibility that there is no genetic contribution was rejected because of the observations of increased frequencies of CHD in family and twin studies, as well as in some studies on animal models. The etiologic contribution of single-gene defects suggested by familial aggregation of ASD, PDA, PS, aortic stenosis (AS) and TOF is presently evaluated as 4%. Chromosomal aberrations (trisomies, monosomies, etc.) underlie about 6% of all CHD. 85% of congenital anomalies of the cardiovascular system are due to gene–environment interactions in the frame of multifactorial etiology (inheritance). The experimental embryology and teratology of the cardiovascular system provide us with some insights into the way environmental and epigenetic factors interact (43). Much less is known about the mechanisms of action of genetic factors (27).

Let us first of all characterize the clinical material for the study of genetic factors. It can be classified in the following groups: 1. familial occurrence of

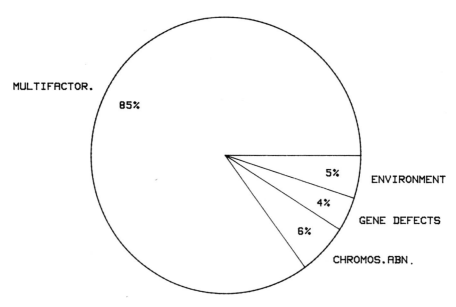

FIG. 1. Etiology of congenital heart disease.

isolated CHD; 2. CHD in syndromes involving abnormal chromosomes; and 3. CHD in syndromes involving normal chromosomes (10,28).

Familial clustering was reported in PDA, ASD (14,51), total anomalous pulmonary venous return (25), coarctation of the aorta (1,46), pulmonary stenosis (1,32), aortic stenosis (19), and in dextrocardia with situs inversus (6).

Whereas CHD was found in 30% of chromosomally abnormal survivors at birth (44), only 1.5% of all ASD, 1.9% of all VSD, 3.7% of all coarctations, and 5% of all aortic stenosis are due to chromosomal abnormalities (11). More important is CHD accompanying specific trisomies. Trisomy 13-15 (D) has a 30 to 97% incidence of CHD composed of dextrocardia, VSD, ASD, DORV, and PDA (31). In trisomy 16-18 (E), the frequency of CHD reaches 80 to 95%, with ASD, VSD, DORV, and PDA as leading lesions (31,34). CHD was observed in 30 to 56% of children suffering trisomy 21. In this particular trisomy, VSD represented 32 to 87%, common atrioventricular ostium 19 to 43%, TOF 6 to 16%, PDA 3 to 6%, and ASD 3 to 76% of all cardiac malformations observed (8,30,31,39,48).

CHD was regularly reported in at least two multiple-malformation syndromes—Di George and Noonan—with normal chromosomes. In the Di George syndrome (partial or complete), concerning the branchial arches and their derivatives, cardiovascular anomalies have been observed in 87% of cases (3,13,17, 21,38,47). Pulmonary stenosis is the predominant lesion of Noonan's syndrome, accompanied in 48 to 100% of cases by CHD (5,7,27,41,50).

Many other syndromes of genetic etiology are accompanied by cardiac defects (34,37). CHD is associated with some of the skeletal-defects syndromes such as Ellis-van Creveld, Laurence-Moon-Biedl, Holt-Oram, Fanconi, and Rubinstein-Taybi. CHD is also observed in syndromes typified by characteristic facies, e.g., Smith-Lemli-Opitz, Cornelia de Lange, Goldenhar, and Williams-Elfin. Among the syndromes in which skin lesions are predominant, CHD was reported in Forney and Leopard syndrome, neurofibromatosis, and tuberous sclerosis. Kartagener and Ivemark syndromes, characterized by situs inversus, also frequently display CHD. Finally, certain anomalies of the cardiovascular system were regularly observed in congenital connective tissue disorders such as Marfan and Ehler-Danlos syndromes, cutis laxa, osteogenesis imperfecta, and pseudoxanthoma tuberosum.

Multifactorial etiology, as recently redefined (15), means "determined by a combination of several genetic factors of unspecific nature and environmental factors." In such instances, the environmental triggers are supposed to act upon developmental thresholds (36). Recently, two new and more or less contradictory and, paradoxically, more or less complementary, concepts have arisen. The first (16) is based on comparison of familial associations of PS, VSD, and TOF with the keeshond dog model (40). In this concept, it is suggested that there is either some nonspecific predisposition (genetic, environmental, or multifactorial) to CHD in general, or that some categories of heart malformations classified as dissimilar are, in fact, similar in etiology. The second concept (52) proposes the possibility that, even within the frame of multifactorial inheritance or etiology, varying types of CHD and the individual families cannot conform with one and the same etiological model.

What is the relevance of these essentially clinically-based observations on the genetic component of CHD to experimental research? First of all, these observations support the multiparametric (multifactorial) concept of heart development as discussed in the organogenesis section of this volume. Furthermore, they provide a background for the rising interest in studies of pathogenesis of CHD of purely genetic etiology (see also p. 389). According to Fraser (15), further progress will certainly depend on identifying the biological attributes of the predisposing factors. This is a specific task for those who study the experimental embryology and teratology of the heart. Some of these studies may perhaps, in a feedback way, help clinicians to identify genetic markers for identifying the family at risk before a CHD is experienced (36).

ACKNOWLEDGMENTS

This work was supported by Grant No. 3.162.0.77 from the Swiss National Science Foundation, and by the Sandoz Foundation.

REFERENCES

1. Bødiker Henriksen, J., Sørland, S. J., and Torp, K. H. (1973): Arv og mdefødte feil i bjerte og sentrale kar. *Tidsskr. Nor. Laegerforen.*, 93:1506-1508.
2. Bound, J. P., and Logan, W. F. (1977): Incidence of congenital heart disease in Blackpool 1957–1971. *Br. Heart J.*, 39:445-451.

3. Cameron, A. H. (1965): Malformations of the thymus and cardiovascular system. *Arch. Dis. Child,* 40:334.

4. Campbell, M. (1973): Incidence of cardiac malformations at birth and later and neonatal mortality. *Br. Heart J.,* 35:189-200.

5. Caralls, D. G., Char, F., Graber, J. D., and Voigt, G. C. (1974): Delineation of multiple cardiac anomalies associated with the Noonan syndrome in an adult and review of the literature. *Johns Hopkins Med. J.,* 134:346-355.

6. Chib, P., Grover, D. N., and Shahi, B. N. (1977): Unusual occurrence of dextrocardia with situs inversus in succeeding generations of a family. *J. Med. Genet.,* 14:30-33.

7. Colloridi, V., Seganti, V., Vestri, A., and Reale, A. (1977): Congenital heart diseases in Noonan's syndrome. *Eur. J. Cardiol.,* 5:291.

8. Cyhlar, M. M., and Wimmer, M. (1976): Congenital heart disease and Downs syndrome. *Paediatr. Paedol.,* 11:254-260.

9. de la Cruz, M. V., Munoz-Castellanos, L., and Nadal-Ginar, B. (1971): Extrinsic factors in the genesis of congenital heart disease. *Br. Heart J.,* 33:203-213.

10. Emanuel, R. (1970): Genetics and congenital heart disease. *Br. Heart J.,* 32:281-291.

11. Emerit, I., de Grouchy, J., Vernant, P., and Corone, P. (1967): Chromosomal abnormalities and congenital heart disease. *Circulation,* 36:886-905.

12. Esscher, E., Michaelsson, M., and Smedby, B. (1975): Cardiovascular malformation in infant death. 10-year clinical and epidemiological study. *Br. Heart J.,* 37:824-829.

13. Finley, J. P., Collins, G. F., De Chadarevian, J. P., and Williams, R. L. (1977): Di George syndrome presenting as severe congenital heart disease in the newborn. *Can. Med. Ass. J.,* 116:641-645.

14. Frantsev, V. I., and Kostylev, E. G. (1971): Familial congenital heart defects. *Vopr. Okhr. Materin. Det.,* 16:23-26.

15. Fraser, F. C. (1976): The multifactorial/threshold concept—Uses and misuses. *Teratology,* 14:267-280.

16. Fraser, F. C., and Hunter, A. D. W. (1975): Etiologic relations among categories of congenital heart malformations. *Am. J. Cardiol.,* 36:793-796.

17. Freedom, R. M., Rosen, F. S., and Nadas, A. S. (1972): Congenital cardiovascular disease and anomalies of the third and fourth pharyngeal pouch. *Circulation,* 46:165-172.

18. Freire-Maia, N., and Arce-Gomez, B. (1971): The epidemiology of congenital cardiovascular malformations. *Hum. Hered.,* 21:209-215.

19. Gaudreault, M., Jean, J. D., Savard, Y., Lapointe, V., and Belanger, M. (1974): Familial supravalvular aortic stenosis. *Union Méd. Canada,* 103:1582-1588.

20. Gautier, M. (1973): Etiology of congenital cardiopathies with malformations. *Rev. Prat.,* 23:4491-4502.

21. Harvey, J. C., Dungan, W. T., Elders, M. J., and Hughes, E. R. (1970): Third and fourth pharyngeal pouch syndrome, associated vascular anomalies and hypocalcemic seizures. *Clin. Pediatr.,* 68:496-499.

22. Heinonen, O. P., Slone, D., Monson, R. R., Hook, E. B., and Shapiro, S. (1977): Cardiovascular birth defects and antenatal exposure to female sex hormones. *N. Engl. J. Med.,* 296:67-69.

23. Hoffman, J. I. E., and Christianson, R. (1978): Congenital heart disease in a cohort of 19,502 births with long-term follow-up. *Am. J. Cardiol.,* 42:641-647.

24. Jackson, B. T. (1968): Review article: The pathogenesis of congenital cardiovascular anomalies. *N. Engl. J. Med.,* 279:25-29, 80-89.

25. Kaufman, R. L., Boynton, R. C., and Harmann, A. F. (1972): Family studies in congenital heart. 3. Total anomalous pulmonary venous connection in sisters and their female maternal 1st cousin. In: *New Syndromes,* edited by D. Bergsma and R. B. Lowry, pp. 88-91. *Birth Defects: Orig. Art. Ser.,* vol. VIII, no. 5. Alan R. Liss, New York.

26. Kenna, A. P., Smithells, R. W., and Fiedling, D. W. (1975): Congenital heart diseases in Liverpool: 1960–1969. *Quart. J. Med.,* 44:17-44.

27. Keutel, J. (1975): Genetic problems in pediatric cardiology. *Klin. Paediatr.,* 187:1-13.

28. Kienast, W., Wagner, G., and Klaube, A. (1975): Hereditary prognosis in congenital cardiopathies. In: *Humangenetische Beratung genetisch belasteter Personen,* edited by H. Bach, pp. 206-211. F. Schiller Univ., Jena.

29. Klimentova, T. (1977): Some genetic aspects of congenital heart defects. *Bratisl. Lék. Listy,* 67:221-226.

30. Laursen, H. B. (1976): Congenital heart disease in Down's syndrome. *Brit. Heart J.*, 38:32-38.
31. Maragos, G. D., and Greene, C. A. (1973): Syndromes association with congenital heart disease and chromosomal aberrations. *Paediatrician*, 2:278-283.
32. McCarron, W., and Perloff, J. K. (1974): Familial congenital valvular pulmonic stenosis. *Am. Heart J.*, 88:357-359.
33. Mitchell, S. C., Sellmann, A. H., Westphal, M. C., and Park. J. (1971): Etiologic correlates in a study of congenital heart disease in 56,109 births. *Am. J. Cardiol.*, 28:653-657.
34. Noonan, J. A. (1978): Association of congenital heart disease with syndromes of other defects. *Pediatr. Clin. North Am.*, 25:797-816.
35. Nora, J. J. (1968): Multifactorial inheritance hypothesis for the etiology of congenital heart disease. *Circulation*, 38:604-617.
36. Nora, J. J. (1974): Genetic counseling in congenital heart disease. *Adv. Cardiol.*, 11:56-66.
37. Nora, J. J., and Nora, A. H. (1978): *Genetics and Counseling in Cardiovascular Diseases*. C. C. Thomas, Springfield.
38. Pabst, H. F., Wright, W. C., Le Riche, J., and Stierm, R. R. (1976): Partial Di George syndrome with substantial cell-mediated immunity. *Am. J. Dis. Child*, 130:316-319.
39. Park, S. C., Mathews, R. A., Zuberbuhler, J. R., Rowe, R. D., Neches, W. H., and Lenox, C. C. (1977): Down syndrome with congenital heart malformation. *Am. J. Dis. Child*, 131:29-34.
40. Patterson, D. F., Pyle, R. L., and Van Mierop, L. (1974): Hereditary defects of the conotruncal septum in Keeshond dogs: Pathologic and genetic studies. *Am. J. Cardiol.*, 34:187-205.
41. Pearl, W. (1977): Cardiovascular anomalies in Noonan's syndrome. *Chest*, 71:677-680.
42. Pentek, E., and Szendrei, E. (1975): Incidence of congenital heart disease in Hungary: Pécs and Baranya County. *Acta Paediatr.*, 16:55-57.
43. Pexieder, T. (1980): Cellular mechanisms underlying the normal and abnormal development of the heart. In: *Etiology and Morphogenesis of Congenital Heart Disease*, edited by R. van Praagh and A. Takao, pp. 127–153. Futura Publ. Co., New York.
44. Polani, P. E. (1968): Chromosomal abnormalities and congenital heart disease. *Guy's Hosp. Rep.* 117:323-337.
45. Rowland, T. W., Hubbell, J. P., and Nadas, A. S. (1973): Congenital heart disease in infants of diabetic mothers. *J. Pediatr.*, 83:815-820.
46. Simon, A. B., Zloto, A. E., Perry, B. L., and Sigmann, J. M. (1974): Familial aspects of coarctation of the aorta. *Chest*, 66:687-689.
47. Stern, A. M., Sigmann, J. M., Perry, B. L., Kuhns, L. R., and Poznanski, A. K. (1977): An association of aorticotruncoconal abnormalities, velopalatine incompetence, and unusual cervical spine fusion. In: *New Syndromes*, edited by D. Bergsma and R. B. Lowry, p. 259. *Birth Defects: Orig. Art. Ser.*, vol. VIII, no. 5. Alan R. Liss, New York.
48. Tandon, R., and Edwards, J. E. (1973): Cardiac malformations associated with Down's syndrome. *Circulation*, 47:1349-1355.
49. Terribile, V., and Pertile, C. (1975): Congenital heart defects, anatomopathological study of 307 cases. *Riv. Anat. Patol. Oncol.*, 40:25-54.
50. Velichkova, D., Atanasova, L., Slavinska, L., Arnaudov, N., and Markova, R. (1977): Cardiac malformations in Noonan's syndrome. *Eur. J. Cardiol.*, 5:290-291.
51. Zer, M., and Levy, M. J. (1971): Familial congenital heart disease. *Harefuah*, 80:535-537.
52. Zetterqvist, P. (1977): Recurrence risk in CHD. *Circulation*, 55:555-556.

Perspectives in Cardiovascular Research, Vol. 5,
Mechanisms of Cardiac Morphogenesis and Teratogenesis,
edited by Tomas Pexieder. Raven Press, New York © 1981

Congenital Heart Disease in Experimental (Fetal) Mouse Trisomies: Incidence

Tomas Pexieder,* Shinichi Miyabara,** and Alfred Gropp**

Institut d'Histologie et d'Embryologie, Université de Lausanne, Lausanne, Suisse
***Institut für Pathologie, Medizinische Hochschule Lübeck,**
Lübeck, Bundesrepublik Deutschland

Our understanding of the etiology and pathogenesis of congenital heart disease (CHD) in human populations is largely dependent on the availability of suitable animal models (35,38). According to Nora (20), 2% of CHD is due to the presence of a single mutant gene and 4% are found associated with chromosomal anomalies. Isolated environmental factors are responsible for 1% of all CHD. A multifactorial etiology underlies the vast majority of human CHD (93%).

Do we have animal models for all four etiologic categories?

Cardiac anomalies in S-line strain of Brown Leghorn (46), Olson-Goss strain of Long-Evans rats (6), blotchy mouse (1), and iv/iv mouse (14) represent animal models of single-gene defect etiology. The different situations in which an extrinsic environmental factor was used to produce CHD have been reviewed by Le Douarin (15), Okamoto (21,22), Hörnblad (10), and, recently, by one of us (39). Heart malformations reported in particular dog breeds (19,24,25,26,27, 28,29,45) are considered to be animal models of CHD of multifactorial inheritance and perhaps also of multifactorial etiology. Particular attention was paid to studies of poodles (4,12,30,31), Keeshond (31,49,50), and Newfoundland dogs (42).

Until 1977, there was no animal model for CHD associated with chromosomal anomalies. Using the recently developed technique for experimental production of trisomy in mice (7), we have discovered and made preliminary reports (36, 40,41) on the presence of heart malformations in trisomic mice. In the present chapter, we will report on and discuss in detail the incidence of various abnormalities of heart development on the 15th e.d. in experimental fetal mouse trisomy.

MATERIALS AND METHODS

Since all of our experience with morphogenesis and teratogenesis of the heart was based on our previous work with chick embryo (34,37), we had to start with an analysis of normal cardiac morphogenesis in the mouse. Preliminary studies were performed and the methods elaborated on A/JAX mice. When we learned that the background for experimental production of trisomies was the strain NMRI, we performed supplementary studies on this strain. Finally, just as the trisomic mice were bred in Lübeck and transported by rail to Lausanne for analysis, we completed the controls with normal NMRI mice bred in Lübeck and transported by railway to Lausanne. Our aim for this control group was to see if the stress of railway transport of a pregnant female has any effect on heart formation. Taken together, the control groups were comprised of 22 pregnant females, with 212 living fetuses (Table 1). The experimental trisomies were obtained by mating NMRI females to males with defined Robertsonian translocations, a method developed by Gropp (7,8). For instance, to obtain trisomy 12 a male that was a double heterozygote with Robertsonian translocation on chromosomes 9 and 5—Rb(8.12)5/Rb(4.12)9Bnr—was used. We analyzed trisomies 10, 12, 13, 14, 16, and 19. The trisomy group totaled 86 females, with 585 living fetuses. The day at which the vaginal plug appeared was considered in all series as Day 1 of gestation. On the 15th e.d., females were injected i.p. with 0.2 ml Colcemid to facilitate the forthcoming karyotyping. Thirty min later the females were killed by cervical dislocation and the uterine horns exposed by laparotomy for inspection. Following statistics of resorptions, the fetuses were removed and fetal membranes sampled for karyotyping. Once removed, each fetus was weighed. Using a dissecting microscope, the thoracic cavity and the pericardium were opened. External inspection of the heart was followed by microdissection of the right ventricular cavity. Malformed hearts were fixed by 2% glutaraldehyde and 1% formaldehyde in 0.1 M cacodylate buffer adjusted to 330 mOsm and further processed for SEM. For illustration, some other malformed specimens were left undissected. Such hearts were fixed by microperfusion with the same fixative. Different phases of the dissection were photographed by a Wild P200 photomacroscope. Finally, the independently obtained genetic and cardiologic diagnoses were combined to produce Table 2.

TABLE 1. *Description of the control group at 15 e.d.*

Control	NMRI Lausanne	A/JAX Lausanne	NMRI transported
Pregnant females	4	3	15
Resorptions	0	0	13
Dead fetuses	0	0	4
Malformed fetuses	0	1	1
Living fetuses	45	22	145
Normal heart	32	17	88
FIV	13	5	54
VSD	0	0	3

TABLE 2. Description of the trisomic group at 15 e.d. Heart status uses the number of living fetuses as denominator (equal to 100%).

Trisomy	Tr 10	Tr 12	Tr 13	Tr 14	Tr 16	Tr 19
Pregnant females	11	19	16	21	14	5
Resorptions	14	33	26	55	33	6
Dead fetuses	3	23	0	0	1	0
Living fetuses	61	110	78	193	94	49
Frequency of trisomy	8.8%	28.2%	25.6%	19.2%	16.0%	6.1%
Normal heart	47.5%	83.4%	71.8%	51.8%	64.9%	40.8%
FIV	34.3%	18.0%	2.6%	20.7%	13.8%	24.5%
VSD	18.2%[a]	14.8%[b]	0	19.2%[c]	11.7%[d]	32.6%[e]
Pst	0	0	21.8%	0	0	0
DORV	0	0	2.6%	5.7%	9.6%	2.1%
TGA	0	0	0	2.6%	0	0

[a] 30% trisomic.
[b] 100% trisomic.
[c] 51% trisomic.
[d] 82% trisomic.
[e] 6% trisomic.

RESULTS

Normal Mouse Fetuses (Table 1)

In untransported A/JAX and NMRI 15th e.d. fetuses, there were no resorptions nor dead fetuses. All of the fetuses had externally normal hearts and great vessels. Microdissection revealed that, at this stage of development, 28.9% of NMRI and 22.7% of A/JAX fetuses exhibited a foramen interventriculare (FIV). The railway transport (11 hours) of normal pregnant NMRI females produced an increase in fetal mortality, and increased the frequency of FIV to 37.2%. In 2.1% of living fetuses, a ventricular septal defect (VSD) was found. There was no other cardiac abnormality in any of the three control groups.

Trisomic Fetuses (Table 2)

Trisomy 10 was present in only a small proportion of surviving fetuses (8.8%). 18.2% of the living fetuses suffered a VSD, but only 30% of VSD-afflicted fetuses were trisomic.

Trisomy 12, comprising 28.2% of the trisomies, had the best rate of survival. In 14.8% of all survivors, a VSD (Fig. 1b) was found. All of the VSD showed the trisomic karyotype.

Trisomy 13 was the second highest frequency of the trisomies (25.6%). Very characteristic of this trisomy was pulmonary stenosis (Fig. 2) with VSD and overriding aorta. 2.6% of the living embryos with this trisomy presented with a double outlet right ventricle (DORV).

Trisomy 14 frequency was 19.2%. 19.2% of the living fetuses in this experiment have displayed VSD. 51% of all VSD occurred in trisomic fetuses. There were also some cases of DORV and of transposition of the great vessels (Fig. 6).

Trisomy 16 was present in 16% of living fetuses. There was an 11.7% frequency of VSD, of which 82% displayed the trisomic karyotype. This trisomy had the highest frequency (9.6%) of DORV (Fig. 1c).

Trisomy 19 was almost nonexistent on the 15th e.d. (6.1%). There was a 32.6% frequency of VSD, but only 6% of them occurred in trisomies. There were some cases (2.1%) of DORV.

Heart Anomalies in Fetuses with "Normal" or "Undetermined" Karyotype

Seven embryos with trisomy 14 and 2 embryos with trisomy 16, with apparently normal karyotype, presented with VSD. Problems with preparation artifacts prevented us from precisely determining the karyotype in one fetus from the trisomy 16 series. This embryo presented a DORV. We were unable to determine the karyotype of 7 embryos from the trisomy 14 series. Four of them suffered VSD and three had a DORV.

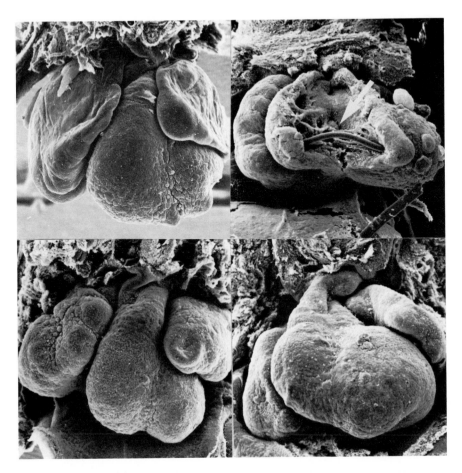

FIG. 1. SEM of normal and trisomic mouse hearts at 15 e.d. **a (top left):** normal NMRI heart, x 33. **b (top right):** ventricular septal defect *(arrow)* in trisomy 12, x 50. **c (bottom left):** double-outlet right ventricle in trisomy 16, x 39. **d (bottom right):** transposition of great vessels in trisomy 14, x 39.

DISCUSSION

We chose embryonic day 15 in mouse for our incidence study as a compromise between a reasonable survival of trisomic fetuses and a stage representing the end of heart organogenesis, which is closure of the interventricular foramen. In the absence of any reliable data on embryonic development of the mouse heart, we established that, at 15 e.d., 77.3% of A/JAX and 71.1% of NMRI fetuses closed their IVF. According to the statistical analysis performed by Professor R. G. Carpenter from the London School of Hygiene and Tropical Medicine, the proportions of closed FIV in the two strains are not significantly different. The weight differences between the A/JAX and NMRI fetuses with terminated heart organogenesis, previously reported (36), were highly significant.

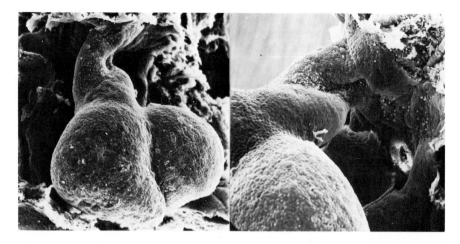

FIG. 2. SEM of pulmonary stenosis in trisomy 13 at 15 e.d. **left:** frontal view after removal of both atria, x 50. **right:** left lateral view of the same heart, x 90.

It should be stressed that, with the exception of exencephaly in trisomy 12, and a weak edema in trisomy 13 and 14, no other external malformations were found in trisomic fetuses. This underlines the importance of careful microdissection in diagnosing fetal anomalies. Variations in the frequency of trisomic fetuses (6.1 to 28.2%, Table 2) depend on individual metacentric combinations and trisomy-dependent sequential elimination of aneuploid embryos (7). With the exception of trisomy 19 (51,52), trisomic fetuses die in earlier or later stages of prenatal ontogenesis. Mouse fetal trisomy is therefore different from that in humans, in whom some types of trisomy can survive into postnatal or even adult life. The extremely low frequency of trisomy 19 in our studies is in contrast to figures given previously by Gropp (7). This may possibly be explained by the limited number of pregnant females with this particular trisomy investigated in the present study.

The interpretation of cases with "normal" or "undetermined" karyotype deserves particular attention. Analysis of the 145 fetuses from pregnant NMRI mice exposed to transport stress does not show, with the exception of VSD, any cardiac anomalies found in the trisomy series, such as pulmonary artery stenosis, DORV, or TGA. VSD found in embryos with normal karyotype in trisomy 14 and 16 experiments can therefore be considered as trisomy-unrelated. By the same token, in the group of fetuses with undetermined karyotype, the fetuses with DORV were probably trisomics. As has been already reported in cleft palate studies (2,3,17,33), transport-related stress is an important teratogenic agent. In our studies, the transport of pregnant females on 8 to 10 e.d. resulted in 9% resorption. Development of the heart was delayed, and the proportion of FIV not yet closed rose from 29% in untransported to 37% in transported NMRI mice.

There have been remarkable manifestations of maternal (litter-bound) factors in trisomy 14 and 16. In one lot of 17 females in the trisomy 14 experiments, two mice had 33 and 38% frequency of trisomic fetuses. These litters were responsible for 75% of all cases of TGA and 40% of all DORV (expected frequencies 8.3%). Similarly, in the trisomy 16 series, of 11 females one produced a litter with a frequency of trisomy as high as 37%. This litter was responsible for one-third of all VSD (expected frequency 9%).

When we look at the heart anomalies found in the trisomy group (Table 2), we can distinguish between trisomy-specific and trisomy-unspecific malformations. Whereas VSD is a trisomy-unspecific anomaly, pulmonary stenosis is highly specific, occurring only in trisomy 13, as is TGA in trisomy 14. DORV is not very specific, since we can see this defect in trisomy 13, 14, 16, and 19. VSD can be considered as a typical anomaly of trisomy 12 only. The percentage of VSD in fetuses with normal karyotype from progeny of Rb heterozygotes (Table 2) is always higher than the percentage seen in transported controls (2%). We suggest, as an explanation, the interaction of an instable genetic background with the teratogenic action of transport stress.

Although the series of anomalies in trisomy 14 (VSD, DORV, TGA) may be interpreted as a continuous spectrum, the coexistence of DORV and pulmonary stenosis in trisomy 13 does not support such a theory. On the other hand, the increased frequency of VSD was accompanied by an increased occurrence of FIV in all of the trisomies studied.

Let us compare fetal mouse trisomy with other established models of congenital heart disease, in frequency and primary lesion. With the exception of trisomies 10 and 19, 95 to 100% of trisomic mouse fetuses had a heart anomaly. The iv/iv strain of mice has a 78% frequency of CHD. The most frequent lesions were atrial anomalies, followed by endocardial cushion defects, VSD, and TGA (14). In 76.9% of the S-line of Brown Leghorn, a VSD was present (43,44). 58.3% of specially bred poodles presented a patent ductus arteriosus (30). The Keeshond strain of dogs also had a reasonable high frequency (53.7%) of conotruncal defects (50). Discrete subaortic stenosis was present in 30.2% of Newfoundland dogs (42). A much lower frequency (9%) of left heart hypoplasia was found in minipigs (48).

Some of the human trisomies are known to be accompanied by congenital heart disease. About 50% of all trisomy-21 children suffer from some form of heart anomaly. Most frequent are VSD (36.7%), endocardial cushion defects (37.7%), tetralogy of Fallot (11.2%), and patent ductus arteriosus (4.4%) (5, 13,23,47). Other human trisomies reported have been trisomy 13–15, with 70.3% of CHD (dextrocardia, VSD, atrial septal defect, DORV, patent ductus arteriosus) and trisomy 16–18, with 89.7% of CHD (atrial septal defect, DORV, patent ductus arteriosus) (11,16). It is interesting that in our trisomic mouse, in the iv/iv mouse (14) and in human trisomies 13 and 18, DORV is more frequent than in the human population in general, in which the frequencies of TGA and tetralogy of Fallot are higher (9,18). We must also speculate about the possibility that the DORV we see at 15 e.d. in mouse fetuses may develop further into another kind of anomaly, which at birth would no longer be diagnosed as DORV.

We would like to close the discussion by analyzing the prospective importance of fetal mouse trisomy as an animal model of human congenital heart disease. Even if not all fetuses from a litter can be made trisomic, the high liability of fetal mouse trisomics to heart anomalies make them, together with the dog models mentioned, a most suitable system to study. In spite of the fact that congenital heart disease in the dog is of multifactorial etiology, and therefore resembles etiologically the vast majority of human CHD, fetal mouse trisomy seems to be the best model of cardiac malformations found in human chromosomal aberrations. It has also the advantage of easier breeding, embryo staging, bigger litter size, and lower cost. We can take advantage of the presence of a marker, which is the trisomy as seen in a karyotype, to detect the abnormal embryos. This is of importance in identifying the very early stages of pathogenesis. We believe that the future use of genetic backgrounds other than NMRI might eventually extend the viability of trisomic fetuses behind birth, and so increase the degree of analogy with human trisomies. Reexamination of some of the trisomies in the absence of the transport stress would certainly aid our insight into gene–environment interactions in the genesis of congenital heart disease. We are most interested to learn whether the teratogenic mechanisms operating under purely genetic influences are the same as those found with extrinsic teratogens. We consider this model to be very promising for forthcoming studies of pathogenesis of selected anomalies of the heart and great vessels.

ACKNOWLEDGMENTS

This study was supported by the Swiss National Science Foundation Grant No. 3.162.0.77, the Sandoz Foundation, and the Deutsche Forschungsgemeinschaff (Gr 71/43).

REFERENCES

1. Andrews, E. J., White, W. J., and Bullock, L. P. (1975): Spontaneous aortic aneurysms in blotchy mice. *Am. J. Path.,* 78:199-210.
2. Barlow, S. M., McElhatton, P. R., and Sullivan, F. M. (1975): The relation between maternal restraint and food deprivation, plasma corticosterone, and induction of cleft palate in the offspring of mice. *Teratology,* 12:97-104.
3. Brown, K. S., Johnston, M. C., and Niswander, J. D. (1972): Isolated cleft palate in mice after transportation during gestation. *Teratology,* 5:119-124.
4. Buchanan, J. W. (1978): Morphology of the ductus arteriosus in fetal and neonatal dogs genetically predisposed to patent ductus arteriosus. In: *Morphogenesis and Malformation of the Cardiovascular System,* edited by G. C. Rosenquist and D. Bergsma, pp. 349-360. *Birth Defects: Orig. Art. Ser.,* vol. XIV, no. 7. Alan R. Liss, New York.
5. Cyhlar, M. M., and Wimmer, M. (1976): Congenital heart disease and Downs syndrome. *Paediatr. Paedol.,* 11:254-260.
6. Fox, M. H. (1967): Genetic transmission of congenital membranous ventricular septal defects in selectively inbred substrains of rats. *Circ. Res.,* 20:422-433.

7. Gropp, A. (1975): Chromosomal animal model of human disease. Fetal trisomy and developmental failure. In: *Teratology, Trends and Applications,* edited by C. L. Berry and D. E. Poswillo, pp. 17-33. Springer-Verlag, Berlin.

8. Gropp, A., Kolbus, U., and Giers, D. (1975): Systematic approach to the study of trisomy in the mouse. II. *Cytogenet. Cell Genet.,* 14:42-62.

9. Hoffman, J. I. E., and Christianson, R. (1978): Congenital heart disease in a cohort of 19,502 births with long-term follow-up. *Am. J. Cardiol.,* 42:641-647.

10. Hörnblad, Y. (1971): Experimentally induced malformation of heart and vessels. *Opusc. Med.,* 16:110-120.

11. Keutel, J. (1975): Genetic problems in pediatric cardiology. *Klin. Paediatr.,* 187:1-13.

12. Knight, D. N., Patterson, D. F., and Melbin, J. (1973): Constriction of the fetal ductus arteriosus induced by oxygen, acetylcholine, and norepinephrine in normal dogs and those genetically predisposed to persistent patency. *Circulation,* 47:127-132.

13. Laursen, H. B. (1976): Congenital heart disease in Down's syndrome. *Br. Heart J.,* 38:32-38.

14. Layton, W. M. Jr. (1978): Heart malformations in mice homozygous for a gene causing situs inversus. In: *Morphogenesis and Malformation of the Cardiovascular System,* edited by G. C. Rosenquist and D. Bergsma, pp. 277-293. *Birth Defects: Orig. Art. Ser.,* vol. XIV, no. 7. Alan R. Liss, New York.

15. Le Douarin, G. (1964): Les malformations cardiaques expérimentales. *Erg. Anat. Entw.-Gesch.,* 37:167-193.

16. Maragos, G. D., and Greene, C. A. (1973): Syndromes association with congenital heart disease and chromosomal aberrations. *Paediatrician,* 2:278-283.

17. Michel, C., and Fritzniggli, H. (1978): Induction of developmental anomalies in mice by maternal stress. *Experientia,* 34:105-107.

18. Mitchell, S. C., Sellmann, A. H., Westphal, M. C., and Park, J. (1971): Etiologic correlates in a study of congenital heart disease in 56,109 births. *Am. J. Cardiol.,* 28:653-657.

19. Mulvihill, J. J., and Priester, W. A. (1973): Congenital heart disease in dogs: Epidemiologic similarities to man. *Teratology,* 7:73-78.

20. Nora, J. J. (1974): Genetic counseling in congenital heart disease. *Adv. Cardiol.,* 11:56-66.

21. Okamoto, N. (1969): Experimental production of congenital cardiovascular anomalies (1). *Cong. Anom.,* 9:45-59.

22. Okamoto, N. (1969): Experimental production of congenital cardiovascular anomalies (concluded). *Cong. Anom.,* 9:117-132.

23. Park, S. C., Mathews, R. A., Zuberbuhler, J. R., Rowe, R. D., Neches, W. H., and Lenox, C. C. (1977): Down syndrome with congenital heart malformation. *Am. J. Dis. Child.,* 131:29-34.

24. Patterson, D. F. (1965): Congenital heart disease in the dog. *Ann. N.Y. Acad. Sci.,* 127:541-569.

25. Patterson, D. F. (1968): Epidemiologic and genetic studies of congenital heart disease in the dog. *Circ. Res.,* 23:171-202.

26. Patterson, D. F. (1971): Canine congenital heart disease: Epidemiology and etiological hypotheses. *J. Small Anim. Pract.,* 12:263-287.

27. Patterson, D. F. (1973): Pathologic and genetic studies of congenital heart disease in the dog. In: *Advances in Cardiology 13,* edited by F. Homburger and I. Lucas, pp. 210-249. Karger, Basel.

28. Patterson, D. F. (1976): Congenital defects of cardiovascular system of dogs—Studies in comparative cardiology. In: *Advances in Veterinary Science and Comparative Medicine, vol. 20,* edited by C. A. Brandly, C. E. Cornelius, and W. I. B. Beveridge, pp. 1-38. Academic Press, New York.

29. Patterson, D. F. (1978): Lesion-specific genetic factors in canine congenital heart disease: Patent ductus arteriosus in poodles, defects of the conotruncal septum in the Keeshond. In: *Morphogenesis and Malformation of the Cardiovascular System,* edited by G. C. Rosenquist and D. Bergsma, pp. 315-347. *Birth Defects: Orig. Art. Ser.,* vol. XIV, no. 7. Alan R. Liss, New York.

30. Patterson, D. F., and Detweiler, D. K. (1967): Hereditary transmission of patent ductus arteriosus in the dog. *Am. Heart J.,* 74:289-290.

31. Patterson, D. F., Pyle, R. L., Buchanan, J. W., Trautvetter, E., and Abt, D. A. (1971): Hereditary patent ductus arteriosus and its sequelae in the dog. *Circ. Res.,* 29:1-13.

32. Patterson, D. F., Pyle, R. L., and Van Mierop, L. (1974): Hereditary defects of the conotruncal septum in Keeshond dogs: Pathologic and genetic studies. *Am. J. Cardiol.,* 34:187-205.

33. Peters, S., and Strassburg, M. (1969): Stress als teratogener Faktor. Tierexperimentelle Unter-suchungen zur Erzeugung von Gaumenspalten. *Arzneimittel Forsch.,* 19:1106-1110.
34. Pexieder, T. (1975): Cell death in the morphogenesis and teratogenesis of the heart. *Adv. Anat., Embryol. Cell Biol.,* 51/3:1-100.
35. Pexieder, T. (1977): Pathogenie des malformations cardiaques. *Bull. Fond. Suisse Cardiol.,* 8:42-48.
36. Pexieder, T. (1978a): Development of the outflow tract of the embryonic heart. In: *Morphogenesis and Malformation of the Cardiovascular System,* edited by G. C. Rosenquist and D. Bergsma, pp. 29-68. *Birth Defects: Orig. Art. Ser.,* vol. XIV, no.7. Alan R. Liss, New York.
37. Pexieder, T. (1978b): Heart anomalies in fetal mouse trisomy. In: *Morphogenesis and Malforma-tion of the Cardiovascular System,* edited by G. C. Rosenquist and D. Bergsma, pp. 387-390. *Birth Defects: Orig. Art. Ser.,* vol. XIV, no. 7. Alan R. Liss, New York.
38. Pexieder, T. (1979): Changing scene in cardiac embryology. *Herz,* 4:73-77.
39. Pexieder, T. (1980): Cellular mechanisms underlying the normal and abnormal development of the heart. In: *Etiology and Morphogenesis of Congenital Heart Disease,* edited by R. van Praagh and A. Takao, pp. 127–153. Futura Publ. Co., New York.
40. Pexieder, T., and Gropp, A. (1977): Cardiac malformations in mouse fetal trisomy. *Exc. Med. Internat. Congr. Ser.,* 426:38-39.
41. Pexieder, T., Miyabara, S., and Gropp, A. (1979): La trisomie foetale de souris—un modèle animal des cardiopathies congénitales humaines. *Acta Anat. (Basel),* 105:120.
42. Pyle, R. L., Patterson, D. F., and Chacko, S. (1976): Genetics and pathology of discrete subaortic stenosis in Newfoundland dog. *Am. Heart J.,* 92:324-334.
43. Rychter, Z., and Lemež, L. (1978): Development of hereditary ventricular septal defects in Siller's strain of chick embryos. In: *Morphogenesis and Malformation of the Cardiovascular System,* edited by G. C. Rosenquist and D. Bergsma, pp. 377-386. *Birth Defects: Orig. Art. Ser.,* vol. XIV, no. 7. Alan R. Liss, New York.
44. Rychter, Z., Lemež, L., and Siller, W. G. (1960): Descriptive morphogenesis of hereditary ventricular septal defects in Brown Leghorn chick embryos. *Cs. Morfol.,* 8:379-404.
45. Shive, R. J., Hare, W. C. D., and Patterson, D. F. (1965): Chromosome studies in dogs with congenital defects. *Cytogenetics,* 4:340-348.
46. Siller, W. G. (1958): Ventricular septal defects in the fowl. *J. Path. Bacter.,* 76:431-440.
47. Tandon, R., and Edwards, J. E. (1973): Cardiac malformations associated with Down's syn-drome. *Circulation,* 47:1349-1355.
48. Van der Linde-Sipman, J. S. (1977): Het links hypoplastisch hart bij de minipig. Een morfologisch en morfogenetisch onderzoek. (thesis). E. J. Nijkamp & Zn., Gouda.
49. Van Mierop, L. H. S., and Patterson, D. F. (1978): The pathogenesis of spontaneously occurring anomalies of the ventricular outflow tract in Keeshond dogs: Embryologic studies: In: *Morpho-genesis and Malformation of the Cardiovascular System,* edited by G. C. Rosenquist and D. Bergsma, pp. 361-375. *Birth Defects: Orig. Art. Ser.,* vol. XIV, no. 7. Alan R. Liss, New York.
50. Van Mierop, L. H. S., Patterson, D. F., and Schnarr, W. R. (1977): Hereditary conotruncal defects in Keeshond dogs—Embryologic studies. *Am. J. Cardiol.,* 40:936-951.
51. White, B. J., Tjio, J. -H., van de Water, L. C., and Crandall, C. (1974): Trisomy 19 in the laboratory mouse. I. Frequency in different crosses at specific developmental stages and relation-ship of trisomy to cleft palate. *Cytogenet. Cell Genet.,* 13:217-231.
52. White, B. J., Tjio, J. -H., van de Water, L. C., and Crandall, C. (1974): Trisomy 19 in the laboratory mouse. II. Intrauterine growth and histological studies of trisomics and their normal littermates. *Cytogenet. Cell Genet.,* 13:232-245.

DISCUSSION

Clark: One reason that you have such a low incidence of trisomies in a certain group is not because of the lethality of a particular trisomy *per se,* but because the cardiovascular system is not capable of supporting the embryo further in development. It might be necessary to clarify this picture, to go back and obtain embryos especially from the early-death group prior to the critical period that you investigated.

Pexieder: I have been able to dissect dead but not yet autolyzed fetuses. I believe that the principal reason for the low incidence of trisomy 10 and 19 is early death of those fetuses preceding by 2 or 3 days the day of dissection, i.e., between the 10 and 12 e.d.

De Vries: Are you planning to do some teratogenic experiments on these mice? We are interested in strains having high ratios of spontaneous congenital heart anomalies. This increases the probability of getting a reasonable number of phenocopies.

Pexieder: The fetal mouse trisomy can be used this way. We were more interested in obtaining a system in which congenital heart disease will be more or less of purely genetic etiology. One of the primary aims with this model is to answer the question; are the mechanisms acting in these hereditary abnormalities the same as those observed in cardiac anomalies induced by epigenetic, e.g., environmental, factors?

Laane: Do you not think that the presence of tetralogy of Fallot only in trisomy 13 may be contradictory to the hypothesis of Drs. Krediet and Klein, which stresses the importance of hemodynamics in the etiology of heart anomalies?

Pexieder: As our approach has, until now, been essentially epidemiologic, no inference in this sense is allowed. What is important in the contribution of Drs. Krediet and Klein is to realize that we can obtain the same phenocopy by different ways. The tetralogy of Fallot may be due to a primary pulmonary stenosis, or it may be a secondary stenosis due to hemodynamic causes located somewhere in the periphery.

Clark: As the term "tetralogy of Fallot" is a very specific anatomic diagnosis, it should perhaps be avoided in initial characterization studies. Would you rather say "hypoplastic right heart syndrome"?

Pexieder: Actually, only the hypertrophy of the right ventricle is missing, which is obviously related to the fetal aspect of the circulation and respiratory physiology at 15 e.d. The exact anatomic diagnosis would be pulmonary stenosis with ventricular septal defect and overriding aorta.

Hurle: Were all the hearts studied only by scanning electron microscopy?

Pexieder: The vast majority of the fetal mouse hearts were studied by microdissection, under a dissecting microscope, for the presence of external *and* internal anomalies. Some malformed hearts were prepared for illustrative purposes, for SEM.

Dor: Did you find any symptoms of adherences on the heart which might explain the double-outlet right ventricle?

Pexieder: No, we have never seen them. Furthermore, I am convinced that the cause is directly or indirectly related to the chromosomal aberrations, and is certainly not of infectious or other epigenetic origin.

Epigenetic Control of Cardiac Morphogenesis

Perspectives in Cardiovascular Research, Vol. 5,
Mechanisms of Cardiac Morphogenesis and Teratogenesis,
edited by Tomas Pexieder. Raven Press, New York © 1981

Introduction

Zdenek Rychter

Department of Histology, Faculty of General Medicine, Charles University,
Prague, Czechoslovakia

Recent meetings devoted to heart morphogenesis and/or teratogenesis (Grand Canyon, 1977; Munich, 1978; Macclesfield, 1979; Lausanne, 1979) bear witness to the increasing amount of research activity in this field. This trend may be expected to continue and even to extend itself to cover all phases of prenatal ontogenesis of the heart. These scientific meetings are designed to improve mutual understanding and respect among researchers. They should stimulate the dissemination of published and personally communicated data and increase the preciseness of these data. However, the frequent failure to accomplish these aims adds to another negative feature of research into cardiac morphogenesis: the absence of integration. Individual papers are seldom adequately related to other relevant communications, and a hierarchy of all the facts reported is lacking.

Heart development is a complex multifactorial morphogenetic process. Despite its complexity, there is still a tendency to oversimplify reality by reducing the dimensions of its explanation to a single causative factor. It is always dangerous to promote a single factor or event to the status of an all-explaining cause, without taking into account the level at which such a factor operates. Morphogenetic processes at certain levels depend upon other morphogenetic processes working on higher levels, and at the same time influence processes operating on lower levels.

Comparative and functional approaches are not adequately respected in the majority of morphological studies. This can easily be demonstrated, for example, by the variety of interpretations of the fate of the bulbus cordis in heart development (page 431). Often, the problems discussed have been created by a loss of general perspective. In such cases, an isolated morphologic feature of a final (definitive) structure has been used as a criterion for characterization of the entire organ and its development. Another source of error is the overly heavy dependence of certain authors on their previous literature experience in interpretation of previously observed facts, or even in the process of observation.

What do "epigenesis" and "epigenetic control" mean? They mean that genetic information provides only a departure point for the repertory of possible developmental outcomes of an organism and its structures. Consequently, each group of cells maintains its own micromilieu. Further on in development, neighboring groups of cells interact mutually. Local interactions among such cell populations are the first steps in a chain of epigenetic events that will influence the choice of developmental pathways. These interactions represent, at the same time, the first possibility for intervention by an environmental factor, such as a particular experiment. Such experimental intervention can either be very simple, based on a simple hypothesis, or very sophisticated, emerging from a deep understanding of the embryonic development of the structure under study.

We should bear in mind that genetic control codes only for developmental processes, and not for isolated morphological details. This was stressed by the late W. Landauer (personal communication), at the end of his fruitful scientific life. Genetic control of the timing and modulation of developmental processes seems to be a sufficient explanation for many principal features of normal and abnormal ontogenesis, such as sex determination or polydactyly.

Each developing structure in an embryo represents a morphogenetic system (2). The functioning of this system leads to embryonic growth and shape changes. There are two essential aspects of morphogenesis, a general quantitative and a specialized qualitative side of a given morphogenetic event. These aspects are mutually interdependent; one of them may reflect or even determine the other. Each morphogenetic system can be studied by multilevel analysis. The morphogenetic processes of a certain level of biological organization are dependent upon those working at a higher level, and, simultaneously, they determine those working on a lower level.

Each morphogenetic system makes use of a fairly limited number of basic developmental processes. The system is composed of a cell population whose members divide, migrate (or are distributed), integrate with other populations, and finally die. Each step in the development of a morphogenetic system is determined, or at least mediated, by previous stages, and determines or mediates the later stages.

The interactions among elements of an early morphogenetic system are quite simple, in number as well as in quality. Interactions among elements of late morphogenetic systems, on the other hand, are much more complex. It is usually very difficult to state their number and to identify and analyze their characteristics.

How can these considerations be reflected in the design of our experiments? The simplest experimental intervention involves disturbing the course of development of an embryonic structure in some way. (We must bear in mind that our goal is to produce malformation, not deformation!) More advanced experimental design consists in changing some of the links in the chain of morphogenetic processes that precedes the phase of morphogenesis under study. The aim of such experiments is to explain the epigenetic interactions of subsequent stages of development of a structure and to gain detailed, step-by-step understanding of the corresponding developmental mechanism. This understanding can then improve our further experimental study. The most advanced experimental design requires an exact quantitative description of cell population dynamics within a given morphogenetic system. Only then can we precisely determine the timing and the kind of experimental intervention. When xenobiotics or drugs are to be used in our experiments, we must follow strictly defined guidelines. First, we must know the morphogenetically effective concentration of the substance. This information can be quickly obtained (24 hours) by the CHEST screening method for embryotoxicity (1). Second, we can select the appropriate stage for experimental intervention on the basis of the growth curve of the morphogenetic system studied. This choice will direct the outcome of our intervention, either by preventing development of the embryonic structure, by disturbing its development, or by changing its cytophysiology without alteration of form and shape. Finally, we must take into account the possibility of the existence of a specific receptor for the substance used. In such a case, the sensitivity of the morphogenetic system increases by two orders of magnitude. This last experimental design is very pretentious. At the same time, however, it represents a condition without which further progress in analysis of heart development, with respect to possible clinical implications, cannot be made.

REFERENCES

1. Jelinek, R., Rychter, Z., and Peterka, M. (1976): *Cs. Author's Certificate No. 2170.*
2. Rychter, Z. (1979): Properties of morphogenetic systems. In: *Evaluation of Embryotoxicity, Mutagenicity and Carcinogenicity Risks in New Drugs,* edited by O. Benešova, Z. Rychter, and R. Jelínek, pp. 25-34. Universita Karlova, Prague.

Perspectives in Cardiovascular Research, Vol. 5,
Mechanisms of Cardiac Morphogenesis and Teratogenesis,
edited by Tomas Pexieder. Raven Press, New York © 1981

Cardiac Function in the Embryonic Chick

Roger N. Ruckman, Robert J. Cassling, Edward B. Clark, and
Glenn C. Rosenquist

Department of Pediatrics, Section of Pediatric Cardiology, University of Nebraska College of Medicine, Omaha, Nebraska 68105

Over the past 50 years, the embryonic chick heart has been the subject of investigations of both form and function. Most of the recorded observations have been in embryos of more than 48 hours gestation (or more than 19 somites). Studies of younger embryos have involved inspection without measurement of function. Over the past 10 years, reliable indices of function have been established that are applicable to the developing heart. There has recently been great interest in characterizing the unique properties of fetal myocardial function, as compared to the function of the mature heart. Very little is known about the function of fetal myocardium in the earliest stages, after initiation of the heartbeat. This chapter presents an evaluation of ventricular function in the chick during these early developmental stages, and reviews the work that bears on our understanding of embryonic cardiac function.

MATERIALS AND METHODS

Embryos were removed from White Leghorn eggs incubated 43 to 53 hours at 37.8°C. The vitelline membranes to which the embryos remained attached were secured to a glass ring and suspended over a pool of albumin (15) and staged, using the Hamburger and Hamilton technique (4), being 13 to 24 somites (4,5,21). A micropipette was advanced from the ventral side at about a 45° angle toward the anterior intestinal portal, entering first the ventral endoderm and then the junction of the right and left omphalomesenteric veins. Entering at this position did not cause damage to the cardiac jelly, nor was there leakage afterwards. Paraffin oil (Saybolt viscosity 125/135) was injected by the micropipette into the cardiac lumen (14) (Fig. 1). The beating hearts containing the oil droplets were filmed, using transmitted light at 18 frames/sec, with a 16 mm Bolex reflex camera, with bellows at constant film-to-subject distance with × 1.6 enlargement. Filming was continued during distal migration of the oil droplet from the primitive ventricle. Since no red blood cells are present within the lumen at this stage of development, the presence of the droplet within the ventricle allowed definition of the endocardial surfaces (Figs. 2 and 3). Nine

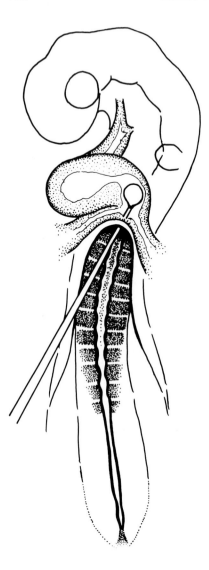

FIG. 1. Technique of oil droplet injection. A micropipette is introduced into the junction of the right and left omphalomesenteric veins. Paraffin oil is injected into the cardiac lumen, thus defining the endocardial surfaces of the primitive ventricular cavity.

of the twelve embryos had hearts that lay at a suitable angle for measurement. Three of the embryos had overlapping cardiac borders that precluded measurement. Measurements were made on frames without droplets, to ensure that no artifact was introduced by the presence of the droplet within the lumen. Cinephotographs were prepared at peak diastole and peak systole for each of the twelve embryos. Each photograph was enlarged 23 times. Initial enlargement by the movie camera was $\times 1.6$. Hence, measurements were made at an overall enlargement of $\times 37.4$ the actual embryo size. Measurements of maximum end diastolic dimension (EDD) and peak end systolic dimension (ESD) were made

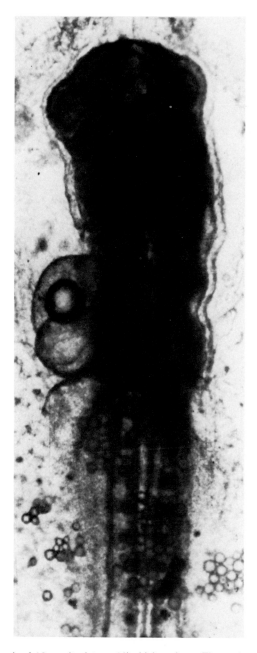

FIG. 2. Cinephotograph of 16-somite (stage 12) chick embryo. The embryo has been injected with an oil droplet which has migrated through the primitive ventricle into the conus. The primitive ventricle is shown in peak diastole.

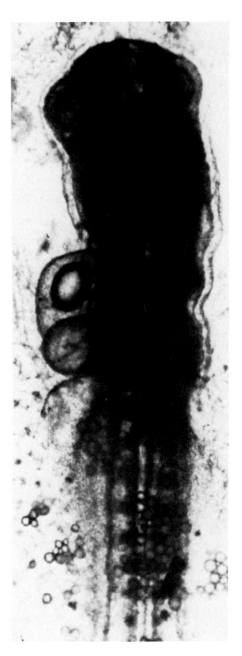

FIG. 3. Cinephotograph of 16-somite (stage 12) chick embryo. The embryo is the same as shown in Fig. 2. The ventricle is shown in peak systole. Note the compression of the oil droplet in the distal conus.

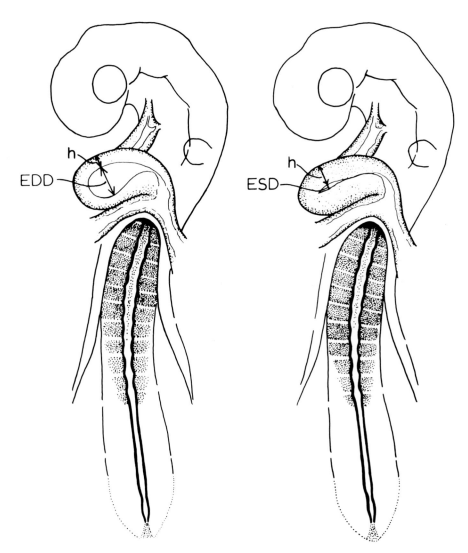

FIG. 4. Technique of measurement of ventricular dimensions in the embryonic chick heart. **Left:** Measurement of end diastolic dimension (EDD) and wall thickness (h). **Right:** Measurement of end systolic dimension (ESD) and wall thickness (h).

independently by each of three observers, and reproducible results were obtained (Fig. 4). Heart rate was determined by frame counting of intervals from peak systole to peak systole over at least six sequences of contraction for each embryo. The formulae used for calculation of indices of cardiac function are summarized in Table 1.

TABLE 1. *Determinants of cardiac function*

End Diastolic Volume[a] (ml) $= (\pi/3)$ (EDD)^3
End Systolic Volume[a] (ml) $= (\pi/3)$ (ESD)^3

Shortening Fraction (%) $= \dfrac{\text{EDD--ESD}}{\text{EDD}} \times 100$

Ejection Fraction (%) $= \dfrac{\text{EDV--ESV}}{\text{EDV}} \times 100$

Stroke Volume (ml/beat) $=$ EDV--ESV
Cardiac Output (ml/min) $=$ HR $\times$ SV
Mass[a] (gm) $= [(\text{EDD} + 2\text{hd})^3 - (\text{EDD})^3][1.05]$

[a] Equations for volume and mass assume ventricular geometry of prolate ellipse.
Abbreviations: EDD, end diastolic dimension; ESD, end systolic dimension; EDV, end diastolic volume; ESV, end systolic volume; HR, heart rate; SV, stroke volume; hd, wall thickness in diastole.

RESULTS

The three measured and five calculated indices of cardiac function are shown in Table 2. The relationship between parameters was assessed by linear regression analysis. Significant correlations are shown (Table 3). As the embryos matured, heart rate increased. Associated with this was a proportionate increase in stroke volume and, accordingly, of cardiac output. The primary determinant of the increased stroke volume is the EDD. Shortening fraction, an easily calculated index of contractility, was found to correlate with the more complex function of ejection fraction. Mass was found to be an unreliable calculation.

Observation of the embryonic heart demonstrated, as the numerical results confirm, that, in the maturing embryo, there is an increase in heart rate and an increase in diastolic volume. All the embryos show nearly complete obliteration of the primitive ventricular lumen at end systole through the action of cardiac jelly. This was noted even in embryos with reduced duration of systole associated with fast heart rates.

DISCUSSION

Previous investigations of embryonic chick heart function have focused on heart rate (18) and blood pressure (7,8). Hill (7) examined the 2 to 3 e.d. chick embryo and found that the capillary pressure necessary to sustain delivery of nutrients is very low (0.5 cm water). Hughes (8) later showed that older embryos increase blood pressure gradually until late gestation, at which time pressure rises more rapidly. Other investigators found structural properties of the embry-

TABLE 2. Determinants of cardiac function in the 13–24 somite chick

Embryo	Stage (somites)	Heart rate	End-diastolic dimension (cm)	End-systolic dimension (cm)	Shortening fraction (%)	Ejection fraction (%)	Stroke volume ($\times 10^{-5}$ cm^3)	Cardiac output ($\times 10^{-5}$ cm^3)	Mass ($\times 10^{-4}$ gm)
1	14(21)	108	.049	.005	89	98	8.2	88.24	2.8
2	14(22)	180	.053	.012	77	99	15.2	2,736.0	1.3
3	13(19)	72	.032	.010	68	97	3.4	244.1	5.2
4	15(24)	215	.049	.012	76	99	11.8	2,537.0	4.7
5	14(22)	180	.039	.005	87	99	6.2	116.0	3.5
6	11(13)	29	.019	.0034	77	99	0.7	19.9	1.78
7	12(16)	33	.0187	.0034	81	99	0.7	22.3	2.5
8	13(19)	68	.037	.0118	68	97	5.1	349.5	3.2
9	12(16)	35	.034	.0118	65	98	3.9	137.9	3.8

TABLE 3. *Relationship between determinants of cardiac function in the 13–24 somite chick (correlation coefficient determined by linear regression analysis)*

	HR	EDD	ESD	SF	EF	SV	CO	Mass
HR	—	.8158[b]	.3167	.3806	.3235	.8516[b]	.9161[b]	.1329
EDD	.8158[b]	—	.5500	.1895	−.0591	.9350[b]	.8226[b]	.0818
EDS	.3167	.5500	—	−.6973	−.6259	.5519	.4520	—
SF	.3806	.1895	−.6973	—	.7791[a]	.1752	.2359	−.3679
EF	.3235	−.0591	−.6259	.7791[a]	—	.1391	.3255	−.5158
SV	.8516[b]	.9350[b]	.5519	.1752	.1391	—	.9545[b]	−.0902
CO	.9161[b]	.8226[b]	.4520	.2359	.3255	.9545[b]	—	−.0745
Mass	.1329	.0818	—	−.3679	−.5158	−.0902	−.0745	—

[a] $p < .05$.
[b] $p < .01$.

Abbreviations: HR, heart rate; EDD, end diastolic dimension; EDS, end diastolic dimension; SF, shortening fraction; EF, ejection fraction; SV, stroke volume; CO, cardiac output.

onic chick heart that allowed this efficiency of function. Barry (1) presented evidence that increases in cardiac output must be explained by increases in stroke volume. Heart rate, after 50 hours gestation, increases relatively slowly. The presence of cardiac jelly appears to facilitate the development of maximum end diastolic volume and the transmission of the force of myocardial contraction during systole. Patten (17) further showed that the initial jerky progression of blood in the early tubular heart develops through a phase of peristaltoid contraction to an ultimately uniform forward flow. Such development of smooth progression depends on the appearance of heaped-up endocardium in the atrioventricular canal, which serves as a "valve." This is noted early in the third day of incubation. From the standpoint of structure, it is important to note that the cellular migration that leads to formation of definitive endocardial cushion tissue occurs through the cardiac jelly. Similar development is noted in the truncal region. Patten (17) also demonstrated functional contraction of the primitive ventricle at 10 somites, confirming Sabin's earlier work (20). These young embryos initially show a heart rate as low as 8 beats per minute. Only small areas of the myocardium contract at the 9-somite stage. There is then rapidly progressing development of a sustained regular rhythm which involves the whole ventricle. Cross-banded myofibrils and glycogen are noted microscopically at this time.

There remains a need to understand the contractile properties of the myocardium that lead to the flow patterns described above. Rychter (19) demonstrated that circulating blood volume increases uniformly with gestational age in the chick. Could such increase in volume lead to distention of the myofibrils, with resultant increase in stroke volume? Understanding of such function depends on a closer analysis of structure. With the advent of electron microscopy, more details of myofibril development were elucidated. Hibbs (6) noted that the myocardium initially shows a network of loosely arranged cells which, by 24 to 30 hours incubation, assume a more compact arrangement. By 30 to 36 hours incubation, the myofilaments begin to become organized into loose bundles. Next, filaments become attached by Z-bands. At this point, the first contractions are noted. Between 48 and 60 hours, the bundles become more compact, and A-substance, H-bands, and M-bands are noted. Manasek (11) noted that the early tubular heart (stage 13) is only 3 cells thick. The first myofibrils are observed at 8 to 10 somites. The myofibrils subsequently increase in number, but lack alignment by 5 days. Between 5 days and hatching, the principal changes in myocyte development are the formation of more fibrils and the reorganization of cell contents. Of importance to the understanding of early embryonic chick heart function is the fact that well-developed fibrils containing organized myofilaments and Z-bands are present at the time of the first heartbeat (10 somites). How, then, does the early cardiac muscle contract? The young myocardial cell is secretory, and filamentous precursor material gives rise, through this secretory function, to definitive myofibrils. Up to 15 somites, there is development of the basal cell layer, as well as orientation and packing of cells such that myocardium shows a thickness of 2 to 3 cells (10). Myofibrils shorten and, although well-oriented fibrils are not observed at these early stages, coordinated contraction does occur. The development of myocardial blood vessels also depends on the secretory function of early myocardial cells, as well as transformation of fibroblasts (12,13). Additional observations in the mouse support the concept of cell transformation, emphasizing the importance of pericardiac coelom epithelial cells as the precursors of definitive heart muscle cells (23). The basis for cell movement which leads to the well-packed and oriented myocardium is a subject of controversy. Some experimental evidence suggests it may be the result of changing cell-to-cell adhesiveness during development (9).

Recent work by Paff (16), Van Mierop (22), and Faber (2,3) has placed renewed emphasis on the importance of direct measurement of cardiac function. In a group of embryos of 3 to 7 days gestation, blood pressure was measured by direct puncture of the primitive ventricle. In the isovolumically beating ventricle, it was found that peak systolic pressure depended strongly on end diastolic pressure. Hence, the Frank–Starling mechanism was observed to function as early as 3 days and 4 hours. Ventricular pressures were found to increase with increasing gestational age. The overall mechanical behavior of the primitive ventricle was found to be analogous to the adult ventricle, except that the forces generated were less. In addition, cardiac regulatory mechanisms, innervation, and circulating catecholamines are absent prior to 4 days gestation. The most recent study by Faber et al. (3) looks more specifically at the determinants of cardiac output, i.e., heart rate and stroke volume, using a cinema technique similar to our study. Forward flow only is confirmed in the 3 day embryo. It is then demonstrated that the key determinant of cardiac output is stroke volume. This is consistent with the findings of increasing blood volume noted during development (19). By injection of Ringer's solution or Dextran, it was also found that stroke volume and cardiac output increase as the result of increases in end diastolic volume.

In summary, the early embryonic heart begins initial contractions at a slow rate. As heart rate increases, there is a rise in stroke volume, with ejection fraction 95% or higher. Contractility, as measured by shortening fraction, is uniformly high, greater than 65% in all embryos studied. Measurement of function in each case is greatly facilitated by the use of cine photoanalysis.

REFERENCES

1. Barry, A. (1948): The functional significance of the cardiac jelly in the tubular heart of the chick embryo. *Anat. Rec.,* 102:289-298.
2. Faber, J. J. (1968): Mechanical function of the septating embryonic heart. *Am. J. Physiol.,* 214 (3):475-481.
3. Faber, J. J., Green, T. J., and Thornburg, K. L. (1974): Embryonic stroke volume and cardiac output in the chick. *Dev. Biol.,* 41:14-21.
4. Hamburger, V., and Hamilton, H. L. (1951): A series of normal stages in the development of the chick embryo. *J. Morphol.,* 88:49-92.
5. Hamilton, H. L. (1952): *Lillie's Development of the Chick,* 3rd ed. Holt, Rhinehart, and Winston, New York.

6. Hibbs, R. G. (1956): Electron microscopy of developing cardiac muscle in chick embryos. *Am. J. Anat.,* 99:17-35.
7. Hill, L., and Azuma, Y. (1927): Blood pressure in the two-three-day chick embryo. *J. Physiol.* (Lond.), 62:27-28.
8. Hughes, A. F. W. (1942): The blood pressure of the chick embryo during development. *J. Exp. Biol.,* 19:232-237.
9. Lesseps, R. J. (1973): Developmental change in morphogenetic properties: Embryonic chick heart tissue and cells segregate from other tissues in age-dependent patterns. *J. Exp. Zool.,* 185:159-168.
10. Manasek, F. J. (1968): Embryonic development of the heart. I. A light and electron microscopic study of myocardial development in the early chick embryo. *J. Morphol.,* 125:329-366.
11. Manasek, F. J. (1970): Histogenesis of the embryonic myocardium. *Am. J. Cardiol.,* 25:149-168.
12. Manasek, F. J. (1971): The ultrastructure of embryonic myocardial blood vessels. *Dev. Biol.,* 26:42-54.
13. Markwald, R. R., Fitzharris, T. P., and Manasek, F. J. (1977): Structural development of endocardial cushions. *Am. J. Anat.,* 148:85-121.
14. Masica, D. N., and Rosenquist, G. C. (1969): Early valve function in embryonic hearts injected with oil droplets: cine photoanalysis. *Circulation,* 40:141.
15. New, D. A. T. (1955): A new technique for the culture of the chick embryo in vitro. *J. Embryol. Exp. Morphol.,* 3:326.
16. Paff, G. H., Boucek, R. J., and Gutten, G. S. (1965): Ventricular blood pressures and competency of valves in the early embryonic chick heart. *Anat. Rec.,* 151:119-124.
17. Patten, B. M., Kramer, T. C., and Barry, A. (1948): Valvular action in the embryonic chick heart by localized apposition of endocardial masses. *Anat. Rec.,* 102:299-311.
18. Patten, B. M. (1949): Initiation and early changes in the character of the heart beat in vertebrate embryos. *Physiol. Rev.,* 29:31-47.
19. Rychter, Z., Kopecky, M., and Lemež, L. (1955): A micromethod for determination of the circulating blood volume in chick embryos. *Nature,* 175:1126-1127.
20. Sabin, F. R. (1920): Studies on the origin of blood-vessels and of red blood corpuscles as seen in living blastoderm of chicks during the second day of incubation. *Carnegie Inst. Contrib. Embryol.,* 9:213.
21. Sissman, N. J. (1970): Developmental landmarks in cardiac morphogenesis: comparative chronology. *Am. J. Cardiol.,* 25:141-148.
22. Van Mierop, L. H. S., and Bertuch, C. J. (1967): Development of arterial blood pressure in the chick embryo. *Am. J. Physiol.,* 212 (1):43-48.
23. Viragh, S., and Challice, C. E. (1973): Origin and differentiation of cardiac muscle cells in the mouse. *J. Ultrastruct. Res.,* 42:1-24.

DISCUSSION

DeHaan: Can you work out, from your calculations of cardiac output, the total volume of circulating blood?

Rosenquist: It certainly could be done, but the application of the Fick principle will do much better. What method did you use, Dr. Rychter, in estimating the total circulating volume after the 1st e.d.?

Rychter: Using the Fick principle, we did an intravenous injection of Evans blue, with subsequent photometric dosage.

Pexieder: Can you correlate the development of ventricular pressure studied by others with the development of cardiac output or other physiological parameters you have studied?

Rosenquist: No, we did not try to measure the ventricular pressure or make such correlations.

DeHaan: The presence of tight junctions in the early heart might contribute to creation of a transmural ionic difference. Would not a measure of the total ionic concentration in the blood contribute to understanding of the cardiovascular physiology at that stage?

Manasek: The role of tight junctions in maintaining an ionic gradient was never well proven. Older hearts are exquisitely sensitive to potassium, at the time of initiation of contraction hearts will beat very often in 100 mM potassium.

Perspectives in Cardiovascular Research, Vol. 5,
Mechanisms of Cardiac Morphogenesis and Teratogenesis,
edited by Tomas Pexieder. Raven Press, New York © 1981

Spectrum of Pulmonary Venous Connections Following Lung Bud Inversion in the Chick Embryo

Edward B. Clark, D. Richard Martini, and Glenn C. Rosenquist

Cardiopulmonary Embryology Laboratory, Department of Pediatrics, University of Nebraska Medical Center, Omaha, Nebraska 68105

The embryologic mechanisms responsible for anomalies of pulmonary venous return have not been clearly defined. It has been suggested that the underlying cause may be either failure of the connection of the pulmonary splanchnic plexus with an outgrowth of the common pulmonary vein from the left atrium, or obliteration of established splanchnic–atrial connections, with subsequent reopening of secondary pathways (1,2,3). We have sought to clarify these mechanisms by evaluating the effect of disruption of previously established pulmonary venous connections, combined with a change in lung position, on the reestablishment of pulmonary venous connections.

MATERIALS AND METHODS

Fertile White Leghorn chicken eggs were incubated at 37.8°C to stage 27 (4). Access to the embryo was gained by opening a window in the shell and removing the outer and inner shell membranes. The embryonic chorion was incised and the embryo turned left side upwards. An incision was then made in the left thoracic wall ventral to the wing, and the thoracic cavity entered. A glass or wire loop was inserted into the cavity and the left lung bud gently withdrawn, amputated close to its base, and removed from the chest cavity (Fig. 1).

In the stage 28 chick embryo, the left lung bud is 1.8 mm in length. After measurement with a micrometer eyepiece, the size of the amputated lung bud fragment was expressed as a percentage of the normal length. The lung bud was then inverted 180° in the cephalo-caudal axis and returned to the thoracic cavity. To be sure of the cephalo-caudal inversion, an India ink-impregnated gelatin mark was placed on the severed surface of the lung bud in 17 experimental embryos (5). The shells were sealed with Parafilm and reincubated. Embryos surviving to stage 36 or older were fixed in 10% formol and chick Ringer's.

In the chick embryo, the pulmonary veins develop from the splanchnic plexus which lies between the lung bud and the left atrium. Two pulmonary veins,

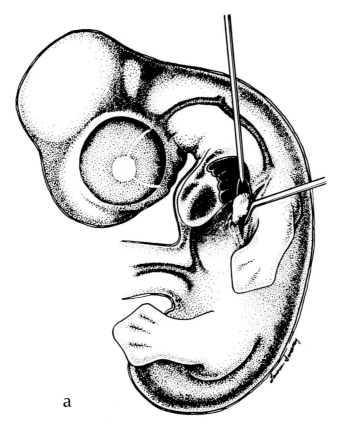

a

FIG. 1. Drawing of a stage 28 chick embryo viewed from the left side. **a:** Withdrawal of the left lung bud before amputation. **b:** Insertion of left lung bud after cephalo-caudal inversion. Black dot represents the position of the India ink marker.

one on each side, form in the dorsal mesocardium and connect with the venous channels developing in the mesenchyme surrounding the subdivisions of the bronchial bud. The two pulmonary veins coalesce to form a right and a left pulmonary vein, which then join as the common pulmonary vein. The common pulmonary vein enters the left atrium adjacent to the posterior aspect of the interatrial septum (6).

Following microdissection of the intrathoracic contents, particular attention was paid to the lungs. In the 17 marked lungs, the India ink mark was at the caudal aspect of the lung, confirming axial inversion. The pulmonary venous drainage from the right and left lungs was determined, and the arterial connections ascertained. After the embryonic heart was evaluated by gross inspection, the free walls of the right and left ventricle were removed and the internal anatomy studied, particularly for the presence and location of ventricular septal defects.

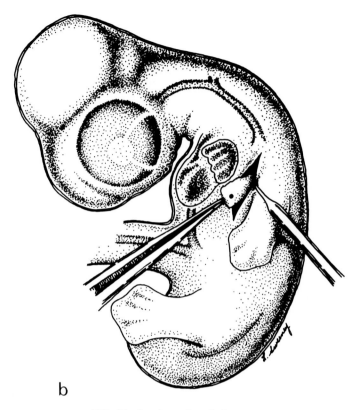

b

FIG. 1.b. See legend on facing page.

A second group of sham-operated embryos underwent left thoracotomy and withdrawal of the lung bud without amputation, return of the lung bud to the thoracic cavity, and reincubation. In total, 1,052 embryos underwent lung bud inversion; 60 embryos survived to stages 36 through 42. Of the 96 sham-operated embryos, 30 survived to stages 36 to 42, and served as controls.

RESULTS

Five patterns of pulmonary venous connection resulted (Table 1). In type I connection, the pulmonary venous blood from the inverted amputated lung bud returned to the left atrium in one of three ways. First, in 21 embryos, the venous connection from the inverted lung bud was directly to the left lung stump, a small amount of remaining lung tissue (Fig. 2a). In 8 embryos, the pulmonary vein from the inverted lung joined the vein from the stump along its course to the left atrium (Figure 2b). Finally, in 12 embryos, the pulmonary vein from the inverted lung joined directly to the left atrium lateral to the insertion of the common pulmonary vein (Figure 2c). In this group, 3 embryos

TABLE 1. *Arterial supply*

Venous drainage		N.	%	L-Pul Art	L-Brachio	Intercostal	Mixed	Associated defects
I.		41	68	31	5	0	7	
	a.	21		18	2	0	1	VSD, int. RAA
	b.	8		5	2	0	1	Persist. LAA
	c.	12		9	1	0	2	None
II.		6	10	0	2	2	2	None
III.		6	10	0	0	4	2	VSD
IV.		4	7	0	0	0	4	VSD
V.		3	5	0	0	0	3	None

Abbreviations: VSD, ventricular septal defect; int RAA, absent right fourth aortic arch; persist LAA, persistent left fourth aortic arch.

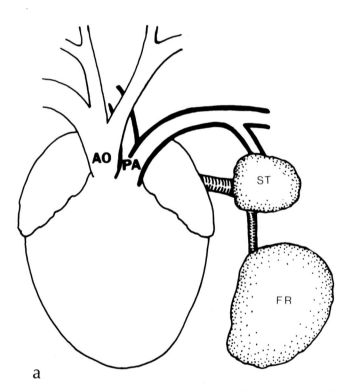

a

FIG. 2. Drawing showing anterior view of the embryo heart, and type I drainage of the pulmonary vein (stippled) from the inverted lung fragment. **a:** Vein coursing to the lung stump. **b:** Vein joining the left pulmonary vein. **c:** Vein joining directly to the left atrium. AO, aorta; PA, pulmonary artery; ST, lung stump; FR, inverted lung fragment; PV, pulmonary vein.

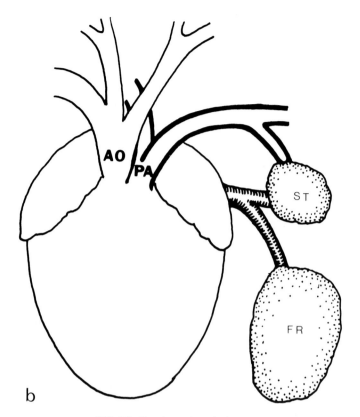

FIG. 2.b. See legend on facing page.

had associated cardiac defects: a supracristal VSD, an absent right fourth aortic arch, and persistence of the left fourth aortic arch. The arterial supply for the inverted lung came from the left pulmonary artery in 31 of the embryos, either as a separate branch or as a continuing vessel from the lung stump. In the remaining embryos, arterial connections arose from the left brachiocephalic or intercostal vessels.

In the second type of drainage pattern (type II) the pulmonary vein joined a systemic venous vessel, the left superior vena cava (Fig. 3). All 6 embryos in this group also demonstrated arterial branches from either the left brachioce-phalic artery or the intercostal arteries, and none had associated intracardiac defects.

Type III drainage was noted in 6 embryos, in which the pulmonary vein joined the paraesophageal venous plexus (Fig. 4). In these 6 cases, the arterial supply was from intercostal arteries. There was only one embryo with a supracris-tal ventricular septal defect.

In type IV drainage (Fig. 5), pulmonary veins from the inverted lung fragment connected with the intercostal veins; the arterial supply similarly arose from

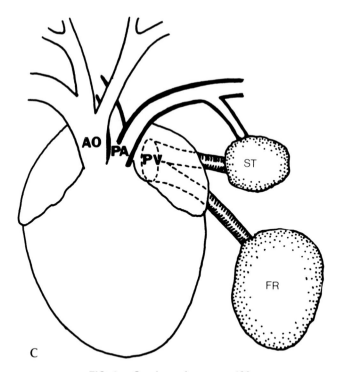

C

FIG. 2.c. See legend on page 422.

the intercostal arteries. One of the 4 embryos in this group had a ventricular septal defect, which was in the supracristal position.

In the final group (type V), mixed venous drainage was observed in 3 embryos, including connections with left superior vena cava, paraesophageal veins, and left atrium (Fig. 6). The arterial supply was also mixed, with branches arising from the left pulmonary artery, left brachiocephalic artery, and intercostal arteries.

The influence of lung bud fragment size was correlated with the pattern of pulmonary venous return. The highest incidence of anomalous venous connections was observed when 70 to 80% of the lung bud had been inverted. In this group, the highest incidence of anomalous arterial supply was also noted.

DISCUSSION

These results suggest that lung polarity at stage 28 is not a major factor in determining the pattern of lung vascular connections. Rather, proximity of the inverted lung fragment to the splanchnic plexus and/or lung bud seems to be of more importance, since the majority of vascular connections were via these

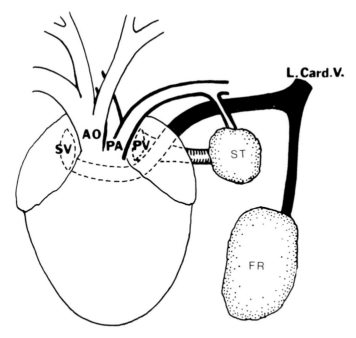

FIG. 3. Type II pulmonary venous drainage from the inverted left lung bud to the left cardinal vein. View as in Fig. 2. AO, aorta; PA, pulmonary artery; SV, sinus venosus; PV, pulmonary vein; ST, lung stump; FR, inverted fragment.

areas. Directional growth of nerve axons is, in part, influenced by chemical substances (7). A similar chemotactic substance may be present in the chick lung, promoting connection between the splanchnic plexus and the developing lung bud. Another factor influencing blood vessel formation may be induction mediated by the embryonic lung mesenchyme (8).

Another important finding is low incidence of ventricular septal defects among the experimental embryos. The observed incidence of VSD is similar to that noted in the human clinical population with partial anomalous pulmonary venous return (9,10), and is in contradistinction to the 75% incidence observed following lung bud amputation in the chick (11). This observation suggests that early reestablishment of vascular connections may result only in minor hemodynamic changes which, in the heart, would not alter the molding of ventricular septation (12,13,14).

The spectrum of anomalous pulmonary venous connections observed in our study group is similar to that noted in humans. This suggests that the etiologic mechanism may be related, particularly since connections to the left superior vena cava and inferior vena cava via the paraesophageal channels are two of the most common types of partial anomalous pulmonary venous return (9).

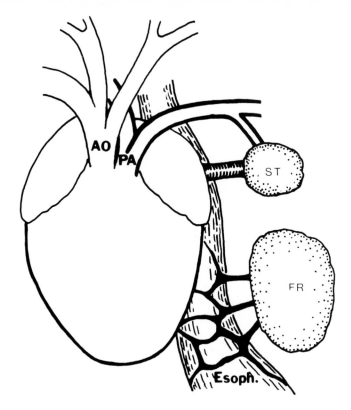

FIG. 4. Type III embryo demonstrating pulmonary vein coursing from the inverted lung bud and joining the paraesophageal plexus of veins. (View and abbreviations as in Fig. 2.)

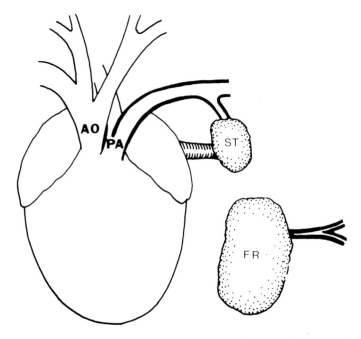

FIG. 5. Type IV pulmonary venous return demonstrating pulmonary vein coursing laterally to join the intercostal veins. (View as previously described, abbreviations as in Fig. 2.)

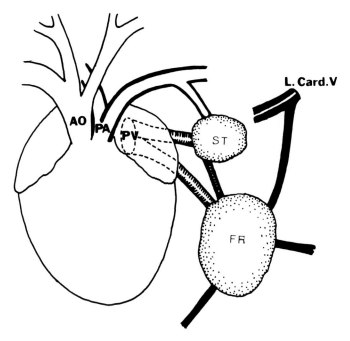

FIG. 6. Type V embryo demonstrating mixed pulmonary venous drainage to the left atrium, intercostal veins, paraesophageal plexus, and left cardinal vein. (View and abbreviations as in Fig. 2.)

We believe these data support the concept that anomalies of pulmonary venous connection may be primary congenital lung defects. This view reemphasizes the need for further investigation of the morphogenetic relationship between the heart and lung.

ACKNOWLEDGMENTS

This investigation was supported by Grant HL20132 from the National Institute of Health.

REFERENCES

1. Neill, C. A. (1956): Development of the pulmonary veins. *Pediatrics,* 18:880-887.
2. Edwards, J. E., and Helmholz, H. F. (1956): A classification of total anomalous pulmonary venous connection based on developmental considerations. *Mayo Clin. Proc.,* 31:151-160.
3. Auer, J. (1948): The development of the human pulmonary vein and its major variations. *Anat. Res.,* 101:581-594.
4. Hamburger, V., and Hamilton, H. L. (1951): A series of normal stages in the development of the chick embryo. *J. Morphol.,* 88:49-92.
5. Seichert, V. (1965): Study of the tissue and organ anlage shifts by the method of plastic linear marking. *Folia Morphol. (Praha),* 13:228-238.
6. Romanoff, A. L. (1960): *The Avian Embryo.* Macmillan, New York.
7. Yamada, K. (1977): Cell morphogenetic movements. *Handbook of Teratology,* edited by F. C. Fraser, and J. G. Wilson. Plenum Press, New York.

8. Wolff, E. (1968): Specific interactions between tissues during organogenesis. *Curr. Top. Dev. Biol.,* 3:65-94.
9. Blake, H. A., Hall, R. J., and Manson, W. C. (1965): Anomalous pulmonary venous return. *Circulation,* 32:406-414.
10. Carlson, R. G., Ferlic, R. M., Kalke, B. R., Lillehei, C. W., and Sellers, R. D. (1967): Partial anomalous pulmonary venous connection. *Am. J. Cardiol.,* 20:91-101.
11. Clark, E. B., Martini, R. D., and Rosenquist, G. C. (1978): Effect of lung bud excision on cardiopulmonary development in the chick. In: *Morphogenesis and Malformation of the Cardiovascular System,* edited by G. C. Rosenquist and D. Bergsma, pp. 423-429. Alan R. Liss, New York.
12. Rychter, Z. (1962): Experimental morphology of the aortic arches and heart loop in chick embryo. *Adv. Morphogenes,* 2:333-371.
13. Clark, E. B., and Rosenquist, G. C. (1978): Spectrum of cardiovascular anomalies following cardiac loop constriction in the chick embryo. In: *Morphogenesis and Malformation of the Cardiovascular System,* edited by G. C. Rosenquist and D. Bergsma, pp. 431-442. Birth Defects: Orig. Art. Ser., vol. XIV, no. 7. Alan R. Liss, New York.
14. Jaffee, O. (1962): Hemodynamics and cardiogenesis. I. The effects of altered vascular patterns on cardiac development. *J. Morphol.,* 110:217-221.

DISCUSSION

Rychter: Your experiments seem to represent an excellent experimental model of lung sequestration. Did I understand you well that the hemodynamic relationship of embryonic lung and heart is less important?

Clark: No, I believe the opposite. Complete removal of the lung bud is followed by a 75% incidence of ventricular septal defects.

Los: There are two pulmonary venous sprouts in the embryo, the real one and the spurious. When you reimplant your lung graft, it can use whatever it likes. Is it not rather dangerous to compare heart defects in chicken and in man because of the interspecific differences in cardiac anatomy?

Clark: I agree with you that the stage we chose for intervention was after completion of pulmonary vein reaching the lung bud. We were specifically addressing the second hypothesis, that the interruption of a previously established pulmonary connection will result in opening of alternative channels.

DeHaan: Could you design an experiment to decide how much of a lung mass is necessary to prevent the formation of the defect?

Clark: It is in the group of 75 to 85% of normal total lung bud volume that you have the highest incidence of anomalous connections.

DeHaan: No, I was asking about ventricular septal defects.

Clark: We did not yet ask this question.

DeHaan: How long can you store your fragment before reimplantation?

Clark: We performed all these manipulations within five minutes, because of the difficulties in manipulation of the chorionic membrane enveloping the embryo.

DeHaan: In fact, you may sometimes come later with a lung bud from another donor and place it back into the thoracic cavity. In this way, you can study how long you have to leave this cavity empty in order to produce ventricular septal defects.

De Vries: In human lung sequestrations I have seen, whether the arterial blood came off the aorta or some other systemic vessel, the venous return was always normal.

Clark: The point is that if the venous return is via left atrium, the arterial supply would be from the pulmonary artery. If the venous return takes another path, then the arterial supply would be from a systemic vessel.

Laane: About 80% of the operated embryos died. Did you see in this particular group results different from the group of survivors?

Clark: All but 10% of the embryos died within the first 24 hours after the operation, because of hemorrhage into the thoracic cavity. In the embryos investigated at earlier stages than HH36 (e.g., HH30 to 35), we have seen the same spectrum of venous return.

Morse: What was the incidence of heart defects in the control embryos?

Clark: About 3%.

Perspectives in Cardiovascular Research, Vol. 5,
Mechanisms of Cardiac Morphogenesis and Teratogenesis,
edited by Tomas Pexieder. Raven Press, New York © 1981

Angio- and Myoarchitecture of the Heart Wall Under Normal and Experimentally Changed Morphogenesis

Zdeněk Rychter and Vlasta Rychterová

Department of Histology, Faculty of General Medicine and Department of Pathology, Faculty of Medical Hygiene, Charles University, Prague 2, Czechoslovakia

We would like to start our chapter with an illustration of the comparative and functional approaches to the analysis of heart development.

The morphogenesis of the heart bulbus will be used as an example. From the comparative point of view, the heart bulb is a structure which, as a separate heart cavity, progressively disappears with advances in phylogenetic status (1). In *Chondrichthyes,* the bulb is a large cavity. In *Amidae,* it begins to shorten. This shortening is even more pronounced in *Osteichthyes* (Fig. 1). The bulb contains parallel rows of valves, increasing in number with age. In *Amphibia,* the number of valves decreases and the cavity of the bulb contains either the spiral ridge or the spiral septum (Fig. 2). Even the histological structure of the bulbar wall changes in phylogenesis, the musculature being replaced by elastic tissue. The bulb is first included in the ventricular compartment of the heart in *Reptilia.*

During the embryonic period in mammals and in birds, the heart bulb functions as a separate heart chamber. This chamber is separated from the ventricular portion of the heart loop by proximal bulbar cushions and from the heart trunk by distal bulbar cushions. In its early development, the bulbus lengthens (Fig. 3). Its cushions function as a valvular device and grow concomitantly (17,19). During later development, the heart bulb progressively shortens (Fig. 3d), to be taken finally into the ventricular portion of the heart, as in phylogenesis. The bulbar cushions are remodeled by the blood flow into spiral ridge-like anlages of the bulbar septum.

The exact position of the boundary between the bulb and the right ventricle is not yet known, not only in the definitive heart, but also during the period when the bulb is fully functional as an individual heart chamber. According to Streeter (35), the ventriculobulbar border seems to be the border between the trabecular and smooth part of the wall in the ascending portion of the heart loop (Fig. 4). This presumption sometimes leads to the conclusion that the opening between the ascending and descending portions of the heart loop

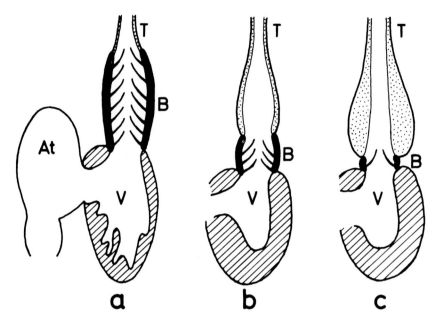

FIG. 1. The first principal trend in phylogenetic development of the heart bulb: progressive shortening. **a:** *Selachoidei;* **b:** *Amiidae;* **c:** *Teleostei.* At, atrium; V, ventricle; B, bulb; T, trunk. (According to Benninghoff, 1933.)

corresponds to the border between the ventricle and the bulbus. It is then falsely termed the foramen ventriculobulbare. The increase in volume of the trabeculated part of the heart wall might be the result of growth of the right ventricular anlage and of the concomitant change in the proportions of different segments

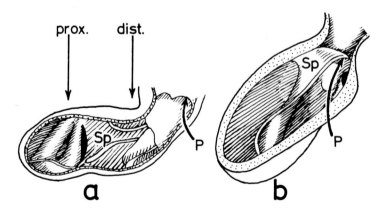

FIG. 2. The second principal trend in phylogenetic development of the heart bulb: reduction of the number of the valves and transformation of the valves in the spiral ridge or septum. **a:** *Salamandra;* **b:** *Rana.* Prox–dist, proximal and distal row of valves; Sp, spiral fold; P, pulmonary part of aortic arches. (According to Boas, 1882.)

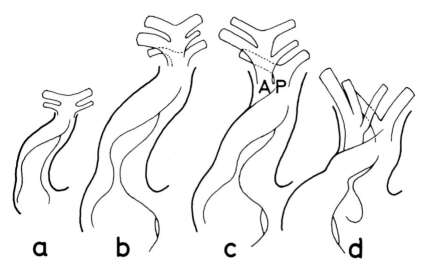

FIG. 3. Growth and reduction of the heart bulb in the chick embryo. **a:** 3 e.d.; **b:** 4 e.d. 16 h; **c:** 4 e.d. 20 h; **d:** 6 e.d. A, P, aortic, pulmonary portion of the heart trunk. (According to Rychter, 1959.)

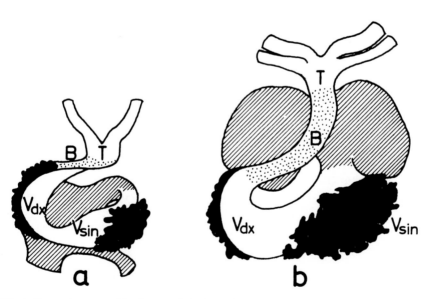

FIG. 4. Reconstruction of the lumen of the heart loop of the human embryo. **a:** 2 to 3 mm (approx. 24 e.d., horizon XI); **b:** 4 to 5 mm (approx. 27 e.d., horizon XIII). $V_{dx,sin}$, right, left ventricle; B, bulb; T, trunk. (According to Streeter, 1948.)

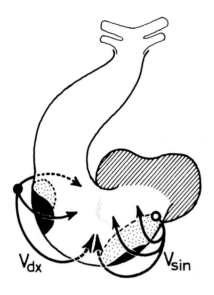

FIG. 5. Directions of the marks' shifts from the proliferation centers in the wall of the right and left ventricle of the chick embryo (older than 3 e.d.). $V_{dx,sin}$, right, left ventricle.

of the heart loop, largely due to the growth of the heart bulb. We do not consider the exact definition of the border between the bulb and the right ventricle to be the most important question of heart morphogenesis. There is a simple marking method available which enables one to follow the development of the bulbar and the ventricular portions of the heart. A glass rod covered with an India ink-colored gelatin sheet (31), when inserted into various parts of the right ventricle, behaves in different ways. The marks pricked in the ventral and dorsal parts of the right ventricle move to the left in the same horizontal plane (Fig. 5). A mark inserted into the lateral part of the right ventricle moves conspicuously to the apex. This may lead to the false interpretation that the bulb becomes part of the right ventricle. Analyses and interpretations of results obtained by marking are impossible without detailed knowledge of the proliferation structure of the heart loop wall. The wall of the right ventricular anlage differs from the wall of the bulb by the presence of a proliferation center. It therefore grows from its own sources, but the bulb does not (19). The right and left ventricular proliferation centers (Fig. 5) are necessary for the development of the interventricular septum (22,23,26). Bulbus growth is accomplished by addition of materials from the embryonic body to its distal part. A knowledge of the proliferation structure of the wall of the heart loop is very important for the understanding of the morphogenetic processes in heart development.

DESCRIPTIVE STUDIES

Myoarchitecture

Development of the heart in the chick embryo will be followed from the stage at which regular contractions begin (9 to 10 somites (15), 1 e.d. 5 h to 1 e.d. 6h, stage 9). A new and important morphogenetic factor enters into heart development—the blood flow. The heart is a tube, irregularly dilated and bended and heterogenous in structure (16). Rulon (16) noted in 1935 that various portions of the heart tube differently reduce Janus green. Maximum reduction was seen at the venous end and convexities. Sissman (32) studied the heart tube by autoradiography. He observed a heterogeneity of ^{3}H-thymidine incorporation (Fig. 6). He could not decide, however, whether the different labeling indices result from variable percentages of cells in S-phase or are the result of varying durations of the cell cycle. Sissman (32) arrived at the conclusion that the changes in configuration of the heart tube are the necessary consequences of different expansions of cell populations in circumscribed portions of the heart tube. Unfortunately, exact mapping of mitoses was not performed, so that the proliferation structure was only approximated and could not be related to the looping of the heart tube. We do not believe that the uneven contribution of the material from the right and left sides of blastoderm is sufficient for elucidation of this looping, as considered by Stalsberg (33).

The proliferation structure of the ventricular portion of the early heart loop was studied by Rychter et al. (26). These authors have seen diffuse proliferation, with exceptions noted on the atrioventricular and ventriculobulbar borders, at which accumulations of mitoses occurred (Fig. 6). To learn how the heart loop grows, it is necessary to identify the location of the proliferation foci and the direction in which the divided cells move.

More information on the proliferation structure of the later stages of the

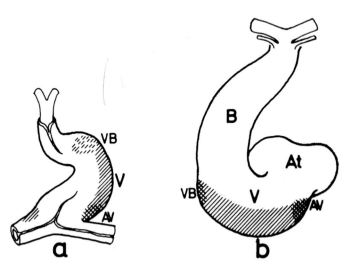

FIG. 6. Localization of DNA synthesis in the wall of the heart tube and heart loop in the chick embryo. **a:** heart tube; stage 12, posterior view (according to Sissman, 1966); **b:** heart loop, 2 e.d. 18 h, anterior view (according to Rychter et al., 1979). At, atrium; V, ventricle; B, bulb; AV, atrioventricular boundary; VB, ventriculobulbar boundary; hatched area, high mitotic activity; cross-hatched area, the highest mitotic activity.

heart loop is also available (10,15). Goerttler's (10) reason for estimation of proliferation activity (Fig. 7) was not to study morphogenesis and morphogenetic movements. He presumed an increased vulnerability of those portions of the heart wall with high mitotic activity. The discovery of these vulnerable portions of the heart loop would provide an explanation for the more frequent occurrence of certain types of congenital heart defects.

To ascertain the direction of movement (22,23), Rychter et al. (26) marked the morphogenetic movements by Seichert's method (31). They confirmed the existence of the right and left ventricular proliferation centers (Fig. 5), and explained their function in formation of the interventricular septum, which develops passively as a common wall of the quickly expanding ventricles. This could be deduced from the direction of the shifts of marks and of their deposition in the interventricular septum (see also Harh and Paul, 11). Asymmetry exists in localization of the proliferation centers and in the direction of cell movements away from them. The marks, situated in the right proliferation center at the ventriculobulbar boundary, move ventrally and dorsally in the right ventricular wall and to the apex of the heart loop (Fig. 8). The apical shift of marks is the greatest. The left ventricular proliferation center is situated lower and more dorsally than the right. The marks move mostly to the ventral wall of the left ventricle. The closer the mark is situated to the apex, the more it moves upward to the heart base (Fig. 8).

What is the meaning of the asymmetry in the proliferation centers, and especially of the asymmetrical growth of the left ventricular wall? The interventricular septum is not oriented in the sagittal plane, but its ventral portion is rotated to the left (Fig. 8). We suppose that the distance myocytes originating from the left ventricular proliferation center must travel is greater on the ventral wall than the distance from the right one. The material from the left ventricular proliferation center is not only directed towards the interventricular septum, but also upwards along it.

The difference in the position of the ventricular proliferation centers and the different mode of outgrowth of the ventricular walls might be responsible for the difference in ventricular myoarchitectonics, especially in the trabecular portions. The trabeculae in the right ventricle are situated radially, as can be seen both on transverse and frontal histological sections (Fig. 9). Their arrangement is congruent with the mode of growth from the right ventricular proliferation center. The largest trabeculae are found in the apical part of the right ventricle. The arrangement of the trabeculae in the left ventricle shows great heterogeneity. In the apical part, parallel large trabeculae are arranged as sagittally oriented lamellae (15). The trabeculae in the more basal part are oriented radially. The inner relief, therefore, is characteristic for each ventricle. The basoapical gradient in the size of the intertrabecular spaces (24) seems also to correlate with the described mode of growth of the heart wall.

As can be seen in Goerttler's picture (Fig. 7), a relatively great degree of proliferation activity also appears on the convexities of the atrial anlage. Rychter

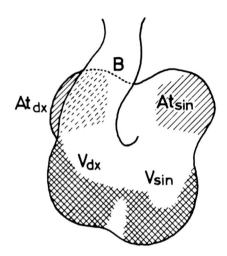

FIG. 7. Localization of mitotic activity in the wall of the heart loop in the chick embryo on 4th e.d. $AT_{dx,sin}$, right, left atrium; $V_{dx,sin}$, right, left ventricle; B, bulb; hatched area, high mitotic activity; cross-hatched area, the highest mitotic activity. (According to Goerttler, 1957.)

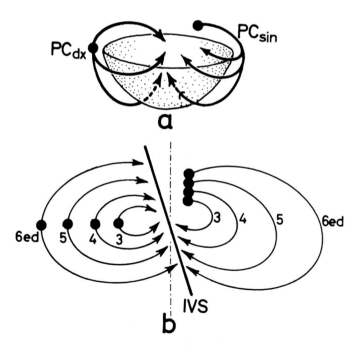

FIG. 8. Contribution of the right and left ventricular proliferation centers to the formation of the interventricular septum and its spatial orientation in the chick embryo. **a:** direction of the marks' shifts in the heart wall on 3rd e.d.; **b:** trajectories of the marks to the interventricular septum (horizontal section). $PC_{dx,sin}$, right, left ventricular proliferation center; IVS, interventricular septum.

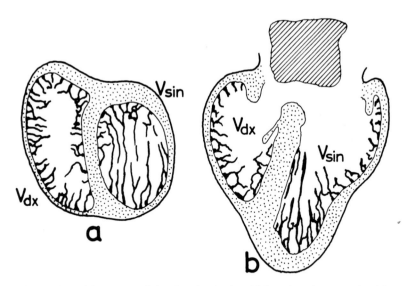

FIG. 9. Orientation of the myocardial trabeculae in the chick embryo heart on the 6th e.d. **a:** horizontal section; **b:** frontal section. $V_{dx,sin}$, right, left ventricle.

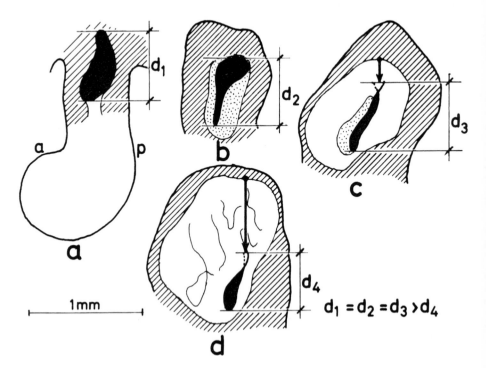

FIG. 10. Mode of formation of the early interatrial septum and the height of foramen primum in the chick embryo. **a:** 2nd e.d.; **b:** 3rd e.d.; **c:** 4th e.d.; **d:** 5th e.d. a, p, anterior, posterior side; d_1—d_4, height of foramen primum. *Arrows* in **c, d** indicate the distance between the upper border of the interatrial septum and the upper border of foramen primum.

and Pexieder (unpublished data) observed that the foramen interatriale does not change in craniocaudal diameter (Fig. 10, between 2 and 5 e.d.), in spite of the fact that the interatrial septum nearly doubles in diameter. They concluded that the interatrial septum, like the interventricular one, develops passively as a common wall of the quickly expanding atrial anlages. Progressive closure of the foramen primum is followed by the appearance of multiple dehiscences (Fig. 11) in the growing interatrial septum (foramina secunda).

Let us return to consideration of the heart bulb. Rychter (17) observed that the heart bulb grows in length until the arterial trunk begins to divide into pulmonary and aortic portions. Growth of the bulb is accomplished by apposition of material from the embryonic body at its distal end (19), not from its own sources. This material is shifted along the caudal margin of the ventral part of the 6th aortic arch, like a wedge from behind, between the 6th and the 4th aortic arches. It separates the aortic and pulmonary part of the trunk as an aorticopulmonary septum. The source of this material was also identified. The original experiment (19) was repeated in two variations, with three Seichert's marks inserted on the 3rd e.d. into both sides of the 4th branchial clefts (Figs. 12,13) and under the still-forming 6th aortic arch. In the first variation, the marks were located in the ventral part of the branchial cleft; in the second variation, they were located in its dorsal part. From the displacement of labels, it was concluded that growth of the aortic arches is concentrated mostly in their ventral halves, and that the mesenchymal material shifts from the hypobranchial region along the lower border of the 6th aortic arches. These arches keep the caudal mark in a more ventral position. Its gelatin mantle with India ink is shifted to the aorticopulmonary septum between the 4th and 6th aortic arches (Fig. 14). The hypobranchial region was studied by Seichert's marks inserted at every angle of an imaginary square and in its middle (Figs. 15,16). From the shifting of marks, we conclude that the material for the distal part of the bulb originates approximately at the middle of the hypobranchial region, as

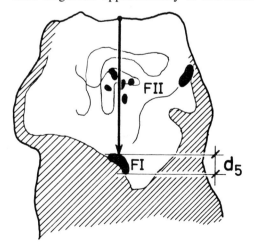

FIG. 11. Size of foramen primum and foramina secunda of the interatrial septum in the chick embryo on the 6th e.d. F I, II, foramen primum, secundum. *Arrow* indicates the distance between the upper border of the interatrial septum and the upper border of the foramen primum.

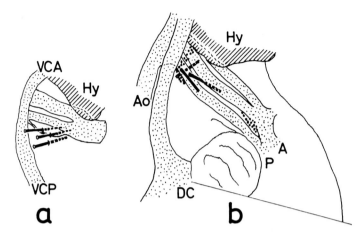

FIG. 12. Marking of the branchial region above (in the 4th branchial cleft) and below the 6th aortic arch on the right side of the chick embryo. **a:** marks inserted in the posterior half of the branchial cleft on the 3rd e.d.; **b:** position of the marks and their pigment on the 5th e.d. Pigment from the mark inserted below the 6th aortic arch is incorporated into the aorticopulmonary septum. VCA, VCP, anterior, posterior cardinal vein; Hy, hyoid opercle; A, P, aortic, pulmonary part of the trunk; Ao, dorsal aorta; DC, Cuvier's duct.

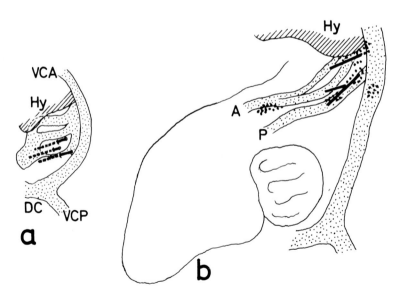

FIG. 13. Marking of the branchial region above (in the 4th branchial cleft) and below the 6th aortic arch on the left side of the chick embryo. **a:** marks inserted in the posterior half of the branchial cleft on the 3rd e.d.; **b:** position of the marks and their pigment on the 5th e.d. Pigment from the mark inserted below the 6th aortic arch is situated on the anterior side of the aorticopulmonary septum. For abbreviations, see Fig. 12.

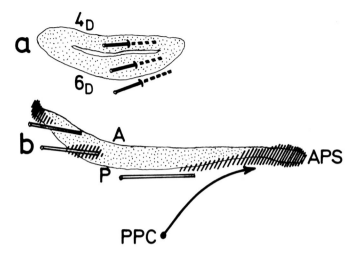

FIG. 14. Scheme of the shifts of the marks and their pigment after their insertion into the anterior half of the 4th branchial cleft and below the 6th aortic arch. Right side of the chick embryo. **a:** insertion of marks on the 3rd e.d.; **b:** position of marks on the 5th e.d. 4_D, 6_D, area occupied by the right 4th and 6th aortic arches; A, P, aortic and pulmonary rims of the aorticopulmonary septum (APS); PPC, peripulmonary proliferation center.

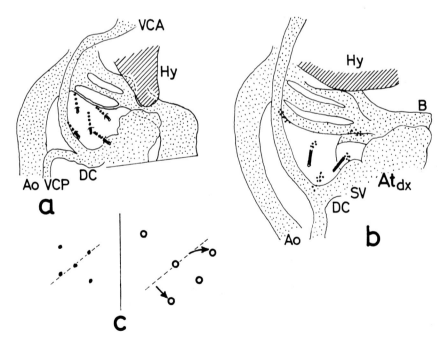

FIG. 15. Marking of the hypobranchial region on the right side of the chick embryo. **a:** 3rd e.d.; **b:** shifts of marks and their pigment observed on the 4th e.d.; **c:** schema of the marks' shifts. SV, venous sinus; At_{dx}, right atrium; B, bulb. For other abbreviations, see Fig. 12.

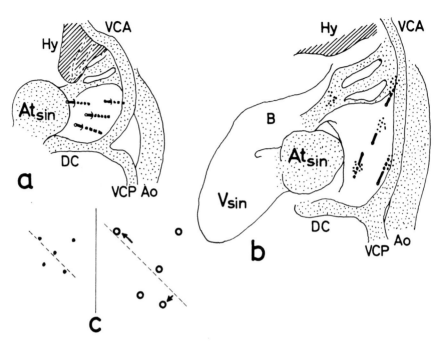

FIG. 16. Marking of the hypobranchial region on the left side of the chick embryo. **a:** 3rd e.d.; **b:** shift of the marks and their pigment observed on the 4th e.d.; **c:** schema of the marks' shifts. At$_{sin}$, left atrium; V$_{sin}$, left ventricle; B, bulb. For other abbreviations, see Fig. 12 and 15.

viewed from the side. In reality, this is the proliferating mesenchyme, surrounding the anlagen of the lungs and separating from them. This material moves cranioventrally and arrives at the bulb via the porta arteriosa of the heart loop. The described movements of mesenchyme can also be followed in serial sections presented by Los (13). The rapid growth in length of the aortic arches, together with rapid coalescence of the bulbar cushions in the direction against the blood flow, as the result of proliferation (15) of the bases of the ridges developing from the bulbar cushions, terminates the existence of the bulb as a separate heart chamber.

We also studied the possible persistence of the ventricular proliferating centers after the end of ventricular septation. Higher proliferation activity could be seen on the heart bases up to the 10th e.d. (30). Following this stage, proliferation activity becomes diffuse, i.e., the ventricles and the ventricular septum grow evenly.

Angioarchitecture

When development of the interventricular septum is finished and the slit between its upper bulbar and lower ventricular portion is closed, development of coronary arteries begins (24). The buds of the coronary arteries, two or

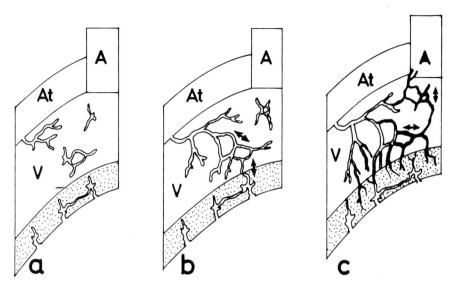

FIG. 17. Development of the coronary bed on the heart surface in the chick embryo. Dotted area, cross-section of the heart wall. **a:** formation of veins and *in situ* differentiated vessel channels; **b:** developing veins incorporate the *in situ* differentiated blood channels and mesh and communicate with intertrabecular spaces; **c:** buds of coronary arteries find the communications with primitive venous network and *in situ* differentiated blood channels; part of venous bed is transformed into arterial bed.

more in number, arise from aortic valvular sinuses and join the preformed venous plexuses (Fig. 17). These plexuses develop mainly in atrioventricular grooves between the ventricles and the atria, and also in the ventricular septum. Development of the coronary arteries can be considered as parasitic. Parts of

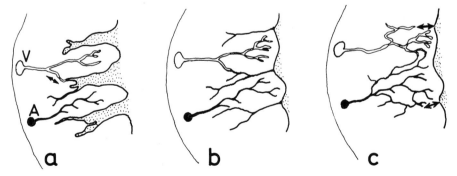

FIG. 18. Disappearance of the intertrabecular spaces and incorporation of the thin endothelial slits into the coronary capillary bed. **a:** communication of veins with the intertrabecular spaces and penetration of arteries into the trabeculae of the myocardium; **b:** situation after the narrowing of the intertrabecular spaces to endothelial slits; **c:** incorporation of the intertrabecular endothelial slits into the coronary capillary bed. *Arrows,* possible communications with the ventricular cavity. A, artery; V, vein.

the primitive venous plexuses are transformed into arteries. During their further growth, a network of vascular channels differentiated *in situ* (in the loose epicardial connective tissue) is incorporated into the coronary bed. This parasitic type of growth further continues within the heart wall by incorporation of the diminished intertrabecular spaces (Fig. 18). These spaces change into narrow slits between muscular trabeculae which become capillaries (29). The process of formation of the capillary bed within the heart wall illustrates the mutual relationship in the development of the angio- and myoarchitectonics. The trabecular compartment gradually disappears (25,28) by a process called compaction of the trabeculae.

Development of the coronary bed occurs at about the same time, 7 to 10 e.d., in various animal species. Differences exist only in its growth on the heart

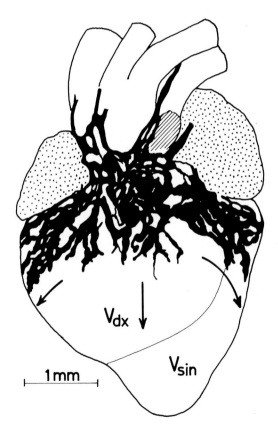

FIG. 19. Three main directions of the expansion of the lymphatic bed on the heart surface in the chick embryo on the 10th e.d. $V_{dx,sin}$, right, left ventricle.

surface, depending on the relations and the modes of ramifications of the parietal and the septal branches of the coronary arteries. This must be taken into account when extrapolating data from one species to the other.

Development of the lymphatics is delayed in comparison with development of the coronary bed. The main lymphatic stems grow through the loose connective tissue along the great arteries on the heart base on the 9th e.d. in chick embryo (27). They can be seen in the aorticopulmonary sulcus and used for contrast injection of the lymphatic bed. On the ventral part of the heart, the lymphatics grow in three directions (Fig. 19): along the right atrioventricular groove, on the ventral wall of the right ventricle in the direction of the interventricular groove, and from the left atrioventricular groove to the margo obtusus. Lymphatic capillaries proliferate and join the intercellular spaces of the loose epicardial connective tissue (12). At the end of coronary artery development, valves appear in the lymphatic vessels near the heart base. They become an obstacle for color injection, so that the lymphatic bed must be filled by repeated partial injections. By extrapolation, development of the lymphatics is assumed to be finished on the 17th e.d. in chick embryo heart, and the coronary bed is already completed on the 14th e.d.

Summarizing data on development of the coronary and lymphatic vessels, it can be stated that their development is almost independent of heart morphogenesis. However, it is influenced by the time sequence and topology of morphogenetic processes within the heart wall.

EXPERIMENTAL STUDIES

Myoarchitecture

Experiments performed by direct intervention on the heart loop were chosen for this chapter. Trials to suppress mechanically the development of the interventricular septum are unsuccessful and give evidence of ignorance of the mechanisms of its development. Suppression of the anlage of the interventricular septum by silver clips (Fig. 20) was performed by Rychter and Lemez (21). The clips were drawn deeply into the ventricular septum, and this led the authors to the idea of marking the heart wall and the discovery of the morphogenetic functions of the ventricular proliferation centers. The experiments of Dor and Corone (8) directed at mechanical suppression of development of the septum interventriculare, and to subsequent production of cor univentriculare, had to be unsuccessful. Moreover they were analogous with the experiments of Rychter and Lemez (20,21), in which we attempted to maintain the bulb in its original relationship to the heart loop and produce transposition of the aorta (Fig. 21) to the right ventricle. The method presented by Dor and Corone (8) is only a variation on the method, elaborated by Stephan (34). Experimental intervention by which the localized proliferation structure can be changed into a diffuse one is not yet available.

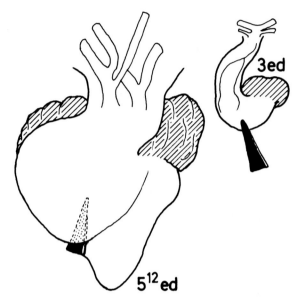

FIG. 20. Clamping of the anlage of the interventricular septum in the chick embryo on the 3rd e.d. Note the incorporation of the silver clip into the interventricular septum 60 hours later.

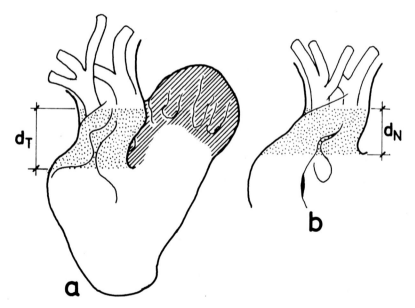

FIG. 21. Length of the bulb in a chick embryo with experimentally produced transposition of the aorta into the right ventricle **(a)** and in normal chick embryo **(b)** on the 6th e.d. d_T, the bulb's length in transposition; d_N, bulb's length in the normal embryo.

The delay in morphogenetic transformation of the bulb is known both from the experiments and from the genetically determined defects. The thin ligature located between the proximal and distal bulbar cushions hinders their coalescence and the bulbar part of the interventricular septum remains incomplete, resulting in a ventricular septal defect (5). A very similar effect was achieved by removal of the lung bud at 5 e.d. 12 h in the chick embryo (4). The amount of material available for growth of the distal part of the bulb was diminished in both experiments. This resulted in insufficient development of the bulbar part of the ventricular septum, producing the septal defect. Rychter tried to influence development of the bulb in younger chick embryos (4 e.d.) and obtained the same defect (Rychter, unpublished data). Van Mierop and Patterson (36) described hereditary VSD in Keeshond dogs. In the embryonic heart of these dogs, the proximal margin of the coalescent bulbar cushions did not grow the entire distance necessary for their fusion with the ventricular (muscular) part of the interventricular septum.

Other experiments were performed in which some effect on the proliferation structure might be expected. Hypoplasia of the left half of the heart was produced by clipping off the anlage of the left atrium in chick embryo (18,20). Study of the proliferation structure of the ventricular walls of operated embryos has shown (up to 10 e.d.) an uneven mitotic activity, as in normal hearts. This is surprising because the shape of the heart is conspicuously changed, with the apex formed by the expanded right ventricle (Fig. 22). Our previous knowledge of the proliferation structure enables us to compare equivalent parts of the ventricular wall in normal and experimental embryos, because localization of the high mitotic activity does not change (Rychterova, unpublished data).

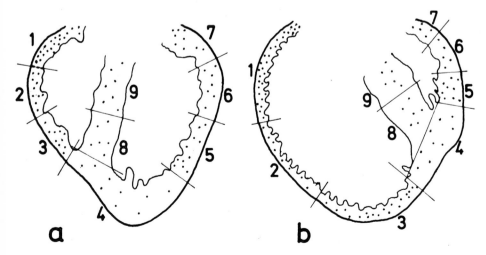

FIG. 22. Distribution of mitoses in the heart wall of the chick embryo on the 8th e.d. Frontal sections. **a:** normal heart; **b:** heart with left hypoplasia. 1 to 9, equivalent segments of the heart wall.

The compaction of the walls of the heart ventricles is expected to be a less rigid process, because it is under the direct formative influence of hemodynamics. In the compensatory enlarged right ventricle of experimentally produced left heart hypoplasia, the usual thickening of the trabeculae, with their subsequent coalescence, does not take place (28). The intertrabecular spaces, with their communications to coronary vessels, persist, and the terminal coronary bed is reduced, because the endothelial changes did not develop from the narrowed intertrabecular spaces. Here, again, the morphogenetic correlation between myo- and angioarchitectonics is evident. The disappearance of the trabecular structure of the heart wall is the result of rearrangement of its proliferation structure.

Angioarchitecture

It has been suggested that development of the coronary bed is independent of heart morphogenesis. The meaning of this sentence must be defined more precisely: development of the coronary bed cannot be suppressed, but can be profoundly changed. In the case of experimental transposition of the aorta (20), the bulbar portion of the heart remains longer than in normal hearts (Fig. 21), because the bulb was not incorporated into the ventricular compartment. Normally originating coronary buds must therefore grow over a greater distance to meet with the venous plexuses. Development of the coronary bed is delayed, and the bed presents a variety of defects: the origin of the coronary arteries

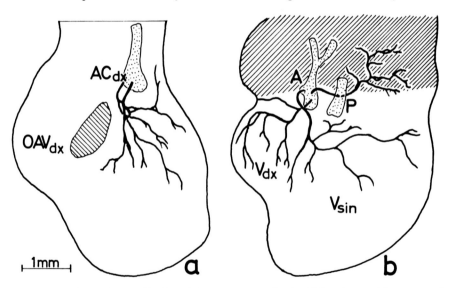

FIG. 23. Variations in the ramification of the coronary arteries in chick embryos with transposed aorta, 14th e.d. **a:** two buds of the right coronary artery with abnormal branching pattern (right profile); **b:** three coronary arteries (frontal view). A, aorta; P, pulmonary artery; AC_{dx}, right coronary artery; OAV_{dx}, right atrioventricular orifice; $V_{dx,sin}$, right, left ventricle.

remains doubled (Fig. 23a), their number multiplies (Fig. 23b), and their origin (Fig. 24a), course, and diameter (Fig. 24b) change. The defects might affect even the terminal bed as a consequence of failure in development of the myoarchitectonics. Development of the coronary arteries and their branching have also been described in experimental hypoplasias of the right and/or left half of the heart (6,7).

We have also studied vessels in hypoplasia of the left half of the heart. We have observed a delay in their development (two days on the 14th e.d.) (Fig. 25). The valves normally present in lymphatic stems did not develop, and lymphatics were absent in the hypoplastic left chamber. Certain areas of the heart wall remained devoid of lymphatic channels. The functional relations between blood and lymphatic vessels were emphasized by Casley-Smith (3) and Elhay and Casley-Smith (9). It remains to be determined how the myocardium differentiates and grows under these circumstances, and how its functional ability is modified. A knowledge of the exact topology of these defective areas will enable us to analyze such regions on the tissue level and to test their functional properties. The discussed alterations at the organ level will make possible further

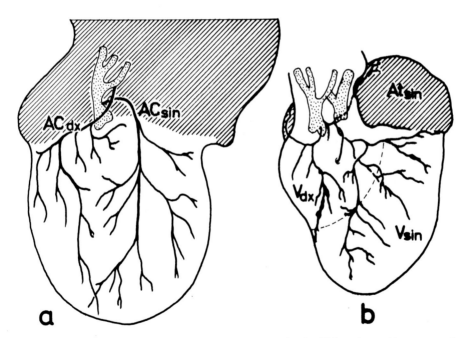

FIG. 24. Variation in the ramification of the coronary arteries in chick embryo with transposed aorta, 14th e.d. **a:** anterior view of abnormal origin of the coronary arteries: the right artery from the left brachiocephalic trunk, the left artery above Valsalva's sinus; **b:** abnormal course of the coronary arteries: the left directly penetrates into the interventricular septum before appearing on the heart surface in the anterior interventricular groove *(dashed line)*. $AC_{dx,sin}$, right, left coronary artery; At_{sin}, left atrium, $V_{dx,sin}$, right, left ventricle.

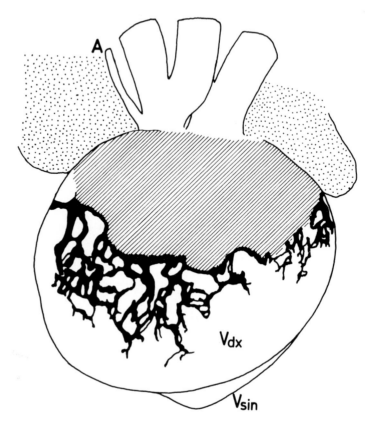

FIG. 25. Lymphatic vessels of the heart wall in the case of left heart hypoplasia, 14th e.d. *Hatched area,* pigment penetrating through the primitive lymphatics' walls and hiding the branching of the lymphatic vessels and nets. A, stenotic ascending aorta; $V_{dx.sin}$, right, left ventricle.

studies on lower levels of the hierarchy of the biological systems, extending even to the subcellular and molecular aspects of cardiac morphogenesis and teratogenesis.

REFERENCES

1. Benninghoff, A. (1933): Herz. In: *Handbuch der vergleichenden Anatomie der Wirbeltiere,* edited by L. Bolk, E. Kallius, and W. Lubosch, pp. 467-556. Urban and Schwarzenberg, Berlin, Vienna.

2. Boas, J. E. V. (1882): Ueber den Conus arteriosus und die Arterienbogen der Amphibien. *Morphol. Jahrb.,* 7:488-572.
3. Casley-Smith, J. R. (1976): The functioning and interrelationships of blood capillaries and lymphatics. *Experientia,* 32:1-12.
4. Clark, E. B., Martini, R., and Rosenquist, G. C. (1978): Effect of lung bud excision on cardiopulmonary development in the chick. In: *Morphogenesis and Malformation of the Cardiovascular System,* edited by G. C. Rosenquist and D. Bergsma, pp. 423-429. *Birth Defects: Orig. Art. Ser.,* vol. XIV, no. 7. Alan R. Liss, New York.
5. Clark, E. B., and Rosenquist, G. C. (1978): Spectrum of cardiovascular anomalies following cardiac loop constriction in the chick embryo. In: *Morphogenesis and Malformation of the Cardiovascular System,* edited by G. C. Rosenquist and D. Bergsma, pp. 431-442. *Birth Defects: Orig. Art. Ser.,* vol. XIV, no. 7. Alan R. Liss, New York.
6. Dbalý, J., and Rychter, Z. (1966): The vascular system of the chick embryo. XVI. Development of branching of coronary arteries in chick embryos with experimentally induced right-half heart hypoplasy. *Folia Morphol. (Praha),* 14:117-129.
7. Dbalý, J., and Rychter, Z. (1967): The vascular system of the chick embryo. XVII. The development of branching of coronary arteries in the chick embryo with experimentally induced left-half heart hypoplasy. *Folia Morphol. (Praha),* 15:358-368.
8. Dor, X., and Corone, P. (1979): Experimental creation of univentricular heart in the chick embryo. *Herz* (Kardiovaskuläre Erkrankungen), 4:91-96.
9. Elhay, S., and Casley-Smith, J. R. (1976): Mathematical model of the initial lymphatics. *Microvasc. Res.,* 12:121-130.
10. Goerttler, K. (1957): Die Stoffwechseltopographie des embryonalen Hühnerherzens und ihre Bedeutung für die Entstehung angeborener Herzfehler. *Verh. Dtsch. Gesellschaft Path.,* 40:181-185.
11. Harh, J. J., and Paul, M. H. (1975): Experimental cardiac morphogenesis. I. Development of the ventricular septum in the chick. *J. Embryol. Exp. Morphol.,* 33:13-28.
12. Klika, E., Antalíková, L., Rychter, Z., and Jelínek, R. (1972): Inception and manner of development of the lymph vessels in the chick embryo heart. *Lymphology,* 5:137-148.
13. Los, J. A. (1978): Cardiac septation and development of the aorta, pulmonary trunk, and pulmonary veins: Previous work in the light of recent observations. In: *Morphogenesis and Malformation of the Cardiovascular System,* edited by G. C. Rosenquist and D. Bergsma, pp. 109-138. *Birth Defects: Orig. Art. Ser.,* vol. XIV, no. 7. Alan R. Liss, New York.
14. Patten, B. M., and Kramer, Th.C. (1933): The initiation of contraction in the embryonic chick heart. *Am. J. Anat.,* 53:349-375.
15. Pexieder, T. (1978): Development of the outflow tract of the embryonic heart. In: *Morphogenesis and Malformation of the Cardiovascular System,* edited by G. C. Rosenquist and D. Bergsma, pp. 29-68. *Birth Defects: Orig. Art. Ser.,* vol. XIV, no. 7. Alan R. Liss, New York.
16. Rulon, C. (1935): Differential reduction of Janus green during development of the chick. *Protoplasma,* 24:346-364.
17. Rychter, Z. (1959): The vascular system of the chick embryo. III. On the problem of septation of the heart bulb and trunk in chick embryo. (In Czech with Summary in English) *Čs. Morfol.,* 7:1-20.
18. Rychter, Z. (1962): Experimental morphology of the aortic arches and the heart loop in chick embryos. *Adv. Morphogen.,* 2:333-371.
19. Rychter, Z. (1978): Analysis of relations between aortic arches and aorticopulmonary septation. In: *Morphogenesis and Malformation of the Cardiovascular System,* edited by G. C. Rosenquist and D. Bergsma, pp. 443-448. *Birth Defects: Orig. Art. Ser.,* vol. XIV, no. 7. Alan R. Liss, New York.
20. Rychter, Z., and Lemež, L. (1960): The vascular system of the chick embryo. VII. The theory of the teratogenetic role of the local disturbance of the heart loop and aortic arches. (In Czech with Summary in English) *Čs. Morfol.,* 8:417-434.
21. Rychter, Z., and Lemež, L. (1963): The significance and methods of experimental malformation research. (In Czech) *Čs. Pediatrie,* 18:432-441.
22. Rychter, Z., and Lemež, L. (1967): Meccanismo della formazione del setto interventricolare nel cuore dell'embrione di pollo. *Arch. Ital. Anat. Embriol.,* 72 (Suppl.):118.
23. Rychter, Z., and Lemež, L. (1978): Development of hereditary ventricular septal defects in Silver's strain of chick embryos. In: *Morphogenesis and Malformation of the Cardiovascular*

System, edited by G. C. Rosenquist and D. Bergsma, pp. 377-386. *Birth Defects: Orig. Art. Ser.*, vol. XIV, no. 7. Alan R. Liss, New York.

24. Rychter, Z., and Ošťádal, B. (1971): On the fate of "sinusoidal" intertrabecular spaces of chick embryo heart wall after the origination of coronary bed. *Folia Morphol. (Praha)*, 19:31-44.
25. Rychter, Z., and Ošťádal, B. (1971): Mechanism of the development of coronary arteries in chick embryo. *Folia Morphol. (Praha)*, 19:113-124.
26. Rychter, Z., Rychterová, V., and Lemež, L. (1979): Formation of the heart loop and proliferation structure of its wall as a base for ventricular septation. *Herz (Kardiovaskuläre Erkrankungen)*, 4:86-90.
27. Rychter, Z., Jelínek, R., Klika, E., and Antalíková, L. (1971): Development of the lymph bed in the wall of the chick embryo heart. *Physiol. Bohemoslov.*, 20:533-539.
28. Rychterová, V. (1971): Principle of growth of the heart ventricular wall in the chick embryo. *Folia Morphol. (Praha)*, 19:262-272.
29. Rychterová, V. (1977): Formation of the terminal vascular bed in the chick embryo heart. *Folia Morphol. (Praha)*, 25:7-14.
30. Rychterová, V. (1978): Development of proliferation structure of the ventricular heart wall in the chick embryo between the 6th and 14th day of embryogenesis. *Folia Morphol. (Praha)*, 26:131-143.
31. Seichert, V. (1965): Study of the tissue and organ anlage shifts by the method of plastic linear marking. *Folia Morphol. (Praha)*, 12:228-238.
32. Sissman, N. J. (1966): Cell multiplication rates during development of the primitive cardiac tube in the chick embryo. *Nature*, 210:504-507.
33. Stalsberg, H. (1969): The origin of heart asymmetry: Right and left contributions to the early chick embryo heart. *Dev. Biol.*, 19:109-127.
34. Stéphan, F. (1949): Sur la ligature des arcs aortiques chez l'embryon de poulet. *C.R. Soc. Biol. (Paris)*, 143:291-293.
35. Streeter, G. L. (1948): Developmental horizons in human embryos. Description of age groups XV, XVI, XVII and XVIII. *Contr. Embryol.*, 32:133-203.
36. Van Mierop, L. H. S., and Patterson, D. F. (1978): The pathogenesis of spontaneously occurring anomalies of the ventricular outflow tract in Keeshond dogs: Embryologic studies. In: *Morphogenesis and Malformation of the Cardiovascular System*, edited by G. C. Rosenquist and D. Bergsma, pp. 361-375. *Birth Defects: Orig. Art. Ser.*, vol. XIV, no. 7. Alan R. Liss, New York.

DISCUSSION

Heitzenberger: The development of coronary vessels in the rat, as we have observed it, seems to be the same as what you have described in the human. Concerning the smaller plexus, how can you differentiate lymphatic and blood vessels?

Rychter: Effectively, there is no difference between rat, mouse, and human, as far as coronary vessel development is concerned. There is a slight difference in the chick embryo, in which the coronary arteries remain in the epicardium and do not penetrate the myocardium. It is also interesting that in different species you need the same amount of time, i.e., 7 to 8 e.d., to develop the coronary vascular bed.

Heitzenberger: How did you determine which is a lymphatic and which is a vein?

Rychter: We have not yet done comparative studies on the development of lymphatics. We differentiate the lymphatics from the coronary veins by their specific injection pattern. On the other hand, we always used the main lymphatic stems lying in the groove between the aorta and the pulmonary artery. The embryos in which we could not inject this main stem were discarded.

Perspectives in Cardiovascular Research, Vol. 5,
Mechanisms of Cardiac Morphogenesis and Teratogenesis,
edited by Tomas Pexieder. Raven Press, New York © 1981

Cono-Truncal Torsions and Transposition of the Great Vessels in the Chick Embryo

Xavier Dor and Pierre Corone

Laboratoire d'Anatomie et d'Organogenèse, C.H.U. Pitié-Salpétrière, Paris 75013, France

An explanation for the transposition of the great vessels is found in two similar sentences concerning the conotruncus. One is by Jane Robertson, written in 1913 (20): "As the distal septum does not twist, its right side joins with the right, and its left with the left proximal bulbar ridge." Bulbar is taken as synonymous with conal. Distal septum designates the truncal septum and the corresponding distal bulbar ridges. The other sentence is by Edward Pernkopf and Wilhelm Wirtinger, and dates from 1935 (17): "Abnormal torsions could bring about various alignments of the (bulbar) ridges prior to their fusion" (as quoted by Grant (10)). Using normal, comparative, and experimental embryology, we will try to demonstrate the correctness of this theory.

Our concept of normal development of the embryonic chick heart is partly based on the work of Pernkopf and Wirtinger (16). A full description can be found in our previous publication (6). Our concept can be summarized as follows: we distinguish three segments (proximal, middle, and distal) in the conus. Proximal and distal ostia connect the conus to the primitive ventricle and the truncus, respectively. The conus contains four main ridges, two proximal and two distal, labeled according to the German nomenclature (16). The ridges are originally straight (6) but are interrupted in the middle segment on the 4 e.d. (13,24) (Fig. 1,2). Together with Pernkopf and Wirtinger (16), we subdivide the primitive ventricle into a right and a left ampulla, separated by an interampular ring (Fig. 4). With progressing development, the proximal and distal conal ridges extend into the middle segment. They next undergo torsions (6) (Fig. 1,2,3). These consist of a proximal torsion 120° clockwise and a distal torsion 150° counterclockwise (6,16,17). The torsions are supposed to start in the middle segment of the conus and extend to both ostia. In the chick embryo, these torsions start at 4 e.d. and terminate at 6.5 e.d. At the same time, the ingrowing aorticopulmonary septum twists 150° counterclockwise. Further displacements occur at the level of the proximal conus ostium as it migrates around the right atrioventricular orifice. The interampullar ring migrates to the left (7,8). A succession of connections characterize this phase of heart morphogenesis. The right tubercle of the medial AV cushions connects with the interventricular septum. The ventral and dorsal horns of the interventricular septum become related to the A and B proximal conal ridges, respectively, by means of expansion of the right tubercle. Proximal conal ridge A becomes connected with distal conal ridge 1, and proximal conal ridge B with distal conal ridge 3. Finally, distal conal ridges 1 and 3 join the aorticopulmonary septum.

The phylogenetic aspects of cardiac development have recently been examined in detail (6). We would like to stress several essential points (Fig. 4). First, the conal ridges are as old as the Vertebrates themselves (2,3,12,20). Conal torsions are first observed in the *Dipnoi,* in which the heart begins to receive separate flows of venous and arterial blood. In the Amphibian, the torsions extend to the conus. This extension continues in Reptiles, in which the conus ostia, the primitive ventricle, and the truncus become involved. The conus preserves only a small part of the torsions.

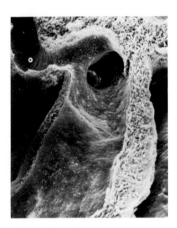
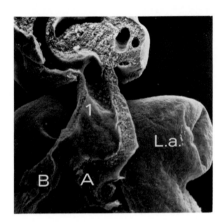

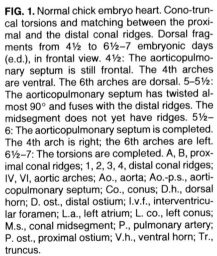
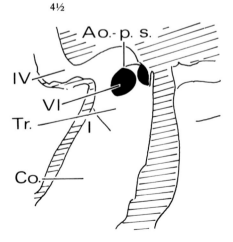

FIG. 1. Normal chick embryo heart. Cono-truncal torsions and matching between the proximal and the distal conal ridges. Dorsal fragments from 4½ to 6½–7 embryonic days (e.d.), in frontal view. 4½: The aorticopulmonary septum is still frontal. The 4th arches are ventral. The 6th arches are dorsal. 5–5½: The aorticopulmonary septum has twisted almost 90° and fuses with the distal ridges. The midsegment does not yet have ridges. 5½–6: The aorticopulmonary septum is completed. The 4th arch is right; the 6th arches are left. 6½–7: The torsions are completed. A, B, proximal conal ridges; 1, 2, 3, 4, distal conal ridges; IV, VI, aortic arches; Ao., aorta; Ao.-p.s., aorticopulmonary septum; Co., conus; D.h., dorsal horn; D. ost., distal ostium; I.v.f., interventricular foramen; L.a., left atrium; L. co., left conus; M.s., conal midsegment; P., pulmonary artery; P. ost., proximal ostium; V.h., ventral horn; Tr., truncus.

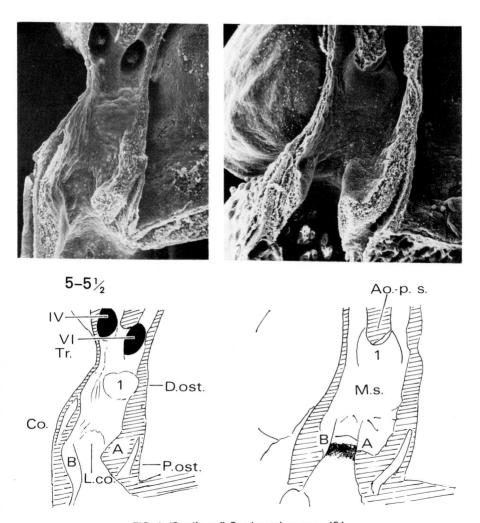

FIG. 1. (Continued) See legend on page 454.

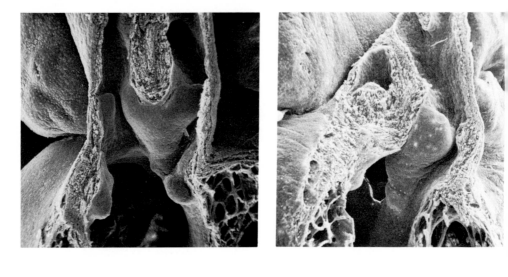

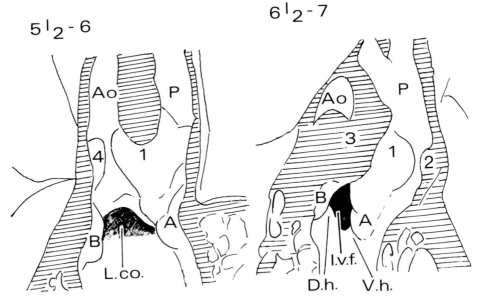

FIG. 1. (Continued) See legend on page 454.

MATERIALS AND METHODS

Leghorn chick eggs were incubated at 38°C in a moist atmosphere. After 48 hours of incubation, 2 or 3 ml of albumin were removed. Intervention took place between 3 and 3½ e.d. 12 h. After opening the shell, the heart was approached through incisions in the amnion and in the pericardium.

A fine lamella was taken from the shell membrane (membrana papyracea).

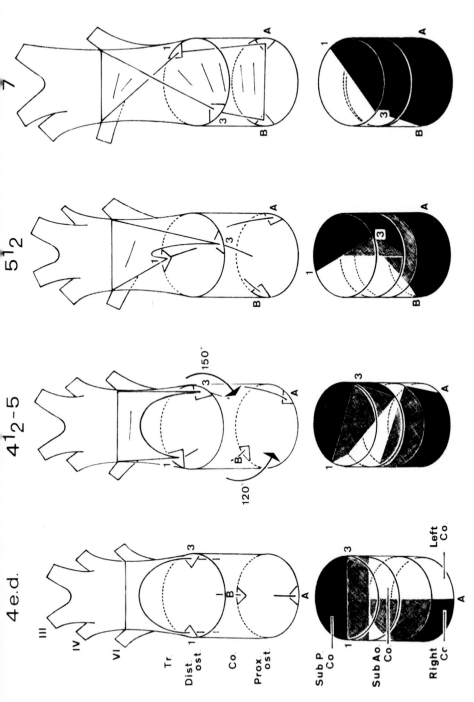

FIG. 2. Normal heart. Cono-truncal torsions and matching between the proximal and the distal conus ridges. Conal concordance: the right conus meets the subpulmonary one, and the left conus meets the subaortic one.

It was applied to one segment of the conus or on the truncus. Sometimes it was difficult to hold the lamella in a constant position. In these cases, it was necessary to repeat its introduction. The lamella could be placed in contact with the cono-truncus or at some distance, near the atrioventricular canal or the primitive ventricle. A piece of mica could also be used. After the intervention, the egg was replaced in the incubator. Within a few hours, adhesions formed around the conus, and these were capable of altering its development at a more or less early stage. For further studies, the embryos were sampled at 6.5 to 7 e.d., after the end of the normal conal torsions. Their hearts were prepared for SEM or for histologic examination. The embryos were submerged in the physiological serum and decapitated. The heart was dissected free and a drawing made. It was then injected with a glutaraldehyde solution (2.5%). After one hour of immersion fixation in this fixative, the heart was placed in a buffer solution and cut with a razor blade in a frontal or transverse plane into two parts. Each fragment was dehydrated by acetone, critical-point dried from liquid CO_2 and metalized by gold–palladium. For histologic studies, the heart was

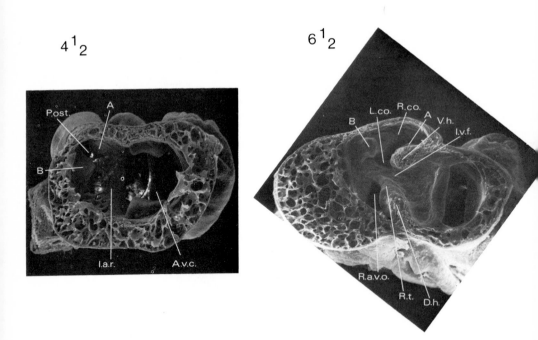

FIG. 3. Normal chick embryo heart. Transverse sections seen from the apex. At 4½ e.d., the conus has begun its migration; ridges A and B have begun their rotation. At 6½ e.d., migration and rotation are completed. At 6½–7 e.d., one can see the normal heart with persisting interventricular communication. l.a.r., interampullar ring; l.v.s., interventricular septum; P.o., pulmonary orifice; R.a-v.o., right atrioventricular orfices; R.co., right conus; R.t., right tubercle; V.h., ventral horn. Remaining abbreviations as in Fig. 1.

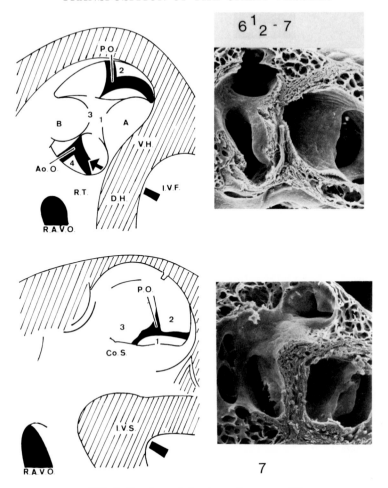

FIG. 3. (Continued) See legend on page 458.

fixed in Bouin's solution, embedded in paraffin, serially sectioned in a frontal or a transverse plane (5 or 10 μm), and stained by hematoxylin–eosin.

RESULTS

Cono–truncal Torsions

According to the proximal or distal location of the lamella, the intervention arrests completely or partially the proximal or the distal cono-truncal torsions. Sometimes they can even be accentuated, or, on the contrary, they can be of an opposite direction. Often the two torsions are simultaneously affected.

An anomaly of proximal torsion cannot be identified by external inspection

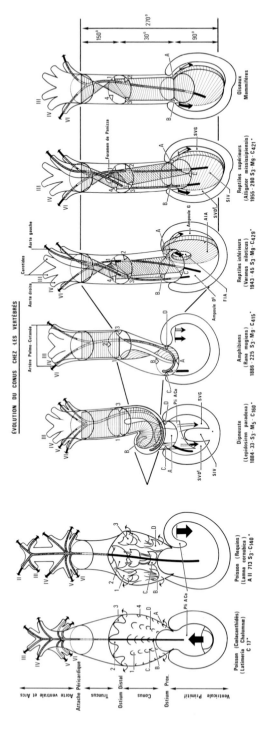

FIG. 4. Schema of conus evolution without a preconceived affiliation among the studied species. *Abbreviations:* A, B, C, D: Distal conal ridges; 1, 2, 3, 4: Proximal conal ridges; A I A: Interampullar ring; A I A: Interampullar foramen; O Ao: Aortic orifice; O P: Pulmonary orifice; Pli A Co: Atrio-conal flange; S I V: Interventricular septum; S V D': Right ventricular sinus; S V G: Left ventricular sinus. From the collection of comparative anatomy at the Museum of Natural History, Paris.

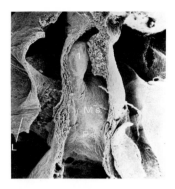

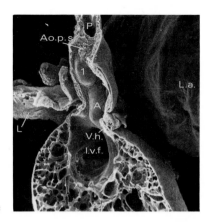

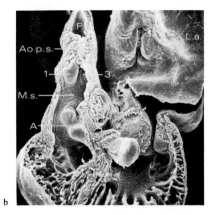

FIG. 5. Experimentally produced malposition of great vessels in the chick embryo. At 3 e.d., a mica lamella has been introduced in the dorsal concavity of the conus. Situation at 7th e.d. Dorsal fragments in frontal view. The lamella is visible on **a** and **c.** The distal ridges have remained in their primitive position (arrested distal torsion). **a:** Absence of fusion of ridges 1 and 3. Absence of the aorticopulmonary septum. Absence of truncus torsion. The proximal and midsegments have no ridges. **b:** Frontal orientation of the aortico-pulmonary septum. The aorta is ventral, and the pulmonary is dorsal. Ridge 1 and ridge 3 are rectilinear. The midsegment has no ridge. It is therefore impossible to diagnose the matching of the proximal and the distal ridges. **c:** Same situation as in **b,** but with spiral disposition of ridge 1 and A. The matching and proximal torsions are therefore normal, whereas the distal torsion is subnormal near the midsegment and absent near the distal ostium. This situation corresponds to an anatomically corrected malposition. L.a., left atrium; P.s., conal proximal segment. Remaining abbreviations as in Figs. 1 and 3.

only, since the great vessels can be in their usual place. Such anomalies must be diagnosed by dissecting the heart (Fig. 9). An anomaly of distal torsion concerns, at the same time, the distal segment of the conus, the truncus, and the origin of the aortic arches. It is obvious at first sight, as the great vessels are not in their usual place. The aorta is ventral, ventral and left, ventral and right, or in lateroposition (Fig. 5,6,7,8).

Matching of the Proximal and Distal Ridges

Matching does not exist if the midsegment remains devoid of ridges. The lamella generally hinders the growth of the ridges (Fig. 5).

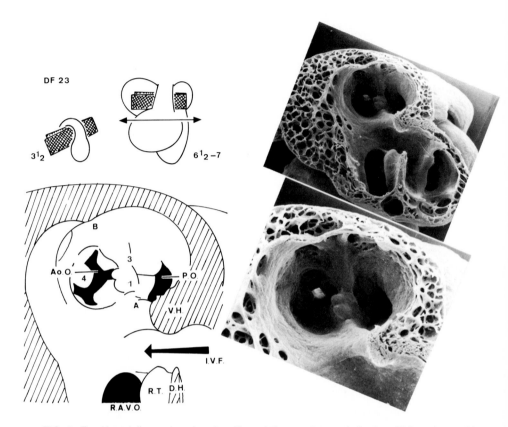

FIG. 6. Experimentally produced malposition of the great vessels in the chick embryo with conal concordance (A–1, B–3). Double-outlet right ventricle. At 3½ e.d., a shell membrane lamella, folded, has been introduced in the atrio-conal sulcus. Situation at 6½–7 e.d. Transverse section, seen from the apex. Excessive proximal torsion. Deficient distal torsion. Normal matching of proximal and distal conus ridges. A ledge separates the conus from the right ventricular sinus. It is caused by the lamella placed in the atrio-conal sulcus, impeding migration of the proximal ostium. The interventricular foramen opens into the right ventricular sinus. For abbreviations, see Fig. 1, 3, and 5.

Normal matching involves A–1 and B–3. In this case, the torsions near the midsegment are normal, but those near an ostium—generally the distal ostium—can be abnormal. The left conus opens into the subaortic conus, and the right conus opens into the subpulmonary conus. The conal distribution is concordant (Fig. 5,6).

Matching can be inverted, as in A–3 and B–1. In this case, the torsions near both an ostium and the midsegment are abnormal. In the midsegment, ridge A can encounter ridge 3, and ridge B can encounter ridge 1. A fuses with 3, B fuses with 1. The left conus opens into the subpulmonary conus, and the right conus opens into the subaortic conus. The conal distribution is

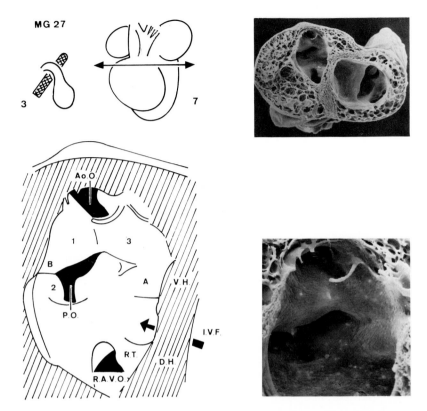

FIG. 7. Experimentally produced malposition of the great vessels in the chick embryo with conal discordance (A–3, B–1). Double-outlet right ventricle. At 3 e.d., a shell membrane lamella has been introduced in the atrio-conal sulcus near the distal segment and has later been lost. Situation at 7 e.d. Transverse section, seen from the apex. Proximal torsion is normal. There is no positive distal torsion. The left or dorsal conus opens into the pulmonary orifice, the right or ventral conus opens into the aortic orifice. Migration of the conus has been insufficient. The interventricular foramen opens into the right ventricular sinus. For abbreviations, see Fig. 1, 3, and 5.

discordant. Matching can be even more different (6), with the accessory ridges participating in the combination (e.g., A–2, B–4, C–3).

Proximal Ostium Migration

In a normal case, the left conus is well aligned with the left ventricular cavity and the interventricular foramen. The right conus remains downstream from the right ventricular cavity. Often an obstacle, the atrio-conal sulcus, impedes this migration. The left conus remains far from the interventricular foramen. The foramen opens into the right ventricular cavity, which opens into the conus as a whole, creating a double-outlet right ventricle (Figs. 6 and 7).

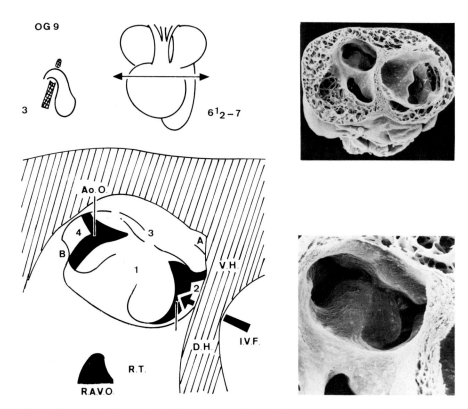

FIG. 8. Experimentally produced distal transposition of the great vessels in the chick embryo with conal discordance (A–3, B–1). Design of experiment as in Fig. 7. Situation at 6½–7 e.d. Transverse section seen from the apex. Proximal torsion is almost normal; distal torsion is deficient. The left conus opens into the pulmonary orifice. The right conus opens into the aortic orifice. Proximal ostium migration and left conus reduction are normal. The interventricular foramen opens directly into the pulmonary orifice. Interventricular communication is similar to that of a 6½–7 e.d. heart. For abbreviations, see Fig. 1, 3, and 5.

Frequently, intervention impedes the closure of the space situated between the conal and the interventricular septum, leaving an interventricular communication to the right of the interventricular foramen.

DISCUSSION

The Cono–Truncal Torsions

Many descriptions lead to the supposition that the conal ridges are initially spiral (4,5,9,13). We do not believe this is true. The conal ridges are rectilinear at their origin. This characteristic is associated with ontogenesis as well as phylogenesis, and can be experimentally reproduced. We can follow the displace-

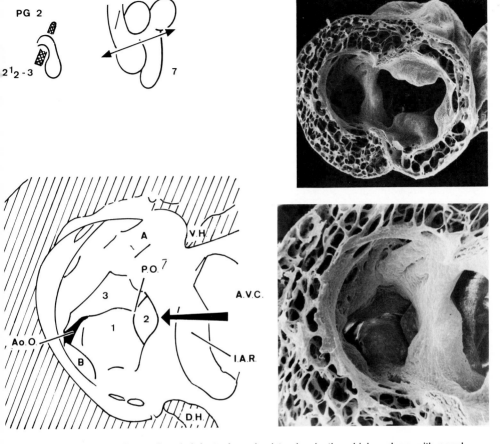

FIG. 9. Experimentally produced defect of proximal torsion in the chick embryo with conal discordance. A shell membrane lamella has been introduced into the atrio-conal sulcus at 2½–3 e.d. Situation at 7 e.d. Transverse section, seen from the apex. The heart is very primitive, like that of a shark. The atrioventricular canal persists. Absent conal migration, insufficient proximal torsion, subnormal distal torsion. The left conus opens into the pulmonary orifice. The right conus opens into the aortic orifice. For abbreviations, see Figs. 1, 3, and 5.

ment of the ridges on histological sections as well as on scanning electron microscope preparations. We can determine its direction, its amplitude, and its timing. Intervention can fix the intermediate stages. Rotation of the ostia in the superior Vertebrates is easy to follow, because the ridges at this level are precociously developed. There also, we can specify the direction, amplitude, and timing of displacement. Taken separately, the rotation of the ostia has no significance. Extension of the torsions to the ostia can be disconcerting, because the conus loses the greater part of its torsions for the benefit of the primitive ventricle and, overall, of the truncus. Thus, the conal ridges are originally rectilinear, then spiral, and finally almost rectilinear. We can see the torsion of the aorti-copulmonary septum when it is not yet well developed, and later on when the truncus is entirely septated before the end of its complete torsion. For us, it is difficult to conceive that the conal ridges and the aorticopulmonary septum are not reference marks. All these formations keep—at least, during certain periods—a definite and characteristic shape: ridge 1 is voluminous and rounded; ridge 3 is large, and divided into two parts in the birds; ridge C is small, triangular, and intercalated between A and B in the right conus; finally, the aorticopulmonary septum is bow-shaped and situated between the 4th and the 6th arches (Fig. 1).

Two mesenchymal condensations of the aorticopulmonary septum (14) can also be used as marks. They are submerged in the cardiac jelly of ridges 1 and 3. They appear at 4 e.d. before the beginning of the torsions. The condensa-tion in ridge 1 is often more precocious and more developed than in ridge 3. These ridges are opposite to each other. They turn, like the distal ridges, 150° counterclockwise. Their rotation ends at 6.5 e.d. (Fig. 10). They fuse together at 5 to 5.5 e.d. However, the following fact seems to contradict any idea of torsion: marking of the conal wall does not show rotation of the marks (18,21,22). Our experiments demonstrate an absence of cono-truncal torsion too, but only for the epimyocardium. A small zone on the ventral side of the mid-conus, cauterized at 3 e.d., remains ventral at 7 e.d.; inside, however, the torsions are normal (Fig. 11). A small zone of the dorsal side of the proximal conus, cauterized at 3 e.d., remains dorsal at 7 e.d., but the torsions inside are normal.

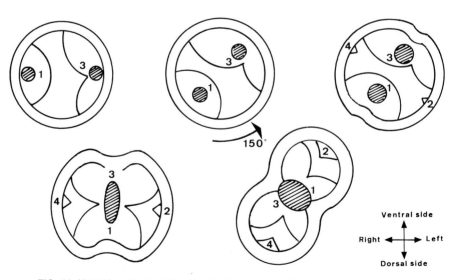

FIG. 10. Natural markers of the distal ostium rotation. For explanation, see text.

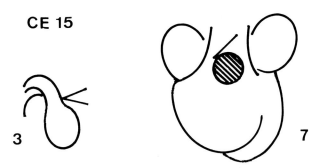

FIG. 11. Do the cardiac jelly and the endocardium turn inside the epimyocardium? Cauterization of the conus ventral side at 3 e.d. Situation at 7 e.d. The cauterized zone remained ventral and the torsions appear normal. On histological sections, the damaged myocardial zone corresponding to the cauterized zone is effectively ventral, and rotations of ridges A, B, 1, and 3 have been effectively correct.

Everything takes place as though the cardiac jelly and the endocardium were independent from the epimyocardium and turned inside it.

Matching Between the Proximal and Distal Conal Ridges

Originally, the conal ridges are interrupted at the level of the midsegment. Such disposition—described by Tandler (24) in human embryos—can be found in all Vertebrate embryos, starting with *Dipnoi*. This disposition is fundamental, because it permits the independence of the proximal and distal ridges and later on enables them to match. These ridges are initially in different planes and then unite in a definite order, ridge A with ridge 1, ridge B with ridge 3.

In our experiments, the proximal and distal ridges join in the midsegment only under two conditions: they must be sufficiently developed, and they must be aligned one with the other. Matching does not seem to be dependent on the identity of the ridges (6), but rather on the position given by the torsions in the midsegment (17). If in this segment the torsions are normal, matching is normal. If in this segment the torsions are abnormal, matching can be inverted (ridge A–ridge 3, ridge B–ridge 1). If the accessory ridges participate in the combination, the matching is different.

Malposition of the Great Vessels

This anomaly can be defined as follows: the great vessels are not in their usual position relative to each other (27). This is due to an anomaly of distal torsion, since the distal segment bears the orifice of the great vessels. Proximal torsion, matching, and proximal ostium migration may be normal or abnormal.

The great vessels can keep their original position, i.e., aorta ventral and pulmonary artery dorsal. More often, however, the aorta is ventral and right, as at 5 to 5.5 e.d., or in lateroposition (Fig. 6), as at 5.5 to 6 e.d. The aorta can become ventral and left even if the heart has no left loop (Fig. 7). All the hearts operated had a right loop. This anomaly is probably caused by adhesions between the great vessels and the ventral wall of the body present in these cases. In our experiments, a malposition is obtained by a lamella located on the distal segment or on the truncus.

Transposition of the Great Vessels

According to Van Praagh (26) and Anderson (1) transposition of the great vessels is characterized by the fact that the pulmonary artery originates from the left ventricle and the aorta originates from the right ventricle. A transposition, in our interpretation, supposes an inverted matching. This inverted matching has also been suggested by Pernkopf and Wirtinger (16,17). It provides a key to the transposition. We do not see any other explanation. Only the continuity A–3 and B–1 makes a communication contrary to the normal, between the right conus and the subaortic conus and the left conus with the subpulmonary conus. The distribution is inverted; there is conal discordance. The experimental proof is illustrated in Figs. 7–9. We believe that the defect of torsion must necessarily involve a zone near the midsegment, because it is at this level that matching occurs. A transposition can be: distal, by a defect of distal torsion. The aorta is ventral, ventral and right, or ventral and left. Such an anomaly is to be distinguished from a simple malposition (Fig. 8); proximal, by a defect of proximal torsion (6). The great vessels can be at their normal position. This anomaly is not obvious. More often, the two defects are associated. The aforesaid definition of transposition requires also a normal or a quasi-normal proximal ostium migration. This allows the left conus to come close to the mitral orifice and to align itself with the interventricular foramen (Fig. 8). The left conus is united with the subpulmonary conus. Its resorption leads to a mitropulmonary continuity. The left ventricle then opens into the pulmonary artery (Fig. 8).

The distal, or the distal and proximal transpositions, is a malposition with an A–3, B–1 combination and a normal proximal ostium migration. It corresponds to the usual form, with a ventral aorta (Fig. 12). The proximal transposition would correspond to the rare form with a dorsal aorta (Fig. 12). Schematically, in our experiments, a distal transposition is obtained by a lamella located on the distal and midsegments (Fig. 8). A proximal transposition is obtained by a lamella located on the proximal and midsegments (6).

Anatomically Corrected Transposition

In this malformation, the aorta is ventral and the pulmonary artery is dorsal. In spite of such an anomaly, the aorta originates from the left ventricle, and

Normal heart : A-1 B-3   Anat. corrected transposition : A-1 B-3

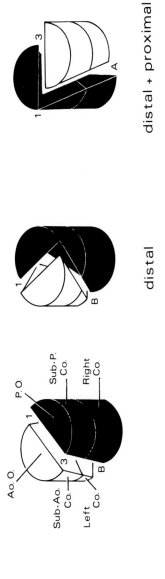

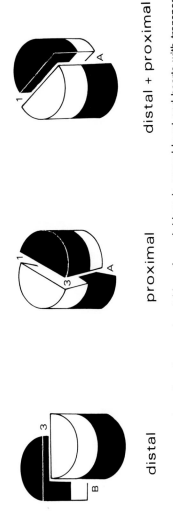

distal   distal + proximal

Transposition : A-3 B-1

distal   proximal   distal + proximal

FIG. 12. Schematic representation of torsions and matching of conal ridges in normal heart and hearts with transposition of great vessels. Normal heart: normal torsions, normal matching. Anatomically corrected transposition: abnormal torsions, normal matching. Transposition: abnormal torsions, inverted matching.

the pulmonary artery originates from the right ventricle (11,25). We do not consider this malformation to be a true transposition, but rather a particular type of malposition (19,23,27). It results from a distal torsion defect limited to the distal ostium, a normal matching of conal ridges, and a normal proximal ostium migration. Such a distal defect makes this particular conus similar to that of the *Dipnoi* or *Batracia,* since both of these keep their torsions without extension to the truncus (Fig. 4). Proximal torsion defect may be associated. Furthermore, another eventuality can be speculated upon (Fig. 4,12): conal torsions could occur in an opposite direction to normal ones, counterclockwise for the proximal segment and clockwise for the distal segment. In this case, the ridges will join more quickly (90°) than usual (270°). In our experiments, an anatomically corrected transposition (or malposition) is obtained by a lamella located on the distal segment or on the truncus.

Malposition of the Conal Ridges

This term could cover all the anomalies of torsions and matching of the conal ridges: the proximal and/or the distal torsions may fail totally or partially, may be exaggerated, or may be in the opposite direction to the normal. Matching may be normal, inverted, or undetermined. The migration of the proximal ostium may or may not be normal. This group seems interesting to individualize, because the previous anomalies concern essentially the distal torsion—the most apparent—and, incompletely, the proximal torsion—the least apparent.

In conclusion, phylogenesis and ontogenesis show that the conal ridges which septate the conus are not initially spiral but become spiral. Early in the chick embryo, they fill the proximal and the distal conus segments, but not the midsegment. Later, they grow, twist, and unite in the midsegment, in the position determined by the torsions. This proceeds according to a definite order, and is always the same. Experimentation can hinder the torsions, and so produce an inverted order, which results in a transposition of the great vessels.

ACKNOWLEDGMENTS

We thank Madame Guillaumin and Madame André, Laboratoire d'Evolution des Etres organisés, and Monsieur Boulekbache and Madame Meury, Laboratoire d'Anatomie comparée for their precious help. We also thank Professor Anthony, and Messrs. Saban and Robineau of the Museum of Natural History of Paris, who permitted us to examine the hearts of various Vertebrates.

This work was supported by an INSERM Grant No. 77-2024-5.

REFERENCES

1. Anderson, R. H., Wilkinson, J. L., Arnold, R., and Lubkiewicz, K. (1974): Morphogenesis of bulboventricular malformations. I. Consideration of embryogenesis in the normal heart. *Br. Heart J.,* 36:242-255.

2. Anthony, J., Millot, J., and Robineau, D. (1965): Le coeur et l'aorte ventrale de "Latimeria Chalumnae". *C. R. Acad. Sci.,* 261:223-226.

3. Bertin, L. (1958): Appareil circulatoire des Poissons. *Traité de Zool. Grasse,* 12:1399.

4. de la Cruz, M. V., and da Rocha, J. P. (1956): An ontogenetic theory for the explanation of congenital malformations involving the truncus and conus. *Am. Heart J.,* 51:782-806.

5. de la Cruz, M. V., Berrazueta, J. R., Arteaga, M., Attie, F., and Soni, J. (1976): Rules for diagnosis of arterioventricular discordances and spatial identification of ventricles. Crossed great arteries and transposition of the great arteries. *Br. Heart J.,* 38:341-354.

6. Dor, X. (1976): Etude des torsions distales de l'ébauche cardiaque. Développement normal et malformations expérimentales réalisées chez l'embryon de poulet. *(Thesis.)*

7. Dor, X., Corone, P., and Cabrol, C. (1978): Création expérimentale de ventricules uniques chez l'embryon de poulet. Etude au microscope électronique à balayage. *Coeur* IX, 6:1131-1156.

8. Dor, X., and Corone, P. (1979): Experimental creation of univentricular heart in the chick embryo. Nosological deductions. *Hertz* 4, 2:91-96.

9. Goor, D. A., Dische, R., and Lillehei, C. W. (1972): The conotruncus. I. Its normal inversion and conus absorption. *Circulation,* 46:375-384.

10. Grant, R. P. (1962): The morphogenesis of transposition of the great vessels. *Circulation,* 26:819-840.

11. Harris, J. A., and Farber, S. (1939): Transposition of the great cardiac vessels with special reference to the pylogenetic theory of Spitzer. *Arch. Path.,* 28:427-502.

12. Hochstetter, F. (1906): Handbuch der Vergleichenden und Experimentellen. Entwicklungslehre der Wirbeltiere. G. Fischer, Jena.

13. Kramer, T. C. (1942): The partitioning of the truncus and conus and the formation of the membranous portion of the interventricular septum in the human heart. *Am. J. Anat.,* 71:343-369.

14. Laane, H. M. (1978): The arterial pole of the embryonic heart. I. Nomenclature of the arterial pole of the embryonic heart. II. Septation of the arterial pole of the embryonic heart. *(Thesis),* Amsterdam.

15. Macartney, F. J., Shinebourne, E. A., and Anderson, R. P. (1976): Connexions, relations discordance and distorsions. *Br. Heart J.,* 38:323-326.

16. Pernkopf, E., and Wirtinger, W. (1933): Die Transposition der Herzostien, ein Versuch der Erklärung dieser Erscheinung. *Z. Anat. Entw.-Gesch,* 100:563-711.

17. Pernkopf, E., and Wirtinger, W. (1935): Das Wesen der Transposition im Gebiete des Herzens, ein Versuch der Erklarung auf Entwicklungsgeschichtlicher Grundlage Virchows. *Arch. Path. Anat.,* 295:143-174.

18. Pexieder, T. (1978): Development of the outflow tract of the embryonic heart. In: *Morphogenesis and Malformation of the Cardiovascular System,* edited by G. C. Rosenquist and D. Bergsma, pp. 29-68. *Birth Defects: Orig. Art. Ser.,* vol. XIX, no. 7. A. R. Liss Inc., New York.

19. Quero Jimenez, M., Casanova Gomez, M., and Perez Martinez, V. (1974): Malposicion anatomicamente corregida de las grandes arterias. *Rev. Esp. Cardiol.,* 27:197.

20. Robertson, J. I. (1913): Comparative anatomy of the bulbus cordis, with special reference to abnormal positions of the great vessels in the human heart. *J. Pathol. Bacteriol.,* 18:191-210.

21. Rychter, Z., and Lemez, L. (1962): Experimental morphology of the aortic arches and the heart loop in chick embryos. *Adv. Morphol.,* 2:333-371.

22. Seichert, V. (1965): Study of the tissue and organ anlage shifts by the method of plastic linear marking. *Folia Morphol.,* 13, 3:228-238.

23. Soret, C. (1976): Malposition anatomiquement corrigée des gros vaisseaux (à propos d'un cas). *(Thesis),* Paris.

24. Tandler, J. (1912): The development of the heart. Sect. II, ch. 18, vol. 2. In: Keibel and Mall, *Manual of Human Embryology,* p. 534.

25. Van Praagh, R., and Van Praagh, S. (1967): Anatomically corrected transposition of the great arteries. *Br. Heart J.,* 29:1, 112-119.

26. Van Praagh, R., Perez Trevino, C., Lopez Cuellar, M., Baker, F. W., Zuberbuhler, J. R., Quero, M., Perez, V. M., Moreno, F., and Van Praagh, S. (1971): Transposition of the great arteries with posterior aorta, anterior pulmonary artery, subpulmonary conus and fibrous continuity between aortic and atrioventricular valves. *Am. J. Cardiol.,* 28:621-631.

27. Van Praagh, R. (1973): Les malformations conotroncales. *Coeur,* No. Spécial:15-77.

DISCUSSION

Rychter: It seems to me that your approach to this problem of heart development is very complicated. You are mixing some observations from embryologic development with some classifications of adult malformed hearts. This can be very misleading. This concept certainly influences the design of your experiments.

De Vries: Have you done earlier manipulations in regard to blood flow or to torsion?

Dor: Three days before the torsion.

Laane: Are the results Dr. Dor showed not contradictory to the experiment of Dr. Rychter, putting marks on the ventral aspect of the outflow tract in the 3 e.d. embryo and not having observed torsion?

Pexieder: The essential difference is in the experimental approach. Dr. Dor has very long intervals, four days or even more, between his intervention and the moment he samples and investigates the operated embryos. Dr. Rychter used repeated observations of the same heart in stages as close as 8 hours, sometimes even 4 hours. Only in this way can you get a more or less complete sequence of events underlying the anomaly seen after the end of heart organogenesis.

Los: Wouldn't it be better to speak about position rather than torsion?

Clark: In what way, Dr. Dor, do you feel your experiments differ conceptually from the work of Dr. Gessner? Can you comment on the importance of the mechanical forces Dr. Gessner thought were most important in the deformation of the outflow tract?

Dor: Unfortunately, I am not sufficiently familiar with Dr. Gessner's work.

Rychter: We have always tried, in our experiments, to apply highly standardized interventions and to use for further analysis only those embryos in which we were sure that this standardized intervention was achieved. If you do not respect this strict quality control, the variability of your results will increase to proportions that will disable any further analysis.

Perspectives in Cardiovascular Research, Vol. 5,
Mechanisms of Cardiac Morphogenesis and Teratogenesis,
edited by Tomas Pexieder. Raven Press, New York © 1980.

The Role of Catecholamines and Other Cardiac Stimulants in Cardiovascular Teratogenesis: Recent Observations and Proposed Mechanisms

Enid F. Gilbert, Harold J. Bruyere, Jr., Shizen Ishikawa, and Matthias O. Cheung

Department of Pathology, University of Wisconsin Clinical Science Center, Madison, Wisconsin 53792

It has been convincingly demonstrated that relatively specific morphologic changes can be induced in the embryonic chick cardiovascular system by modifying normal blood flow patterns (11,12,23,44,47). However, few studies provide significant clinical implications, since hemodynamic alterations were induced primarily by mechanical interference.

We chose physiological agents that induce dramatic hemodynamic changes in the embryonic circulation (19,27) as probes for an extensive study in teratogenesis. The agents selected were among those that stimulated adrenergic nerves and that have been termed by Barger and Dale (3) the *sympathomimetic amines.*

PREVIOUS OBSERVATIONS

Epinephrine: A Cardiovascular Teratogen

We have previously demonstrated that a single exposure to epinephrine (5×10^{-3} M) produces a wide spectrum of aortic arch and associated intracardiac malformations in 3 to 6 e.d. chick embryos (25). The highest frequency of malformations (94%) occurred after treatment at 4 e.d. 12 h. Although this study did not prove a causal relationship between hemodynamics altered during a period of extensive cardiovascular morphogenesis and the occurrence of cardiovascular malformations, it demonstrated that a compound which affected at least one important hemodynamic parameter in the chick embryo, i.e., blood pressure (19,27), was a potent cardiovascular teratogen.

Other Sympathomimetic Agents

Since epinephrine induced cardiovascular malformations both before and after innervation of the chick embryo heart (43), it was apparent that innervation

473

was not essential to the teratogenic action of epinephrine. At the time that we were designing experiments subsequent to the epinephrine study, there was some experimental evidence that cell-surface receptors that respond to sympathomimetic agents were functional in young chick embryos (32,42). This has recently been confirmed by St. Petery and Van Mierop (45).

By exposing chick embryos to one of 4 concentrations (8×10^{-5} M to 4×10^{-3} M) of various sympathomimetic agents, we generated dose-response data which enabled us to produce a hierarchy of teratogenic drug potency: isoproterenol > epinephrine >> phenylephrine ≥ norepinephrine (26). The period of morphogenesis in this study extended from Hamburger-Hamilton (22) stages 20 to 27. Dose-response data from stage 26 corresponded well with results from stages 20 to 27 (17). Furthermore, the frequency of isoproterenol-induced malformations was significantly reduced when embryos were pretreated with propranolol (26), a β-adrenergic receptor blocking agent. At equimolar concentrations, propranolol virtually abolished the teratogenic effect of isoproterenol. Thus, two significant observations—a hierarchy of teratogenic drug potency and the protective effect of propranolol—lent some credence to a hypothesis that β-receptor hyperstimulation and the production of cardiovascular malformations were related (1,10).

Lands et al. (35) have classified β-adrenergic receptors into two types: β-1, which govern chronotropic and inotropic actions of the heart, and β-2, stimulation of which induces bronchodilation and vasodepression. In a previous study (26), propranolol had prevented the induction of cardiovascular malformations by isoproterenol, an equipotent β-1/β-2 stimulant (35). Since propranolol nonselectively blocks both β-1 and β-2 receptors (41), the protective effect exerted by propranolol stimulated an investigation to determine the relative participation by β-1 and β-2 receptors in the teratogenic process.

An equimolar concentration of practolol (8×10^{-4} M), a β-1 blocker (7), reduced the incidence of cardiovascular malformations by isoproterenol from 39% to 4% (14). In concentrations as high as 5 times that of isoproterenol, the β-2 blocker butoxamine (36) could inhibit no more than one-third of the arch anomalies induced by isoproterenol. We have not determined whether this mild protective effect is the result of a weak β-1 receptor blockade, which has been suggested as an action of butoxamine in high concentrations (50), or is caused by β-2 receptor blockade. Probably the most significant result of this study involved the ability of practolol to prevent isoproterenol-induced aortic arch hypoplasia and interrupted aortic arch, anomalies frequently accompanied by relatively large subpulmonary ventricular septal defects (26).

Since propranolol and practolol inhibited the induction of aortic arch and associated intracardiac malformations by isoproterenol, whereas butoxamine had only a mild effect, the inference was made that isoproterenol produced the malformations primarily via hyperstimulation of β-1 adrenergic receptors. Investigations into potential teratogenic effects of other β-1 receptor stimulants and the capacity of various cardioselective drugs to block the effects of these stimulants have been planned in this laboratory.

Synergism with Cocaine

Sympathomimetic amines are metabolized and regulated in mammalian systems by several distinct mechanisms (2). Primary among the terminating processes of these agents is uptake by postganglionic sympathetic neurons. Since such neurons are present in the embryonic chick heart (48,49) and can concentrate epinephrine and norepinephrine in their synaptic terminals as early as 3 days of incubation (28,29), we reasoned that our hierarchy of drug potency might be greatly influenced by this uptake phenomenon.

To formulate a more realistic theory relative to the effects of the sympathomimetic agents on β receptors, we pretreated embryos with cocaine, a drug that blocks the uptake mechanism in young chick embryos (29,30) and apparently allows sympathomimetic agents to persist near receptors of the embryonic heart in higher concentrations. The results of this study (16) demonstrated that cocaine potentiates the teratogenic effect of epinephrine and norepinephrine but has little effect with isoproterenol and phenylephrine. The results with the latter two agents were expected, since isoproterenol is not taken up by postganglionic sympathetic neurons (24) and phenylephrine only weakly stimulates β receptors (31).

Synergism with Methylxanthines

Relatively confident that β-receptor hyperstimulation played a major role in isoproterenol induced teratogenesis, we were inclined to look closely at various biochemical effects of β-receptor activity. One predominant effect is an increase in adenyl cyclase, the enzyme that converts adenosine triphosphate into cyclic $3'5'$ adenosine monophosphate (cyclic AMP) (34). In view of this well-established pathway and the myriad effects mediated by cyclic AMP (18), we felt it was important to determine a possible role of cyclic AMP in the production of catecholamine-induced malformations in chick embryos.

Caffeine and theophylline are methylated xanthines which competitively inhibit at least certain forms of cyclic nucleotide phosphodiesterase, enzymes that catalyze the conversion of cyclic AMP to $5'$ AMP (5). By virtue of their different sites of action, β-receptor stimulants and methylxanthines are synergistic relative to their effects in raising concentrations of intracellular cyclic AMP.

By pretreating embryos with various concentrations of theophylline or caffeine (1×10^{-2} M to 3×10^{-2} M), we demonstrated that methylxanthines potentiate the teratogenic effect of epinephrine and norepinephrine in chick embryos (15). The effect was concentration-dependent. The most striking observation in this study was that theophylline (2×10^{-2} M) potentiated the teratogenic effect of norepinephrine by more than 125-fold, increasing malformation incidence from 2% to 31%.

Inhibition of cyclic AMP phosphodiesterase activity and, consequently, production of high cyclic AMP concentrations (5) and/or promotion of increased calcium movement (39,40), are regarded as the principal actions of methylxanthines. Our results did not determine the primary action of theophylline or caffeine in the chick embryo heart; however, the data raised interesting questions concerning the role of cyclic AMP and/or calcium in biochemical mechanisms of cardiovascular teratogenesis.

RECENT OBSERVATIONS

Calcium: A Cardiovascular Teratogen

It has been shown that catecholamines increase transmembranous calcium ion flow into early chick embryo heart cells (46). This study also demonstrated efficient blockade by calcium antagonists of a cell-surface receptor that mediates calcium influx. Furthermore, pilot studies in our laboratory indicate that verapamil, a potent calcium antagonist, reduces the teratogenic effect of isoproterenol (4). Based on the role of calcium in excitation–contraction coupling and on findings that excessive calcium influx can be cardiotoxic (8), experiments were designed to demonstrate whether or not calcium could mimic the teratogenic effects of catecholamines in the chick embryo cardiovascular system.

The materials and methods were similar to those previously described (25). Calcium chloride dihydrate was dissolved in distilled water and tonicity was adjusted with 0.15 M sodium chloride. The calcium solutions were then dropped onto the extraembryonic membranes of the embryo through an observation window in the eggshell.

Whereas 1 mM, 10 mM, and 50 mM calcium chloride did not change the anomaly rate appreciably from that of the control group, 100 mM calcium chloride increased the frequency of malformations from 1% to 21% (P < .0005). The survival rate was unaffected by high concentrations of calcium chloride.

One question was raised as a result of these data: Can the teratogenic effect of isoproterenol be potentiated by an elevation in extracellular calcium? If the answer to this question were yes, then one might predict a significant increase in cardiovascular malformation frequency if calcium chloride and isoproterenol were both added to the chick egg. At least with 50 mM calcium chloride, which provided the egg albumen with twice as much calcium as is normally present on the 5th day of incubation (9), no enhancement was observed (Fig. 4). Although this is not conclusive evidence, if calcium does play a major role in isoproterenol-induced teratogenesis, the results may indicate that isoproterenol maximizes calcium influx. Apparently, then, we could not force more calcium into cells and increase the probability of a teratogenic effect simply by overloading the extracellular space.

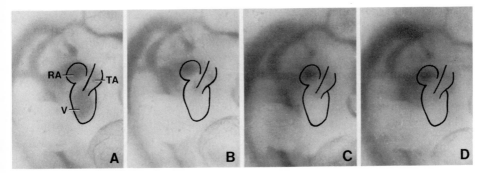

Note: Figures 1 and 2 are microphotographs of a 5-day-old embryonic chick heart (Fig. 1) and an entire embryo (Fig. 2) before isoproterenol treatment **(A)**, and at 2 minutes **(B)**, 5 minutes **(C)**, and 15 minutes **(D)** after treatment with the catecholamine.

FIG. 1. Microphotographs of embryonic heart. Note the loss of blood in the ventricle after isoproterenol treatment. Exposure time was controlled at 5 seconds and, therefore, micrographs are images of 15 to 20 contraction–relaxation cycles. V, ventricle; RA, right atrium; TA, truncus arteriosus/conotruncal area.

The Role of Cardiac Output in the Teratogenic Process

In light of an earlier observation that the positive chronotropic response of embryonic chick hearts *in vivo* to catecholamines was not necessarily related to cardiovascular teratogenesis (6), experiments were designed to determine other cardiovascular effects of isoproterenol in the embryonic chick. Since practolol markedly reduced the incidence of isoproterenol-induced malformations (14), we also attempted to identify the physiological mechanism of the practolol protection.

Figures 1, 2, and 3 demonstrate several major cardiovascular effects of isoproterenol observed in this study. Figure 2 demonstrates that blood flow through the embryonic chick heart is dramatically reduced after treatment with isoproterenol (7.5×10^{-4} M). It also demonstrates a commonly observed "snaking" phenomenon of the anterior vitelline vein. This striking observation was not seen in normal and saline-treated embryos, and may indicate a venous pressure change.

Figure 3 demonstrates representative reduction effects of isoproterenol on impedance cardiographic waves in embryonic chicks, indications that this agent markedly decreased stroke volume. Isoproterenol induced a significant decrease in the amplitude of the waves in 100% of the cases studied (31 cases). Comparatively, practolol-pretreated embryos demonstrated the same phenomenon in only 56% of the embryos tested (15/27). Furthermore, isoproterenol induced a significant decrease in heart rate in 52% of embryos (16/31), in contrast with only 26% (7/27) in the practolol-pretreated group. Combined data indicated that 100% of the embryos treated with isoproterenol showed a significant decrement in cardiac output (after an initial transient increase), compared with only 26%

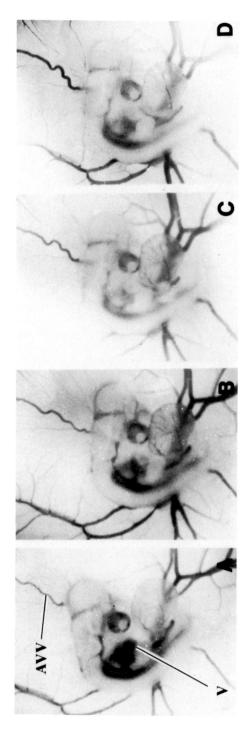

FIG. 2. Microphotographs of embryonic chick *in vivo*. Note, again, the loss of blood in the ventricle after isoproterenol treatment; also, notice the more tortuous path taken by the anterior vitelline vein (AVV), an indication of a pressure change within the vitelline venous system. Photographic exposure time, 5 seconds.

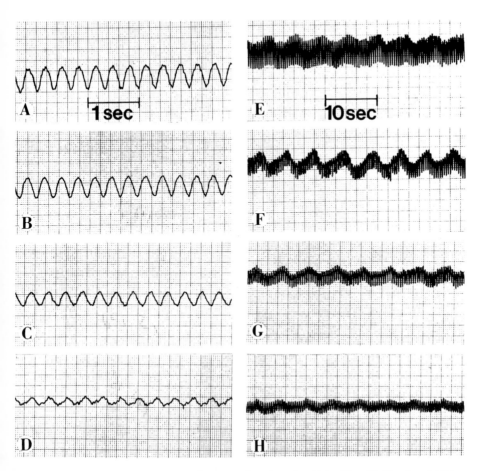

FIG. 3. Bioelectrical impedance cardiograms of embryonic chicks (5 e.d.). The two series A–D (chart speed 25 mm sec⁻¹) and E–H (2.5 mm sec⁻¹) demonstrate patterns in two embryos before exposure to isoproterenol (**A** and **E**), and at 2 minutes (**B** and **F**), 5 minutes (**C** and **G**), and 15 minutes (**D** and **H**) after exposure. Note the progression to smaller waves in both cases, an indication of decreased stroke volume.

(7/27) of practolol-pretreated embryos. These values corresponded with malformation frequencies of 39% and 4%. It was also shown that 45% (14/31) of isoproterenol-treated embryos demonstrated a significantly decreased cardiac output for more than one hour, compared with only 7% (2/27) in the practolol-pretreated group.

The data from this study indicate that a dramatic and prolonged decrease in cardiac output may be involved in at least some of the teratogenic processes initiated by isoproterenol treatment. Such a hypothesis finds support in important observations made by Manhoff and Johnson (37), Stephan (47), Rychter (44), Gessner (11), and Gilani and Silvestri (13). Their findings indicate that markedly

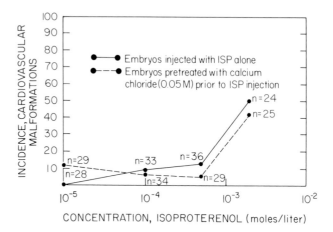

CONCENTRATION, ISOPROTERENOL (moles/liter)

FIG. 4. Dose response of isoproterenol demonstrating the negative effect of high extracellular calcium concentration on cardiovascular malformation incidence. Isoproterenol may maximize transmembranous calcium influx (see text).

reduced blood flow through the developing aortic arches (whether a result of mechanical obstruction or of reduced cardiac output due primarily to bradycardia) may cause cardiovascular malformations in chick embryos. There is some evidence that reduced blood flow may also be involved in the pathogenesis of

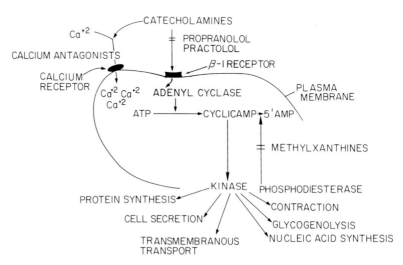

FIG. 5. Schematic diagram of the possible biochemical and physiological events initiated by catecholamines in the embryonic chick heart. Hyperstimulation of cardiac β-adrenergic receptors and high concentrations of cyclic AMP may be especially critical factors. Cyclic AMP mediates a variety of intracellular processes, including contraction–excitation coupling in the heart (troponin). Catecholamines may also increase transmembranous influx of calcium to cardiotoxic concentrations (see text).

certain forms of congenital heart disease (38). Furthermore, Grabowski (20) has recently emphasized that bradycardia and hypotension could be significantly involved in teratogenesis, since they might increase the potential for localized damage through oxygen deficiency.

SUMMARY

Our data suggest that cardiac β-adrenergic hyperstimulation is teratogenic in the chick embryo. Calcium mobilization and/or cyclic AMP, which regulates a wide variety of intracellular processes (Fig. 5), may play crucial roles in the biochemical process of teratogenesis. Furthermore, we have demonstrated that a prolonged depression in cardiac performance, characterized by a substantial decrease in both stroke volume and cardiac rate, is related to cardiovascular malformations. These results appear consistent with the hypothesis that prolonged ischemia, and therefore hypoxia, is teratogenic to the developing aortic arches (21,33) and may ultimately lead to certain types of intracardiac defects.

ACKNOWLEDGMENTS

This research project has been supported primarily by the National Heart, Lung, and Blood Institute, National Institutes of Health, Bethesda, Maryland (NIH Grant HL18050). The American Heart Association, Wisconsin Affiliate, Milwaukee, and the University of Wisconsin Graduate School, Madison, have provided supplementary funds. We also wish to extend our appreciation to Dr. John M. Opitz for his generous support through the Clinical Genetics Center of the University of Wisconsin, Madison.

REFERENCES

1. Ahlquist, R. P. (1966): The adrenergic receptor. *J. Pharm. Sci.,* 55:359-367.
2. Axelrod, J., and Weinshilboum, R. (1972): Catecholamines. *N. Engl. J. Med.,* 287:237-242.
3. Barger, G., and Dale, H. H. (1910): Chemical structure and sympathomimetic action of amines. *J. Physiol. (Lond.),* 41:19-59.
4. Bruyere, H. J., Jr., Gilbert, E. F., Ishikawa, S., and Cheung, M. O. (1979): The roles of calcium and glucose in isoproterenol induced cardiovascular malformations in embryonic chicks. *Teratology,* 19:21A (abstract).
5. Butcher, R. W., and Sutherland, E. W. (1962): Adenosine 3'5'-phosphate in biological materials. *J. Biol. Chem.,* 237:1244-1250.
6. Cheung, M. O., Gilbert, E. F., Bruyere, H. J., Jr., Ishikawa, S., and Hodach, R. J. (1977): Chronotropism and blood flow patterns following teratogenic doses of catecholamines in 5-day-old chick embryos. *Teratology,* 16:337-344.
7. Dunlop, D., and Shanks, R. G. (1968): Selective blockade of adrenoceptive β receptors in the heart. *Br. J. Pharm. Chem.,* 32:201-208.
8. Fleckenstein, A., Janke, J., Doring, H. J., and Leder, O. (1974): Myocardial fiber necrosis due to intracellular calcium overload—A new principle in cardiac pathophysiology. In: *Recent Advances in Studies on Cardiac Structure and Metabolism, Vol. 4, Myocardial Biology,* edited by N. S. Dhalla, pp. 563-580. University Park Press, Baltimore.
9. Freeman, B. M., and Vince, M. A. (1974): *Development of the Avian Embryo: A Behavioural and Physiological Study.* Chapman and Hall, London.

10. Furchgott, R. F. (1967): The pharmacological differentiation of adrenergic receptors. *Ann. NY Acad. Sci.,* 139:553-570.
11. Gessner, I. H. (1966): Spectrum of congenital cardiac anomalies produced in chick embryos by mechanical interference with cardiogenesis. *Circ. Res.,* 18:625-633.
12. Gessner, I. H., and Van Mierop, L. H. S. (1970): Experimental production of cardiac defects: The spectrum of dextroposition of the aorta. *Am. J. Cardiol.,* 25:272-278.
13. Gilani, S. H., and Silvestri, A. (1977): The effect of propranolol upon chick embryo cardiogenesis. *Exp. Cell Biol.,* 45:158-166.
14. Gilbert, E. F., Bruyere, H. J., Jr., Ishikawa, S., Cheung, M. O., and Hodach, R. J. (1977): The effect of practolol and butoxamine on aortic arch malformation in β adrenoreceptor stimulated chick embryos. *Teratology,* 15:317-324.
15. Gilbert, E. F., Bruyere, H. J., Jr., Ishikawa, S., Cheung, M. O., and Hodach, R. J. (1977): The effects of methylxanthines on catecholamine-stimulated and normal chick embryos. *Teratology,* 16:47-52.
16. Gilbert, E. F., Hodach, R. J., Cheung, M. O., and Bruyere, H. J., Jr. (1976): The effects of cocaine in the production of cardiovascular anomalies in β adrenoreceptor stimulated chick embryos. *Experientia,* 32:1026-1027.
17. Gilbert, E. F., Ishikawa, S., and Bruyere, H. J., Jr. (1979): Spectrum of cardiovascular malformations in embryonic chicks induced by β stimulating agents. In: *Proceedings of the Symposium on Etiology and Morphogenesis of Congenital Heart Disease,* edited by R. Van Praagh and A. Takao, pp. 155–175. Futura Press, New York.
18. Gilman, A. G., and Murad, F. (1975): Hormones and hormone antagonists: Introduction. In: *The Pharmacological Basis of Therapeutics,* edited by L. S. Goodman and A. Gilman, pp. 1369-1371. Macmillan, New York.
19. Girard, H. (1973): Adrenergic sensitivity of circulation in the chick embryo. *Am. J. Physiol.,* 224:461-469.
20. Grabowski, C. T. (1977): Altered electrolyte and fluid balance. In: *Handbook of Teratology, Vol. 2, Mechanisms and Pathogenesis,* edited by J. G. Wilson and F. C. Fraser, pp. 153-170. Plenum Press, New York.
21. Grabowski, C. T., and Paar, J. A. (1958): The teratogenic effects of graded doses of hypoxia on the chick embryo. *Am. J. Anat.,* 103:313-348.
22. Hamburger, V., and Hamilton, H. L. (1951): A series of normal stages in the development of the chick embryo. *J. Morphol.,* 88:49-92.
23. Harh, J. Y., Milton, H. P., Gallen, W. J., Friedberg, D. Z., and Kaplan, S. (1973): Experimental production of hypoplastic left heart syndrome in the chick embryo. *Am. J. Cardiol.,* 31:51-56.
24. Hertting, G. (1964): The fate of ^{3}H-iso-proterenol in the rat. *Biochem. Pharmacol.,* 13:1119-1128.
25. Hodach, R. J., Gilbert, E. F., and Fallon, J. F. (1974): Aortic arch anomalies associated with the administration of epinephrine in chick embryos. *Teratology,* 9:203-209.
26. Hodach, R. J., Hodach, A. E., Fallon, J. F., Folts, J. D., Bruyere, H. J., and Gilbert, E. F. (1975): The role of β adrenergic activity in the production of cardiac and aortic arch anomalies in chick embryos. *Teratology,* 12:33-45.
27. Hoffman, L. E., Jr., and Van Mierop, L. H. S. (1971): Effect of epinephrine on heart rate and arterial blood pressure of the developing chick embryo. *Ped. Res.,* 5:472-477.
28. Ignarro, L. J., and Shideman, F. E. (1968): Appearance and concentrations of catecholamines and their biosynthesis in the embryonic and developing chick. *J. Pharmacol. Exp. Ther.,* 159:38-48.
29. Ignarro, L. J., and Shideman, F. E. (1968): Norepinephrine and epinephrine in the embryo and embryonic heart of the chick: Uptake and subcellular distribution. *J. Pharmacol. Exp. Ther.,* 159:49-58.
30. Ignarro, L. J., and Shideman, F. E. (1968): The requirement of sympathetic innervation for the active transport of norepinephrine by the heart. *J. Pharmacol. Exp. Ther.,* 159:59-65.
31. Innes, I. R., and Nickerson, M. (1975): Norepinephrine, epinephrine, and the sympathomimetic amines. In: *The Pharmacological Basis of Therapeutics,* edited by L. S. Goodman and A. Gilman, pp. 477-513. Macmillan, New York.
32. Jaffee, O. C. (1972): Effects of propranolol on the chick embryo heart. *Teratology,* 5:153-157.

33. Jaffee, O. C. (1974): The effects of moderate hypoxia and moderate hypoxia plus hypercapnea on cardiac development in chick embryos. *Teratology,* 10:275-281.
34. Koelle, G. B. (1975): Neurohumoral transmission and the autonomic nervous system. In: *The Pharmacological Basis of Therapeutics,* edited by L. S. Goodman and A. Gilman, pp. 404-444. Macmillan, New York.
35. Lands, A. M., Arnold, A., McAuliff, J. P., Luduena, F. P., and Brown, T. G., Jr. (1967): Differentiation of receptor systems activated by sympathomimetic amines. *Nature,* 214:597-598.
36. Levy, B. (1966): The adrenergic blocking activity of N-tert-butylmethoxamine (butoxamine). *J. Pharmacol. Exp. Ther.,* 151:413-422.
37. Manhoff, L., Jr., and Johnson, M. (1951): The production of cardiovascular anomalies by electrocoagulation in chick embryos. *Am. J. Path.,* 27:751 (abstract).
38. Moore, G. W., and Hutchins, G. M. (1978): Association of interrupted aortic arch with malformations producing reduced blood flow to the fourth aortic arches. *Am. J. Cardiol.,* 42:467-472.
39. Nayler, W. G. (1963): Effect of calcium on cardiac contractile activity and radiocalcium movement. *Am. J. Physiol.,* 204:969-974.
40. Nayler, W. G. (1967): Calcium exchange in cardiac muscle: A basic mechanism of drug action. *Am. Heart J.,* 73:379-394.
41. Nickerson, M., and Collier, B. (1975): Drugs inhibiting adrenergic nerves and structures innervated by them. In: *The Pharmacological Basis of Therapeutics,* edited by L. S. Goodman and A. Gilman, pp. 533-564. Macmillan, New York.
42. Paff, G. H., and Glander, T. P. (1968): The time of appearance of sympathomimetic receptors in the chick embryo heart. *Anat. Rec.,* 160:405 (abstract).
43. Romanoff, A. L. (1960): *The Avian Embryo.* Macmillan, New York.
44. Rychter, Z. (1962): Experimental morphology of the aortic arches and the heart loop in chick embryos. *Adv. Morphol.,* 2:333-371.
45. St. Petery, L. B., Jr., and Van Mierop, L. H. S. (1977): Evidence for the presence of adrenergic receptors in 3-day-old chick embryo. *Am. J. Physiol.,* 232:H250-H254.
46. Shigenobu, K., and Sperelakis, N. (1972): Calcium current channels induced by catecholamines in chick embryonic hearts whose fast sodium channels are blocked by tetrodotoxin or elevated potassium. *Circ. Res.,* 31:932-952.
47. Stephan, F. (1949): Sur la ligature des arcs aortiques chez l' embryon de poulet. *C.R. Soc. Biol.,* 143:291-293.
48. Szepsenwol, J., and Bron, A. (1935): Le premier contact du systeme nerveux vago-sympathique avec l'appareil cardio-vasculaire chez les embryons d'oiseaux (canard et poulet). *C.R. Soc. Biol.,* 118:946-948.
49. Szepsenwol, J., and Bron, A. (1935): L'origine des cellules nerveuses sympathiques dans le coeur des oiseaux (embryons de canard et de poulet). *C.R. Soc. Biol.,* 118:1030-1031.
50. Wastila, W. B., Su, J. Y., Friedman, W. F., and Mayer, S. E. (1972): Blockade of biochemical and physiological responses of cardiac muscle to norepinephrine by N-tert-butylmethoxamine (butoxamine). *J. Pharmacol. Exp. Ther.,* 181:126-138.

DISCUSSION

Klein: I wonder about the diagnostic criteria and techniques used to establish the presence of a malformation. In our opinion, hypoplastic ductus arteriosus and hypoplastic segment of the aortic arch are consequences of other malformations.

Gilbert: Major malformations included large subcristal VSD, DORV, truncus arteriosus, and interruption of the aortic arch. The hypoplastic right ductus was induced by methylxanthines in association with an aortic aneurysm.

De Vries: This is a significant clinical point. In the last six months, we have found four interrupted-aortic arches with the ventricular septal defect. I understand the arch anomaly to be extracardiac and the interventricular septum defect to be a flow phenomenon.

Gilbert: I think that it is a hemodynamic effect, and will agree with Dr. Rychter's interpretation.

Clark: What has the histology of the aortic aneurysm demonstrated?

Gilbert: The walls of the aortic aneurysm show marked thinning of the media. The elastic structure of the media is degenerating.

Oppenheimer-Dekker: What about the specificity of isolated defects?

Gilbert: Specific induction of a single malformation may be modulated by regulating the time at which the insult is given.

Rychter: From the point of view of cell population dynamics, the specificity of an anomaly may depend on the fact that there are two major types of morphogenetic systems. In the first type, all of the developmental mechanisms have equal importance. In the second type, one of the mechanisms is, in a given period, more important than the other. If a teratogen acts by the way of this dominating mechanism, the resulting defect will be rather specific.

Perspectives in Cardiovascular Research, Vol. 5,
Mechanisms of Cardiac Morphogenesis and Teratogenesis,
edited by Tomas Pexieder. Raven Press, New York © 1981

Teratogenetic Considerations Regarding Aortic Arch Anomalies Associated with Cardiovascular Malformations

*A. Oppenheimer-Dekker, **R. J. Moene, †A. J. Moulaert, and *A. C. Gittenberger-de Groot

*Institute of Embryology and Anatomy, State University, 2300 RC Leiden, The Netherlands. ** Department of Pediatric Cardiology, Free University, 1081 HV Amsterdam, The Netherlands. † Wilhelmina Children's Hospital, State University, 3512 LK Utrecht, The Netherlands.*

In considering the mechanisms underlying normal and abnormal embryogenesis from the epigenetic point of view, it is important to keep in mind that embryonic development is the result of a chain of overlapping events, in which the normal and timely completion of a certain process can be the indispensable condition for the start and normal progression of another process. This is one way in which morphologic differentiations are interdependent, and it applies to the development of all organs and organ systems during the period of organogenesis.

In addition, the cardiovascular system has the special characteristic of performing its function at a very early time. At that time, the vessel walls are still very thin and can be remodeled, and heart morphogenesis is not yet terminated. This implies an interaction between embryonic blood flow patterns and cardiovascular development. The significance of this interaction has been very explicitly underlined by Congdon (4). He ascribed the successive disappearance of certain branchial arteries and segments of the dorsal aortae chiefly to changes of flow. If we accept this concept, the next step must logically be the assumption that flow disturbances can interfere with normal development. Thus, in addition to the general pathogenetic mechanisms, the role of hemodynamics in cardiovascular maldevelopment must be taken into consideration. Problems to be solved in this context include the question of what data are available or can be obtained on normal embryonic flow patterns, and of how and where abnormal flow patterns have their origin. Those questions cannot easily be answered in the setting of human embryology. In particular, the first question confronts the human embryologist with problems difficult to come to grips with. The strength of comparative and experimental embryology lies in the fact that many accurate and reliable data can be obtained by measurements of normal circulation and by local interventions that interfere with normal circulation. In the latter field, fruitful work has been done by Rychter (18), and more recently by Pexieder (15,16), who, furthermore gave an excellent review of the literature concerning the links between embryology and teratology.

Despite the undoubtedly great practical advantages of this experimental work and the great progress made in experimental teratology, research in human embryology and teratology should not be completely rejected, since this might imply a loss of potential sources of information. For there are indeed significant possibilities of gaining more insight into the nature of developmental events in the human embryo, and of collecting at least circumstantial evidence for certain hypotheses and theories on human teratology. We shall try to illustrate this by discussing various aspects of the relationship between aortic arch anomalies and cardiovascular malformations.

Development of the Aortic Arch in Relation to Fetoplacental Vasculogenesis

In normal human embryology, a crucial point concerning early embryonic flow patterns is the following hypothesis: During the sixth week, in embryos growing from about 10 to about 20 mm CR length (the midportion of the period of metamorphosis (20)), a significant increase in volume of aortic flow would be responsible for the so-called widening and shortening phenomenon (2,3) in those vessels or segments of vessels which, because of their position, are easily accessible for the increased flow. They rapidly widen at the expense of their length. In turn, these preferential channels cause a "steal phenomenon" in other vessels or vessel segments which, because of their position, provide a less direct route for the blood stream. In such vessels, the blood flow diminishes, resulting in their regression and obliteration. The aforementioned widening and shortening phenomenon might also be involved in certain shifting processes ("migration"). Thus, the relatively great distances separating the innominate, the left common carotid, and the left subclavian arteries in embryos of about 16 to 18 mm CR length disappear in embryos of about 25 mm CR length.

The weak point of this reasoning is, of course, the assumption of a sudden and considerable increase of circulating blood volume during the sixth week of embryonic development. Looking for possible sources of increased blood volume, our thoughts were led to the placenta. The placenta is an organ which must establish, in an early phase, an extensive vascular network for exchange between the maternal and the embryonic organisms. We therefore studied serial sections of villi from the chorions of normal human embryos of 7, 10, 11, 12, 14, 16 and 20 mm CR length (11). In the youngest specimens, plump villi were found, with relatively few and narrow endothelium-lined vascular spaces (Fig. 1a). Comparison with the older embryos showed an increase in number

---

FIG. 1. a: Chorionic villi of a human embryo of 10 mm CR length. Vasculogenesis along the superficial layer (trophoblast) of the villi. Vessel lumina, if present, are very narrow ($\times$ 93).

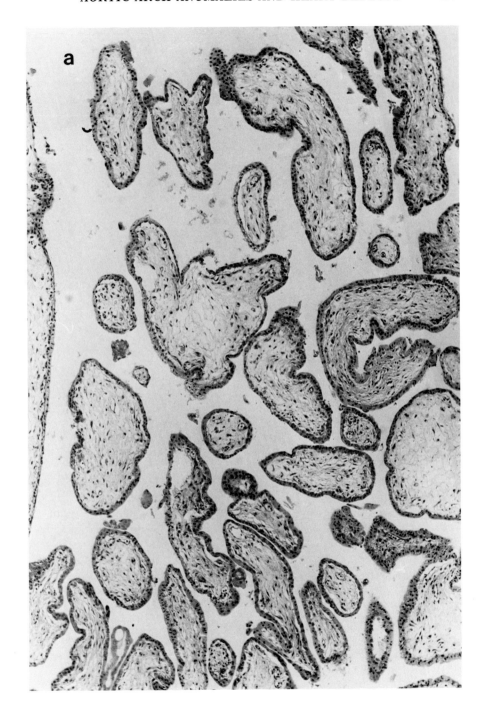

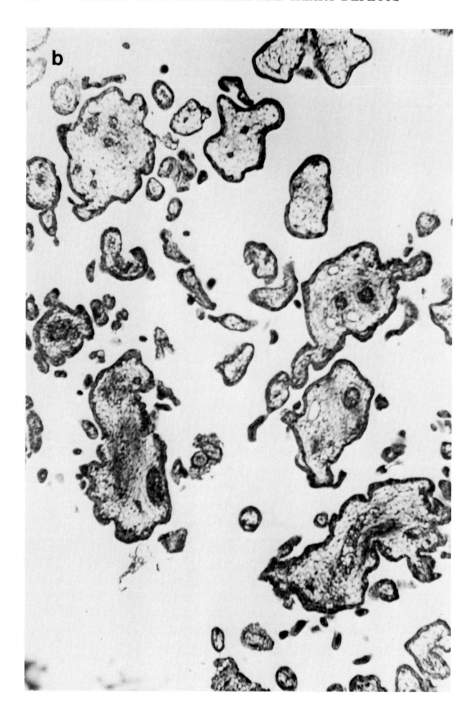

and in width of the chorionic vessels associated with sprouting of the villi (Fig. 1b). Furthermore, the investigations of Boyd and Hamilton (1) on the human placenta have clearly shown that, from Streeter horizon XVI (10 mm CR length) onwards, the area available for the intervillous space, and thus for the extending sprouts, becomes considerably augmented as a result of expansion of the cytotrophoblastic shell. These observations make plausible the concept that there is an explosive development of the chorionic circulation in the sixth week, consequently leading to a significant increase in the volume of circulating blood in the embryo. This supports the above-mentioned hypothesis.

Flow Distribution and Development of the Ventricular Outflow Tracts

Final establishment of adequate junction of the pulmonary and aortic parts of the bulbus with the matching areas of the right and the left ventricle, respectively, occurs in embryos of about 14 to 18 mm CR length. In the usual terminology, these processes are rather loosely identified with the visually most conspicuous result: transfer of the aorta to the left ventricle, with completion of septation. However, in view of the architecture of the outflow tracts, it should be emphasized that this so-called aortic transfer is only part of an intricate complex of events (12). In these processes, a decisive role must probably be assigned to differences in the growth rates and in the directions of growth, coupled with waves of cell-death foci (15,16), in different parts of the bulbar wall, the bulbar ridges (respectively, the bulbar septum), and the bulboventricular transitional zone. These three components cooperate in the shaping of the early embryonic outflow tracts and their common partition. The normal course of this shaping establishes a normal intracardiac flow distribution over the pulmonary channel and the aortic channel, respectively, during the sixth week. Thus, part of the simultaneously increased blood flow will be directed into the developing aortic arch.

Aortic Arch Anomalies and Intracardiac Pathology

In the shaping of the left and right ventricular outflow tracts in the early embryo, loosely arranged and poorly differentiated tissue functions as a matrix for the histogenesis of the developing myocardial muscle bundles. After a normally completed bulbo-ventricular junction is formed, this "muscularization" can proceed according to the specific patterns. In case of failures in the junction of the three components, the matrix will have an abnormal shape, possibly with a defect in the partition. Should this be combined with an excessive bulging of the left part of the bulbo-atrioventricular transitional zone, then intracardiac

FIG. 1. b: Chorionic villi of a human embryo of 16 mm CR length. Same magnification as 1a. The villi branch intensively and contain many wide vessels with blood cells. ($\times$ 93). Courtesy of J. Anat. (11), Cambridge University Press.

flow distribution can be disturbed at the expense of the aortic flow. During subsequent differentiation, the abnormal shape of the matrix, together with the alterations in blood flow, may disturb the muscularization pattern. In particular the ventricular septal defect could deviate the myoblasts, genetically coded for the right ventricular outflow tract, towards the aforementioned left-sided bulge. In terms of teratology, this would mean a deviated infundibular septum continuous with an anterolateral muscle bundle (8,10). This deviation reduces blood flow through the embryonic preductal aorta, and may thus contribute to the pathogenesis of dimensional anomalies of the aortic arch (9,17,19).

An anatomic study of 150 heart specimens combined with dimensional aortic arch anomalies (7) indicated that, apart from the above-mentioned type of outflow tract obstruction, intracardiac anatomy offers various other possibilities of potential obstructive factors with an early morphogenetic background. Among others, special mention should be made of the combination of a posteromedial muscle (21) and an anterolateral muscle clasping the mitral orifice, the leftward deviation of the anterior part of the ventricular septum, sometimes with abnormal trabeculae crossing the aortic outflow tract, and other complex malformations of the ventricular septum (22).

Embryologically, the simplest type of aortic arch anomaly is tubular hypoplasia, i.e. a persisting embryonic pattern in cases of insufficient increase in aortic blood flow. A further decrease in aortic flow could result in cessation of flow across a particular aortic arch segment, eventually leading to atresia or even interruption. This concept implies that the microscopic picture of the atretic segment reflects some primary characteristics of the normal aortic wall structure (13) (Fig. 2). Our microscopic observations do not support the statement of Goor and Lillehei (5) that "in most instances, the atretic segment consists of fibrous tissue not shaped like an obliterated vessel."

"Uncommitted" Developmental Anomalies in the Branchial Arterial System

Overemphasis of hemodynamically induced maldevelopment of the branchial arterial system, located in the section of the aortic arch, should be avoided. In our collection, 5 cases with complex heart anomalies of early embryonic origin were found, in which various malformations of the arterial pole could be interpreted as the result of persistence of parts of the branchial arterial system, which normally disappear, in combination with the regression of parts normally persistent (14). The most conspicuous features were encountered in three specimens with various types of univentricular heart. One of the vascular abnormalities was that one of the neck arteries seemingly originated from the pulmonary trunk. However, serial section investigation revealed that, in each case, the

FIG. 2. Transverse section through an atretic segment of the aortic arch in a specimen of truncus arteriosus persistens with a small aortic part. Concentric arrangement of elastic tissue around a local remnant of a vessel lumen *(arrow)*. Resorcin-fuchsin-iron hematoxylin-picric acid-thiazin red (× 175).

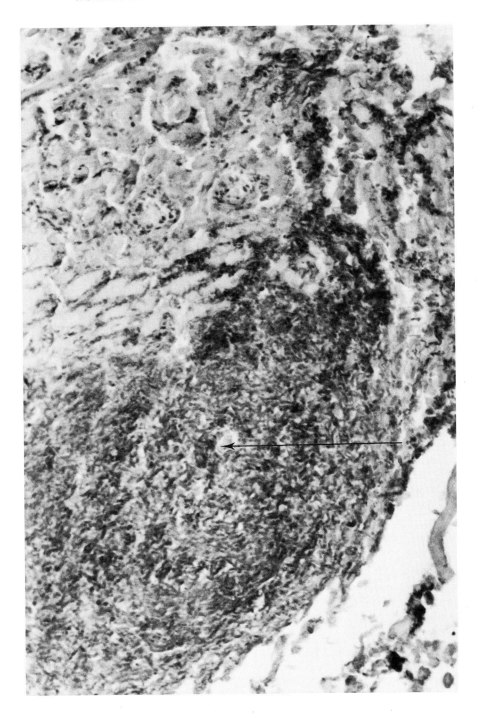

initial part of the artery had the typical wall structure of a ductus arteriosus (Fig. 3), with a change in the elastic type at the cervical level. In all 3 specimens, there was also a persistent ductus arteriosus on the contralateral side, connecting the pulmonary trunk with the descending aorta. The abnormal vessel was the normally disappearing distal part of the right sixth branchial artery (programmed to differentiate a ductus-like histology), continuous with an otherwise isolated neck artery. This would mean that normally persistent parts of the homolateral dorsal aorta had disappeared, in combination with interruption (or maybe primarily incomplete development) of the fourth and third branchial arteries. In such cases, a more diffuse and not only primarily hemodynamically induced anomaly in the transformation of the branchial arterial system seems likely. The combination with severe cardiac anomalies of a primitive type even suggests that both the cardiac and the vascular malformation might be the result of one and the same teratogenic agent, either on the basis of a developmental error as a response to injury, or as the result of a chromosomal abnormality (one of the patients had Down's syndrome) or a single-gene disorder.

Ductus Arteriosus and Abnormalities of the Aortic Arch

The ductus arteriosus closely resembles a muscular artery and consequently has a muscular media without the elastic lamellae typical of the aorta. A marked internal elastic lamina demarcates the intima from the media. After birth, the ductus normally contains intimal thickenings or cushions, consisting of fine elastic fibres and smooth muscle cells which are lacking in the aorta. At the junction with the ductus, the outer two-thirds of the elastic lamellae of the aorta merge into the adventitia of the ductus, without forming an external elastic lamina. The inner third forms the internal elastic lamina of the ductus. Extension of ductus tissue into the aorta is normally not greater than about one-third of its circumference (23).

In cases with dimensional aortic arch anomalies, the relationship between ductus and aorta is different. In local coarctation, the narrowing curtain is partly composed of ductal tissue. In our specimens of young infants, the ductus was usually patent, and the media as well was as the intima continued into the aorta. In some cases, the ductal tissue completely encircled the lumen of the aorta, but the elastic aortic wall always continued in the roof of the coarctation. This situation can be explained by the concept that the aortic arch enters end-to-side into the ductus, although the elastic wall of the aortic arch and the descending aorta remain continuous (Fig. 4). The same concept can explain the ductal involvement in several other forms of aortic arch anomalies. In cases of coarctation with tubular hypoplasia of the isthmus, the situation is similar

---

FIG. 3. a: Ventral view of the heart base with the arterial pole in a case of univentricular heart. An artery (pd), taking its origin from the right side of the pulmonary trunk (P), courses upwards to the neck. A, ascending aorta, D, patent ductus arteriosus. The dotted line indicates the plane of section shown in Fig. 3b.

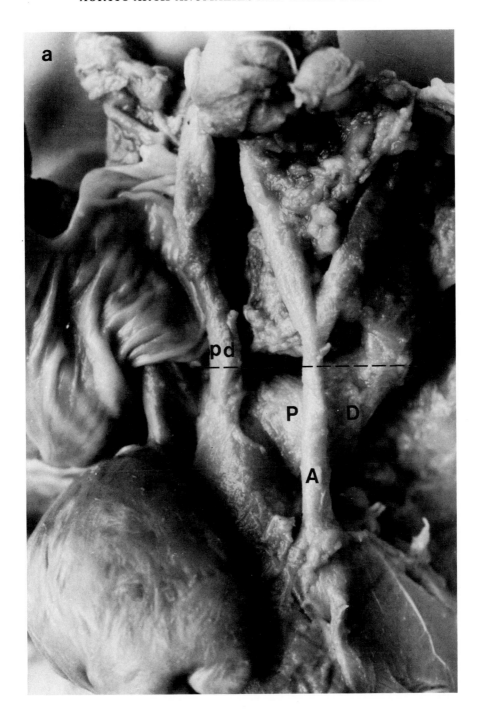

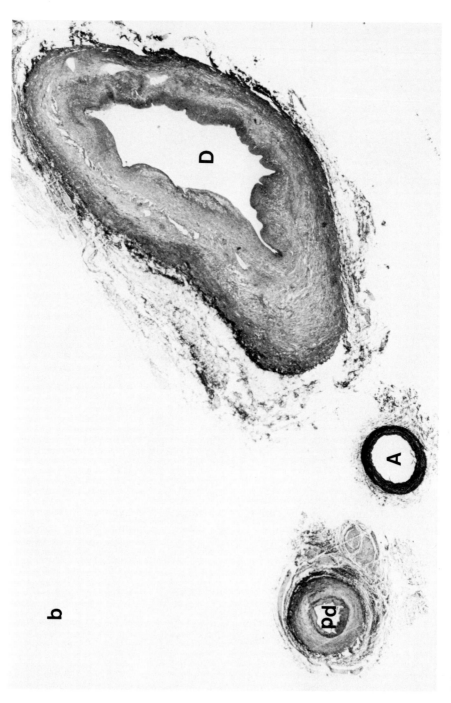

FIG. 3. b: Transverse section through the abnormal vessel (pd), the ascending aorta (A), and the large patent ductus arteriosus (D). Note the ductal wall structure of pd (× 11.6).

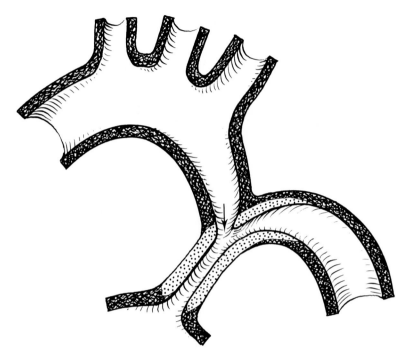

FIG. 4. a: Schematic representation of the aortic arch and the ductus arteriosus in local coarctation. The ductal tissue is indicated by dots; the elastic tissue of the aorta is more dense. The narrowest point of the coarctation is at the entrance of the aortic arch into the side of the ductus *(arrow).*

to local coarctation, in that the rim at the entrance of the hypoplastic isthmus (end-to-side) into the ductus contains ductal tissue. The same thing is true of isthmus atresia. We do not yet have reliable data about the microscopic picture of the channel ductus arteriosus–descending aorta in cases of complete interruption of the isthmus.

As is clearly shown in Fig. 4a, the narrowest point of local coarctation usually lies at the junction of the aortic arch and the ductus. More rarely, the curtain is just opposite the lumen of the ductus, allowing a flow of blood in both directions (3). In these cases, the narrowest point remains exactly opposite the ductal ligament after this is formed.

A situation encountered twice in our studies is that the ductal continuation in the descending aorta had such large intimal cushions that its lumen was almost obliterated (Fig. 4b and 5b). Macroscopically, this presents as though the ductus were continuous with the aortic arch, the coarctation seemingly

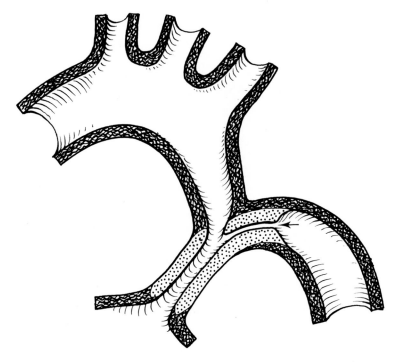

FIG. 4. b: Ductal tissue extending into the descending aorta almost closes off the lumen. The narrowest point of the coarctation now seems to be located distal of the entrance of the aortic arch into the ductus *(arrow)*.

located distal to this junction. This situation is clinically dangerous, because spontaneous closure of the ductus after birth will cause serious circulatory problems. Reopening of the ductus with prostaglandin E_1 can be life-saving (6).

SUMMARY

In summary, the embryological and teratological data so far collected provide ample evidence for the important role of hemodynamics in normal and abnormal morphogenesis. A special accent in this respect was given to the sixth embryonic week, but interaction between flow and morphologic changes in the cardiovascular system during fetal and neonatal development also remains an important factor. The architecture of the two differently curved routes to the descending aorta, with the striking histologic history of the ductal part in the arch pulmonary artery–descending aorta, is just one example of a long-lasting interdependence. Fetal changes in the architecture of the outflow tracts and of the different components of the ventricular septum probably have an important hemodynamic signifi-

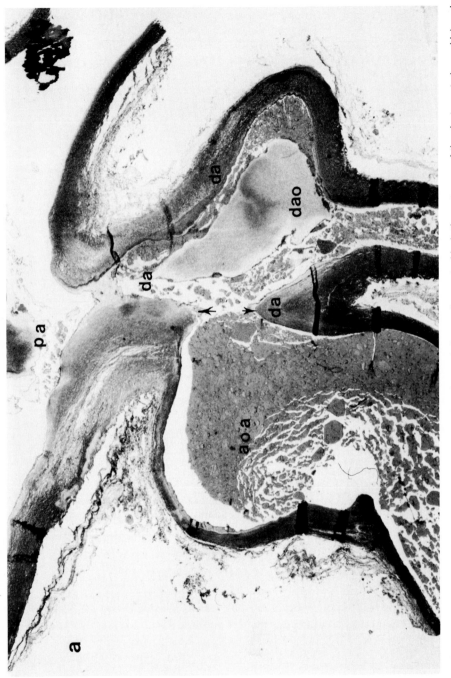

FIG. 5. a: Sagittal section of aortic arch (aoa), coarctation *(arrows)*, descending aorta (dao), the entrance of the ductus arteriosus (da) and the pulmonary artery (pa). Male infant, 5 weeks. Van Gieson elastic tissue stain (× 23).

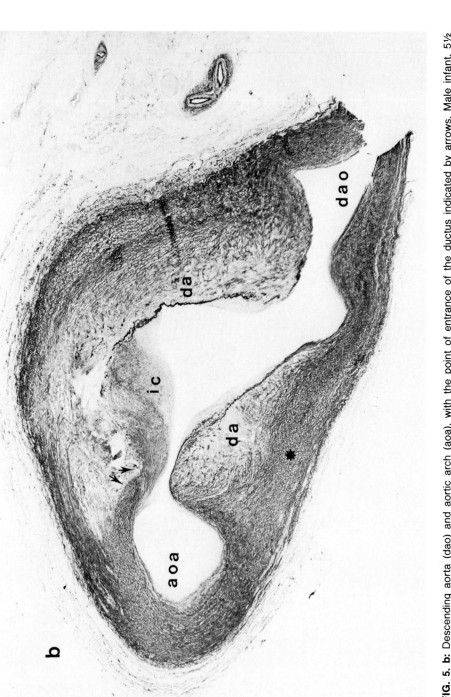

FIG. 5. b: Descending aorta (dao) and aortic arch (aoa), with the point of entrance of the ductus indicated by arrows. Male infant, 5½ weeks. Thick intimal cushions (ic) distal to this point cause a considerable narrowing of the aorta. Ductal intimal and medial tissue (da) is conspicuously present in the aorta. The continuation of the aortic vessel wall in the outer layer is indicated by an asterisk. Van Gieson elastic tissue stain (× 23).

cance. These factors deserve special attention in future work on prenatal development of the heart.

ACKNOWLEDGMENTS

We thank Messrs. van Duyvenbode and Tinkelenberg for photography and art work, and Miss Ria Stokman for preparation of the manuscript.

REFERENCES

1. Boyd, J. D., and Hamilton, W. J. (1970): *The Human Placenta.* Heffer, Cambridge.
2. Bruins, C. L. D. Ch. (1973): *De Arteriële Pool van het Hart. (Thesis)* Groen, Leiden.
3. Bruins, C. L. D. Ch. (1978): Competition between aortic isthmus and ductus arteriosus: Reciprocal influence of structure and flow. *Eur. J. Cardiol.,* 8:87-97.
4. Congdon, E. E. (1922): Transformation of the aortic arch system during the development of the human embryo. *Contrib. Embryol.,* 14:47-110.
5. Goor, D. A., and Lillehei, C. W. (1975): *Congenital Malformations of the Heart.* Grune and Stratton, New York/London.
6. Heymann, M. A., Berman, W. Jr., Rudolph, A. M., and Whitman, V. (1979): Dilatation of the ductus arteriosus by prostaglandin E_1 in aortic arch anomalies. *Circulation,* 59:169-173.
7. Moene, R. J., Oppenheimer-Dekker, A., Moulaert, A. J., Wenink, A. C. G., and Gittenberger-de Groot, A. C.: The concurrence of dimensional aortic arch anomalies and abnormal left ventricular muscle bundles. *Pediatr. Cardiol. (in press).*
8. Moulaert, A. (1974): *Ventricular Septal Defects and Anomalies of the Aortic Arch. (Thesis)* Luctor et Emergo, Leiden.
9. Moulaert, A. J., Bruins, C. C., and Oppenheimer-Dekker, A. (1976): Anomalies of the aortic arch and ventricular septal defects. *Circulation,* 53:1011-1015.
10. Moulaert, A. J., and Oppenheimer-Dekker, A. (1976): Anterolateral muscle bundle of the left ventricle, bulboventricular flange and subaortic stenosis. *Am. J. Cardiol.,* 37:78-81.
11. Oppenheimer-Dekker, A. (1975a): Development of the chorionic vascular network with reference to the transformation of the aortic branchial arteries in 10–20 mm human embryos (sixth week). *J. Anat.,* 120:399-400.
12. Oppenheimer-Dekker, A. (1975b): Normale en abnormale ontwikkeling van de arcus aortae en van de ventrikeluitstroomgebieden in hun relatie tot de foeto-placentaire vaatontwikkeling bij menselijke embryonen in de zesde ontwikkelingsweek (10–20 mm). In: *Thoraxchirurgie Leiden 1950–1975,* edited by C. Hahn and Th. Dirksen, pp. 127-133. Nederlands Drukkerij Bedrijf, Leiden.
13. Oppenheimer-Dekker, A. (1978): Embryogenesis of aortic arch anomalies coupled with ventricular septal defect and subaortic stenosis. *J. Anat.,* 127:198-199.
14. Oppenheimer-Dekker, A. (1979): Maldevelopment of the branchial arterial system in congenital heart anomalies. *J. Anat,* 129:212.
15. Pexieder, T. (1975): Cell death in the morphogenesis and teratogenesis of the heart. *Adv. Anat. Embryol. Cell Biol.,* 51:11-100.
16. Pexieder, T. (1978): Development of the outflow tract of the embryonic heart. In: *Morphogenesis and Malformation of the Cardiovascular System,* edited by G. C. Rosenquist and D. Birgoma, pp. 29–68. *Birth Defects: Original Article Series,* vol. XIV, no. 7, A. R. Liss, Inc., New York.
17. Rudolph, A. M., Heymann, M. A., and Spitznas, U. (1972): Hemodynamic considerations in the development of narrowing of the aorta. *Am. J. Cardiol.,* 30:514-525.
18. Rychter, Z. (1962): Experimental morphology of the aortic arches and the heart loop in chick embryos. *Adv. Morphogen.,* 2:333-371.
19. Shinebourne, E. A., and Elseed, A. M. (1974): Relation between fetal flow patterns, coarctation of the aorta, and pulmonary blood flow. *Br. Heart J.,* 36:492-498.
20. Sissman, N. J. (1970): Developmental landmarks in cardiac morphogenesis: Comparative chronology. *Am. J. Cardiol.* 25:141-148.
21. Wenink, A. C. G. (1978): Considerations pertinent to the embryogenesis of transposition. In: *Embryology and Teratology of the Heart and the Great Arteries,* edited by L. H. S. van Mierop, A. Oppenheimer-Dekker, and C. L. D. Ch. Bruins, pp. 129-135. Leiden University Press, Leiden.

22. Wenink, A. C. G., Oppenheimer-Dekker, A., and Moulaert, A. J. (1979): Muscular ventricular septal defects: A reappraisal of the anatomy. *Am. J. Cardiol.*, 43:259-264.
23. Wielenga, G. (1959): *De relatie tussen coarctatio aortae en ligamentum arteriosum. (Thesis)* Eduard Ijdo, Leiden.

DISCUSSION

De Vries: In the age group 14–16, there is another interesting phenomenon, the involution of the right umbilical vein. Can you comment on this?

Oppenheimer-Dekker: We just happened to start at the other end because we were fascinated by the combination of outflow tract defects with dimensional anomalies of the aortic arch.

Dor: I have the impression that Dr. Rychter could produce tetralogy of Fallot or pulmonary stenosis by elimination of both sixth aortic arches.

Oppenheimer-Dekker: I know that there are many right-sided aortic arches in human beings with Fallot tetralogy. I am not too familiar with this syndrome. I am more interested in the aortic channel.

Clark: Did you find an association of aortic semilunar valves anomalies with aortic arch anomalies?

Oppenheimer-Dekker: Yes, we had a number of bicuspid aortic valves. But I do not know whether this has to be considered as a primary or a secondary anomaly.

Clark: What was the pattern of the aortic valve malformations?

Oppenheimer-Dekker: We have clearly seen bicuspid aortic valves and then normal valves.

Krediet: In the pathogenesis of the tetralogy of Fallot, the aorta takes a more midline position and therefore opens into the aortic arches only from the middle and not, as normally, from the right side. The bloodstream is then obviously directed to the right fourth aortic arch.

Clark: In the tetralogy of Fallot, the two aortic valvular cusps are asymmetric. There is one very large and one normal size cusp.

Subject Index

A-bands in myofibrils, 369-373
Aberrant mitotic divisions, 110
N-Acetylsalicylic acid (NASA) in GAG synthesis, 177
Action potential, rising phase of, 317
Action potential threshold, neuraminidase in, 340-345
β-Adrenergic receptors, types of, 374
β-Aminopropionitrile (BAPN), effects on collagen, 231
Anastomotic shunt, 3-4
Angioarchitecture in heart, 442-445, 448-450
Aorta, semilunar valves of, 135
Aortic arch abnormalities
  cardiovascular malformations and, 485-500
  ductus arteriosus and, 492-496
  fetoplacental vasculogenesis and, 486-496
  intracardiac pathology and, 489-490
Aortic arch system, transformation of, 7
Aortic conus
  formation of, 20
  septation of, 23
Aortic infundibulum
  atrium dextrum connection with, 18
  origin of, 23
  third root of, 24-26, 29-30
Aortic sac
  aortic sinus versus, 47
  development of, 45
Aorticopulmonary septum
  formation of, 268

mesenchymal condensations of, 466
Aorticopulmonary window, pathogenesis of, 30
Arterial pole, in pericardial cavity, 268
Arterial valves
  formation of, 130
  in ventricles, 135-136
Artificial ductus arteriosus, 3
Atrial infundibular duct, 27
Atrial infundibulum, 26
Atrial muscle, ventricular muscle separation from, 169
Atrial septal complex, formation of, 145
Atrial septation, blood flow in, 8
Atrial septum
  closure of, 4
  collagen in, 225
  foramen secundum in, 140
Atrioventricular canal
  blood flow in, 9
  development of, 169
  endocardial cushions in, 10
  extracellular matrix of, 169-176
  malformations related to, 177-178
  myocardium in, 167, 169
Atrioventricular cushion cells, migration of, 207
Atrioventricular cushion tissue, 197-210
Atrioventricular cushions, 17-29, 277
  dead mesenchymal cells in, 159
Atrium, discontinuity between ventricle and, 176-177
Atrium dextrum, aortic infundibulum and, 18

501

Atropine, in DMPP, 356
Autophagocytosis, 94

Blood
  ionic concentration in, 417-418
  total volume of circulating, 417
Blood flow
  deviation from normal, 8, 9-14, 15
  predilectional, 14
  right heart predominance in, 15
Blood vessels, capacity of, 7
Branchial arterial system anomalies,
    490-492
Bulbar cushions, dead mesenchymal
    cells in, 159
Bulbar growth, definition of, 65
Bulbar ridges
  formation of, 20
  in pars membranacea, 24, 27-28
Bulbar width, definition of, 65
Bulbo-auricular canal, closure of,
    18
Bulboventricular foramen, formation
    of, 23
Bulboventricular index, definition
    of, 65
Bulboventricular loop, formation of,
    176
Bulboventricular malformations,
    retinoic acid in, 157-159
Bulbus, 18-19
  distal parts of, 235
  position change in, 52-56
  septation of, 17
  truncus independence from, 18-19
  width of, 56

Calcium, as cardiovascular teratogen,
    476
Calcium exchange
  neuraminidase in, 346
  sialic acid in, 345
Calcium ions, in cardiac develop-
    ment, 327
Canalis infundibulo-atrialis, form-
    ation of, 18

Capillary pressure, in delivery of
    nutrients, 412
Cardiac asymmetry, development of,
    45
Cardiac cytodifferentiation, 72
Cardiac defects
  chicken as model of man in, 428
  genetic and mechanical effect
    in, 16
Cardiac development
  calcium ions in, 327
  deviation from, 8
  loop formation in, 39
  normal, 7-16
  phylogenetic aspects of, 454
  principles of, 8
  reference frame in, 60
  salicylates in, 177-178
  SEM in, 67, 278
  synoptic diagram of, 10-14
Cardiac embryology, 3-5
  historical perspective of, 3
  terminology in, 3
Cardiac function, 407-418
  calculated indices of, 412, 413
  determinants of, 412, 413, 414
  formulae for calculation of, 411, 412
  measurement of, 416
  stroke volume in, 412, 415
Cardiac innervation, 349-365
Cardiac jelly, 128
  cellular debris in, 96
  composition of, 237
  CT cells in, 197
  diastolic volume in, 415
  distribution of, 45
  elaboration of, 96, 176
  endocardial cells in mesenchyme of,
    276
  endocardial cushion cells in, 181,
    415
  extracellular glycoprotein in, 198
  mesenchyme immigration effect on,
    47
  myocardium as source of, 207
  seeding of, endocardial cells in, 74
  shape and structure of, 256
  in zone of fusion, 110

Cardiac loop, 431-434
   myofibril orientation and, 379
Cardiac malformation, retinoic acid
   in, 151, 157
Cardiac morphogenesis
   hypothesis of mosaicism of
      mechanisms of, 73
   research on, absence of integration
      in, 403
Cardiac myocytes, 349-365
   differentiation in, 337
   PAS in, 352
   sympathetic neurons and, 358
   synchrony in, 301
   trypsin and, 369
Cardiac output, in teratogenic process,
   477-481
Cardiac pathology, 3
Cardiac tissue, coupling in, 300-301
Cardioacceleration, DMPP in, 359
Cardiorespiratory bypass, 4
Cardiovascular malformations
   arch anomalies and, 485-500
   hemodynamics in, 485
   β-receptor hyperstimulation of,
      474
Cardiovascular teratogenesis
   catecholamines in, 473-483
   epinephrine in, 473
Catecholamine-induced chronotropy,
   356
Catecholamine sensitivity, in H aggregates, 355
Catecholamine uptake process, 358
Catecholamines
   in cardiovascular teratogenesis, 473-
      484
   in TTX, 356
Cell aggregate systems, advantage of,
   349
Cell death, 93-97
   in aberrant mitotic divisions, 110
   chemical teratogens in, 95-96
   classification of, 93
   in conal ridges, 121-123, 127-137
   in conotruncus, morphogenetic role
      of, 94

cyclophosphamide in, 95-96
dexamethasone in, 95-96
in EEFZ, 108
genetically programmed, 115-126
history of studies on, 93
intracellular organelle quantification of, 123
irradiation in, 96-97
mechanism of, 110
as morphogenetic factor in fusion,
   101
programmed, 108-110
ribosome crystallization in, 110
SEM studies of, 96
as term, 121, 127
time of appearance and disappearance of, 127
tubular heart role of, 101-110
ultrastructure of physiological and
   teratogen-induced, 97
Cell lysis, 121
Cell migration in embryonic systems,
   235
Cell proliferation, 71-72
   cluster analysis in, 87
   DNA synthesis in, 87
   global outflow tract pattern in,
      75-77
   in heart versus skeletal muscle, 71
   mitotic wave traveling in, 86
   in outflow tract, 84, 87
   patterns of, 73-88
      comparison of, in selected localiza-
         tions, 77
      diversification of, 87
      global labeling index in, 77
      index of labeled mitoses in, 77
      two-dimensional graphic recon-
         struction of, 77
   in skeletal muscle versus heart, 71
   structure-related peaks in, 86
Cell surface, 255-265
Cell volume, ratio of DNA content to,
   90
Cells
   in monolayer versus intact heart,
   90

Cells (*contd.*)
  subpopulations of, 94
Cellular decoupling, mechanism for,
  316
Cellular electrogenesis, 317-329
  calcium in, 324-325
  manganese ions in, 324
  potassium in, 319
  recording, 317
  sodium in, 320-324
CHD, *see* Congenital heart disease
Chondroitin sulphate
  in endocardial cushion cells, 177
  synthesis by myocyte, 167
Chronotropic response, 359
Cocaine, synergism with, 475
Coelomic activity, 37
  epithelial lining of, 255
Coelomic primordia, 32
Collagen
  in aging myocardium, 213-214
  antibody reaction with, 225
  atrial septum formation in, 225
  double-staining in, 225
  Ouchterlony in, 225
  types of
    localization of, 213-215
    synthesis of, 219
  ventricular concentration of, 214
Compaction of trabeculae, 444
Conal ridges
  cell death in, 121-123, 127-137
  characteristics of, 464-466
  development of, 128-133
  malposition of, 470
  sheets of condensed tissue in, 128
Conal torsions, arguments for, 66
Congenital heart disease (CHD), 383-
  385
  absence of fusion in, 257
  chromosomal aberrations in, 383
  etiology of, 383
  incidence of, 383
  mouse as model of human, 396
  single-gene defects in, 383
  in skeletal-defects syndrome, 384-385
  surgical management of, 3-4
  in trisomies, 394, 389-399

Conotruncal cushions, fusion of, 176
Conotruncal torsions, transposition of
  great vessels and, 453-472
Conotruncus
  blood flow in, 9
  medial shift of, 49, 61
  morphogenetic role of cell death in, 94
  positional changes versus growth in, 60
Conus
  absorption of, 136
  formation of, 133
  involution of, 131, 133-135
  muscle elements in, 135
  septation in, 9
  shortening of, 136
Corneal endothelium, cell movement in,
  259
Coronary arteries, development of, 442-
  444
Coronary vascular bed development,
  444-445, 448-449
Coronary vessel development, 452
Coupling of heart cells, 299-316
  in absence of gap junctions, 310
  in cardiac tissue, 300-301
  cycloheximide (CHX) in, 310-
    311
  decoupling and, 311
  duration of, 316
  formation of, 284
Coupling resistance (R_c) measurement,
  305-306
Cushion cells (CT)
  in cardiac jelly, 243
  cytoplasmic protrusions in, 241
  DON effects on, 237-251
  endocardial motility and formation
    of, 247-248
  endocardial shape change in, 229
  endocardium as source of, 227
  extracellular macromolecules in, 237
  GAG and collagen in formation
    of, 197-198
  major events in development of, 237
  maldevelopment of, 197
  muscularization of, 248
  potential heterogeneity of origin of,
    228-229

Cushion cells (*contd.*)
   reduction of, due to DON, 243
   seeding of, 229-230
      DON effects on, 239-240
   significance of, 197
Cyanotic heart disease, 3
Cyclic adenosine monophosphate
   (cyclic AMP), in catecholamine-induced malformations,
   475-476
Cycloheximide (CHX), and coupling
   of heart cells, 310-311
Cyclophosphamide, and cell death,
   95-96
Cytochalasin B, effects of, 247-248
Cytokinesis, 90
Cytoplasm
   deformation of, 373-376
   of endocardial cells, 142
   glycogen in, 142
   vacuolization in, 122-123
Cytoplasmic discontinuity, 301
Cytoplasmic hypertrophy of endocardium, 239

D-loop of heart tubes, 153
Dead cells
   in foramina secunda, 148
   programming of, 112
   removal of, 110
   thymidine incorporation in, 88
Deoxyribonucleic acid (DNA)
   in myocytes, 89
   ratio of cell volume to content
   of, 90
   synthesis and polypoidization of,
   89-90
   synthesis localization of, 80,
   81
Depolarization, in pacemaker mechanisms, 339
Dexamethasone, and cell death, 95-96
Dextro-dorsal conal ridge, 118, 133
Dextro-superior truncal swelling,
   118, 128, 131
Diastolic depolarization, in pacemaker mechanisms, 340

Diastolic membrane potential, in embryonic development, 319
6-Diazo-5-Oxo-L-Norleucine (DON), 237-
   251
   CT cell reduction due to, 243
   in CT cell seeding, 239-240
   GSA and, 241-243
   in HA synthesis, 248
   motility suppression by, 247
   toxicity of, 251
DiGeorge syndrome, 384
1,1-Dimethyl-4-phenylpiperazinium
   iodide (DMPP), 356-359
   in cardioacceleration, 359
   chronotropy induced by, 360
Distal and proximal ridges, matching of,
   461-463, 467
Distal infundibulum
   fusion of, 38
   tubular length of, 42
Distal truncus ridges, fusion of, 268
DNA, *see* Deoxyribonucleic acid
DON, *see* 6-Diazo-5-Oxo-L-Norleucine
Dorso-lateral bulbar ridges, 24
Dorsal mesocardium, 103
Double outlet right ventricle, 399
Ductus arteriosus, and aortic arch
   anomalies, 492-496

ECM, *see* Extracellular matrix
Eisenmenger's complex, 50
Electrical coupling, in embryonic
   heart cell aggregates, 301-311
Electrogenesis, changes in action po-
   tential of, 337
Embryonic death, due to DON, 239
Embryonic heart
   in chick and rat, 115-126
      initial change of dying cell in,
      122-123
      primary difference between,
      116-117
   events modifying appearance of, 49
Embryotoxicity, screening method
   for, 405
Endocardial cells
   of AV endocardial cushions, 277

Endocardial cells (*contd.*)
  in cardiac jelly seeding, 74
  characteristics of, 145
  condensation of, 112
  of cytoplasm, 142
  in foramen secundum, 140
  mesenchyme and, 274-276
  microfilaments in, 149
  septal tissue subdivision by, 142
  thymidine incorporation in, 86
Endocardial cushions, 197-210
  cardiac jelly in, 181, 415
  chondroitin sulfate in, 177
  coalescence of, 257-259
  endocardium and, 176, 180
  mesenchymal cell in, 169
  myocardium in formation of, 177
  radioautographic observations
    on, 201
Endocardial expected fusion zone
    (EEFZ), 106
Endocardial fusion, 102-106
Endocardial motility, 247-248
Endocardial shape change
  in CT formation, 229
  in truncus, 227-235
Endocardial structures, fusion of,
    267-280
Endocardial tubes, composition of,
    103
Endocardium
  acid phosphatase activity in, 232
  cytoplasmic hypertrophy of, 239
  endocardial cushion cells and, 176
  flute formation in, 229, 231-232
  hydrolytic activity in, 232
  mitotic index in, 251
    in CT formation, 227-228
  proliferation in, 278
  as source of cushion tissue, 180,
    227
  trabeculation and, 232-233
Endocytosis *in vitro*, in cultured
    heart cells, 193
Endoderm-mesoderm interaction, 256
Endothelial and epithelial surfaces,
    nonadhesiveness of, 261

Endothelial cells
  fusion and detachment of, 149
  lamellipodia in, 261
  and muscle strands, 149
  reorientation of, 234
  ruffling of, 261-262
Epigenesis, as term, 403-404
Epigenetic control, as term, 403-404
Epinephrine, in cardiovascular terato-
    genesis, 473
Epithelial cells, retinoic acid in, 160
Epithelial surfaces, nonadhesiveness
    of, 261
Epithelium, definition of, 255
Experimental intervention, 404-405
Extracellular matrix, 165-180
  of AV canal, 169-176
  in endocardium flute formation,
    230
  fiber tracts of, 230-231
  origin of, 167
  macromolecules in, 167
  myocardial cell migration in, 179-
    180

Fallot's tetralogy, 5, 8, 12, 50
  pathogenesis of, 500
  as term, 399
Fetoplacental vasculogenesis, 486-496
Fiber tracts, of extracellular matrix,
    230-231
Fibroblasts
  lack of purposeful activity in, 335
  muscle cells versus, 332
  polymorphic movement of, 335
  in synchronization, 331-336
  trypsin-dissociated muscle cells and, 335
Fick principle, 417
Flow-dependence rule, 7
Foramen infundibulo-atriale, formation
    of, 24
Foramen interatriale primum, blood
    flow in, 8
Foramen interventriculare persistens,
    10
Foramen primum, 145

Foramen secundum
  atrial septum in, 140
  composition of, 140
  endocardial cells in, 140
  as term, 139
Foramina secunda, 139-149
  appearance of, 145
  dead cells in, 148
  proliferation in, 436-439
Foregut diverticulum, 35
Fracture face area, 289
Frank-Starling mechanism, 416
Fusion
  absence of, in congenital heart
    malformation, 257
  of atrioventricular cushions, 17-29
  cell death as morphogenetic
    factor in, 101
  characteristics of, 276
  of conotruncal cushions, 176
  delayed, interpreting, 279
  of distal infundibulum, 38
  disturbances in process of, 259
  of endocardial structures, 102-106,
    256-257, 267-280
  of endothelial cells, 149
  gap junctions in, 279
  mechanism of, 102-106
  merging versus, 257
  mitotic activity modification and,
    278
  model systems for cellular and
    subcellular, 257
  plasminogen inactivator in, 279
  premyocardial layer in, 103
  secretory organelles in, 259
  as term, 257
  of ventral myocarduim, 113

GAGs, see Glycosaminoglycans
Gap junctions
  with arms, 291
  assembly of, 258-298
  in cardiac muscle development, 286-
    287
  common features of, 300

  coupling in absence of, 310
  distribution of, 287-289
  earliest forms of, 291
  electrical communication in, 296
  formation plaques in, 291
  fracture face area in, 289
  in fusion, 279
  junctional resistance in, 301
  myocardial development in, 294-296
  permeability of, 299-300
  plasma membrane area in, 289
  polypeptides in, 298
  ratio of cell volume and, 296
  ratio of plasma membrane area
    to, 289
  stages of formation of, 298
  types of, 286-287
Global outflow tract cell proliferation
    pattern, 75-77
Glucosamine (GSA), 238
  in cell division and migration, 251
  deficiency of, 237
  DON and, 241-243, 248
Glycocalyx, 181
  turnover of, 195
Glycogen
  in cytoplasm, 142
  in myocytes, 47, 149
Glycopeptides
  distribution of, 181-195
  synthesis of, 181-195
β-Glycopeptides, 193-194
Glycophorin, in lipid bilayer,
    346
Glycoprotein (GP)
  in cardiac jelly, 198, 203
  collagen-associated, 207
  fucosylated, 207
  as tissue-specific extracellular stimu-
    lant, 203
Glycosaminoglycans (GAGs)
  cultured heart cell synthesis of, 189
  distribution of, 181-195
  in infundibular primordium, 39
  mesenchymal cells in, 44
  synthesis by myocytes, 167
  in myoendocardial space, 42

Glycosaminoglycans (GAGs) (*contd.*)
  synthesis of, 181-195
Golgi region, vacuole formation in, 123
GSA, *see* Glucosamine
Guanethidine, in DMPP, 357

H aggregates, *see* Heart aggregates
HA, *see* Hyaluronic acid
Heart, *see also* Cardiac *entries*
  electrophysiological properties
    of, 283
  as epithelial organ, 255
  imbalance of, 15
  normal, definition of, 8
  positional changes of neighboring
    structures in, 60
Heart (H) aggregates
  catecholamine sensitivity in, 355
  in catecholamine uptake process, 358
  contraction rate in, 355
Heartbeat
  initiation of, 110
  potassium and, 418
  synchronization of, *see* Synchronization
Heart bulb, 431
  growth of, 439-442
  as separate heart chamber, 431
Heart cells
  environmental changes and response
    of, 193
  physiology of, 283-284
Heart loop, proliferation in, 435-436
Heart lumen, rounded cells in, 112
Heart-sympathetic ganglion cells (H-SG),
    351-361
  beat rate in, 360
  catecholamine uptake process in, 358
  contraction rate in, 355
Heart tubes, D-loop of, 152, 153
Heart wall, angio- and myoarchitecture
    of, 431-452
Hexamethonium, in DMPP, 356
H-SG, *see* Heart-sympathetic ganglion
    cell (H-SG)
Hurler's syndrome
Hyaluronic acid (HA)
  in motility, 249
  synthesis by myocyte, 167

  synthesis of, 167, 177, 247, 248
Hyperpolarization, in pacemaker mech-
    anisms, 339
Hypoplastic heart, 13, 15, 399, 447, 449

I-bands in myofibrils, 369
IMP, *see* Integral membrane proteins
Infundibular cushions, fusion of, 45
Infundibular septum, deviated, 490
Infundibulo-atrial communication, 24-26
Infundibulum
  evolution of, 31-48
  expansile growth of, 44
Insulin, in TTX sensitivity, 327
Integral membrane proteins (IMP), 299
  CHX in, 311
  in non-junctional membrane, 300
Interatrial septum, proliferation in, 436-
    439
Intercellular channels, 299
Interkinetic nuclear migration, 255
Interventricular communication, closure
    of, 26-29
Interventricular foramen, formation of,
    23-26
Interventricular septum, proliferation
    in, 436
Interventricular septal primordium, 44
Intracardiac surgery, 4
Intraluminal plasma pressure, in heartbeat
    initiation, 110
Intraneural catecholamines, release of,
    356
Ionic concentration in blood, 417-418
Irradiation, and cell death, 96-97
Isoproterenol, teratogenic effect of,
    476-479
Isthmus atresia, 495

Junctional channel, 310
Junctional channel resistance, 299
Junctional conductance, linear versus
    exponential increase in, 310
Junctional resistance, 308-311

L-loop of heart tubes, 153

Lamellipodia, cytoplasmic deformation in, 375
Latency, 305-306
Left-sided defects, incidence of, 15
Looping in tubular heart, 367
Lung bud inversion and pulmonary venous connections, 419-429
Lung fragment, splanchnic plexus proximity to, 424-425
Lymphatics, development of, 445

Macrophage, as term, 113
Malposition of great vessels, 467-468
Manganese ions, 324
Maximum diastolic potential (MDP), 340-345
Merging versus fusion, 257
Mesenchymal cells
    in atrioventricular cushions, 159
    in bulbar cushions, 159
    endocardial cushion coverage in, 169
    in GAG, 44
      locomotive appendage formation in, 248
    retinoic acid in death of, 160
    in truncus arteriosus, 256
Mesenchymal primordia, in infundibulum myocardial wall, 45
Mesenchymal spiral cushions, expansile growth of, 44
Mesenchyme
    endocardial cells and, 274-276
    immigration of, 47
    labeling index of, 84
    myocardium replaced by, 278
Metazoan cell movement, mechanisms of, 255
Methylxanthines, synergism with, 475
Microplicae, as term, 278-279
Microsurgical wounds, repair of, 108
Mitoses
    index of labeled, 77
    two-phase behavior of labeled, 86
Mitotic activity, fusion and modification of, 278
Mitotic index, variations of, 73, 74
Morphogenetic system
    experimental intervention and, 405

mutual interdependence of, 404
types of, 484
Muscle cells, fibroblasts versus, 332
Myoarchitecture of heart, 434-442, 445-448
Myocardial cells
    migration of, 179-180
    in pulmonary anterior semilunar valve, 121
    retinoic acid in, 155-157
    in right ventricular cavity, 121
Myocardial development, gap junction in, 294-296
Myocardial excitation-contraction coupling, 346
Myocardial expected fusion zone (MEFZ), 106
Myocardial mantle, splanchnic fold of, 37-38
Myocardium
    of AV canal, 167, 169
    collagen in, 213-214
    contractile properties of, 415-416
    differentiation of, 167
    downward movement of, 66
    in endocardial cushion matrix formation, 177
    labeling index of, 84
    looping in, 367
    mesenchyme as replacement for, 278
    mitotic indices for, in CT formation, 227-228
    separation of cells of, 169
    as source of cardiac jelly, 207
    stress in, 376
Myocyte cell division, 71
Myocytes
    DNA in, 89
    GAGs in synthesis of, 167
    glycogen in, 47, 149
Myoendocardial glycosaminoglycan, 35, 37
Myofibril orientation
    cardiac looping and, 379
    stress and, 368
Myofibrillogenesis, 367-369
    in stress-free environment, 373-376
Myofibrils
    aberrant patterns of, 377

Myofibrils (*contd.*)
   alignment of, 369
   in core cells versus periphery cells, 316
   packing disorders of, 371

Neural crest cells, grafting of, 245-246
Neuraminidase
   in calcium exchange, 346
   in maximum diastolic potential,
      340-345
Neuromuscular junctions, 365
Nexuses, in heart cells, 283
Noonan's syndrome, 384
Notochordal process in presomite
   embryos, 32
Nucleic acid synthesis, 360

Osmotic pressure, potassium in, 113
Ostium atrioventriculare commune, 8
Outflow tract
   cell proliferation in, 87
   division of, 45
   localizations identified in, 75

Pacemaker mechanisms, 337-348
   cell surface anions in, 345-346
   depolarization in, 339
   diastolic depolarization in, 340
   hyperpolarization in, 339
   voltage clamp analysis of, 339-340
Parietal truncus ridge, 272
Pars membranacea
   bulbar ridges in, 24, 27-28
   formation of, 9, 27
      failure of, 12
PAS, *see* Periodic acid Schiff (PAS)
   staining
Pericardiac surgery, 4
Pericardial cavity, arterial pole in, 268
Pericardial coelom, 32, 45
Periodic acid Schiff (PAS) staining,
   89, 148, 352
Phagocytes
   differentiation of, 94
   kinds of, 113
Phagocytic cell, of septal core, 145
Phagocytosis
   cells capable of, 112

after retinoic acid administration, 157
Physiological cell death, *see* Cell death
Plasma membrane area, 289
Plasminogen inactivator, in fusion, 279
Polymorphic movement, 335
Polypoidization
   DNA synthesis and, 89-90
   of heart muscle *in vivo*, 89-90
Potassium
   heartbeat and, 418
   in osmotic pressure, 113
Practolol, protective effect of, 477-479
Precardiac splanchnic mesoderm, 37
Prechordal plate, 32
Prepharyngeal mesoderm, third arterial
   arches in, 42
Prepharyngeal truncus arteriosus pri-
   mordium, 42
Presomite embryos, 32-35
Primitive node, in presomite embryos, 32
Primordia, asymmetric distribution of,
   47
Programmed cell death, as term, 126
Proliferation, in foramina secunda, 436-
   439
Propranolol, protective effect of, 474
Proximal and distal ridges, matching of,
   461-463, 467
Proximal bulbus angle, straightening of, 61
Proximal ostium migration, 463-464
Pulmonary anterior semilunar valve, 121
Pulmonary circulation, systemic circula-
   tion and, 15
Pulmonary conus, septation of, 23
Pulmonary infundibulum, formation of,
   20
Pulmonary venous connections, 419-429
   patterns of, 421-424
Pyknotic cells
   abundant cytoplasmic vacuoles in, 106
   in FZ, 106-108

Quantitative shape analysis, 49–67

Retinoic acid, 151-161
   in bulboventricular malformation, 157-
      159
   in cardiac malformation, 151, 157

Retinoic acid (*contd.*)
    duration of teratogenic effect of, 159
    in epithelial cells, 160
    in mesenchymal cell death, 160
    in myocardial cells, 155-157
    phagocytosis after effects of, 157
Ribosome crystallization, in cell
    death, 110
Ruffling, as term, 278

Saccus aorticus ventralis
    blood flow in, 9
    dilation of, 20
Salicylates, and cardiac development,
    177-178
Satellite cells, 71
Scanning electron microscopy (SEM)
    in fusion of endocardial structures,
      256-257
    in heart development, 67
    standardization of, 278
Semilunar valves, 135
    formation site of, 46
Septa of heart, differences of, 257
Septal core
    cells of, 145-148
    phagocytic cell of, 145
Septal tissue, endocardial cell subdivi-
    sion of, 142
Septal truncus ridge, 272
Septation, 7
    of aortic conus, 23
    conus ridges in, 9
    critical points in, 10-14
    fundamental points in, 17
    myocardium in, 66
    normal and abnormal, 3
    of pulmonary conus, 23
Septum intermedium, formation of,
    17-18
SG aggregates, *see* Sympathetic ganglion
    aggregates
Shape development in embryo heart,
    49-67
Sinistro-inferior truncal swelling, 118
Sinistro-truncal swelling, 128, 131
Sinistro-ventral conal ridge, 118, 133
Sinus venosus, 8

Skeletal-defects syndromes, 384-385
Sodium permeability, of ventricular cells,
    326
Somatic mesoderm, formation of, 32
Splanchnic folds, and myocardial mantle,
    37-38
Splanchnic mesoderm, formation of, 32
Splanchnic plexus, lung fragment prox-
    imity to, 424-425
Splanchnopleura, 256
Spontaneous cell death, *see* Cell death
Strain
    decreasing gradient of, 376
    in myocardium, 376
    in Purkinje fibers, 368
    strain versus, 379
Sympathetic ganglion (SG) aggregates,
    352-361
Sympathetic neurons, 352-355
    cardiac myocytes and, 358
    clumping of, 358
    in vitro model systems of, 349
Synapse formation, 349-350
Synchronization, 302-305
    fibroblasts in, 331-336
    intermediate rate of, 316
    latency in, 308
    nexal current in, 307
    onset of, 301-302
    partial synchrony of, 304
    phase shift in, 308
Synchrony, definition of, 305
Systemic circulation, pulmonary circ-
    ulation and, 15

Taussig-Bing anomaly, 50
Teratogenesis, cardiac output in, 477-481
Teratogenic drug potency, hierarchy of,
    474
Terminology, accuracy of, 66
Tetraethylammonium (TEA), 325-326
Tetralogy of Fallot, *see* Fallot's tetralogy
Tetrodotoxin (TTX)
    catecholamines and, 356
    in cellular electrogenesis,
    in electrical activity, 283
    insulin sensitivity to, 327
    in monolayer cells versus aggregates, 329

Thymidine incorporation, 88
[3]H-thymidine autoradiography, 73-74
[3]H-thymidine incorporation, 435
Trabeculation, and endocardium, 232-233
Transport-related stress, 394
Transposition of great vessels, 453-472
Transseptal communication, 145
Trisomic fetuses, death in, 394
Trisomies, congenital heart disease in, 384, 389-399
Trisomy, incidence of, 388-399
Trisomy-specific versus trisomy-unspecific malformations, 395
Truncobulbar sulcus, 128
Truncus
  bulbus independence from, 18-19
  endocardial shape change in, 227-235
  evolution of, 31-48
  sections of, 227
  septation of, 17-19
  as term, 126
Truncus arteriosus
  blood flow in, 9-10
  in chick embryo, 116
  internal aspect of, 118
  intrapericardial, 44
  location of, 9
  mesenchymal cells in, 256
Truncus arteriosus persistens, varieties of, 20
Truncus ridges
  development of, 128-133
  fusion process of, 272
Trypsin, and cardiac myocytes, 369
TTX, *see* Tetrodotoxin
Tube-like heart, parts of, 267-268
Tubular heart
  cell death role in, 101-110
  formation of, 8
  looping of, 367
Tubular hypoplasia, 490
Tubular proximal infundibulum, 40
Twins, cardiac structure in, 16

Vacuoles, formation of, 123
Vacuolization, in cytoplasm, 122-123

Vectorial flow and vessel size, 16
Vectorial bulbar torsion, 51
Vectorial bulbus rotation, 49-50, 61, 62, 65-66
Vena cava, blood flow in, 8
Ventral mesocardium, persistence of, 47
Ventral myocardium, fusion of, 113
Ventricle
  arterial valves in, 135-136
  bulbus and, positional changes in, 61
  contribution of left versus right, 47
  discontinuity between atrium and, 176-177
  expansion of right, 61
  position change in right, 52-57
  proliferation center of, 61
  septation of, 17
  width of, 56
Ventricular AP depolarization, 324
Ventricular cavity, myocardial cells in, 121
Ventricular cells
  sodium permeability of, 326
  spontaneous electrical activity of, 283
Ventricular concentration of collagen, 214
Ventricular flow pathways, 17-29
Ventricular growth, definition of, 65
Ventricular muscle, atrial muscle separation from, 169
Ventricular outflow tract
  development of, 489
  flow distribution of, 489
  formation of, 123
  normal development of, 128-136
Ventricular proliferation centers, 436
Ventricular septal defects (VSD), 94
  after lung bud inversion, 425
Ventricular width, definition of, 65
Ventriculo-bulbar index, 56, 59, 60
  definition of, 65
Ventro-medial ridges, 24
Vessel size and vectorial flow, 16
Voltage clamp analysis, automaticity in, 345